T0220093

Inglese per chirurghi

Ramón Ribes • Pedro J. Aranda • John Giba

Inglese per chirurghi

Presentazione di
Lorenzo Capussotti

Edizione italiana a cura di
Giuseppe Zimmitti

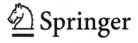 Springer

Ramón Ribes
Reina Sofia University Hospital
Servicio de radiología
14005 Córdoba, Spain

John Giba
C/ Mossèn Cinto Verdaguer
19, 2-7
08181 Sentmenat, Spain

Pedro J. Aranda MD, PhD, ED
Cardiovascular Surgery Department
Hospital Regional Universitario, Carlos Haya
Málaga, Spain

Hanno collaborato all'edizione originale:
Juan Francisco Martinez Canca, Esteban Sarria García, Irene Palomo Gomez, Maria Teresa Gonzalez González, Lorena Rubio Lobato

Titolo dell'opera originale:
Surgical English
Ramón Ribes, Pedro J. Aranda, John Giba
© Springer-Verlag Berlin Heidelberg 2008

Edizione italiana tradotta e curata da:
Giuseppe Zimmitti
Specialista in Formazione presso la S.C. Chirurgia Generale e Oncologica
Ospedale Mauriziano Umberto I
Torino

ISBN 978-88-470-2414-4   e-ISBN 978-88-470-2415-1

DOI 10.1007/978-88-470-2415-1

© Springer-Verlag Italia 2012

Copertina: Ikona S.r.l., Milano
Impaginazione: Graphostudio, Milano
Stampa: Fotoincisione Varesina, Varese

Springer-Verlag Italia S.r.l., Via Decembrio 28, I-20137 Milano
Springer fa parte di Springer Science+Business Media (www.springer.com)

Presentazione all'edizione italiana

La realtà medica scientifica, inclusa quella chirurgica, ha subito negli ultimi decenni una profonda rivoluzione che ha completamente trasformato l'attività e la ricerca del singolo, inserendola in una rete internazionale di contatti e collaborazioni. La formazione dei giovani chirurghi, così come l'aggiornamento di chi già regolarmente pratica la professione, non può prescindere da un continuo, serrato e approfondito confronto con l'esperienza degli altri centri internazionali. La lingua inglese è indubbiamente il mezzo di comunicazione universale di tale scambio. Per tale ragione la sua conoscenza profonda e specialistica è un requisito fondamentale per ogni chirurgo moderno. L'inglese è indispensabile per cogliere pienamente i progressi della chirurgia nella letteratura, per relazionarsi direttamente con i colleghi e per portare la propria esperienza al di là dei confini nazionali contribuendo in prima persona alla ricerca e al progresso.

In tale prospettiva, questa pubblicazione è quanto mai attuale e di particolare interesse. Essa combina le conoscenze di base con le nozioni più complesse rivolgendosi quindi a tutti i chirurghi, anche a coloro che hanno già familiarità con la lingua. L'opera è inoltre stata ideata specificamente per chirurghi, pertanto raccoglie vocaboli tecnici e fornisce competenze specialistiche altrimenti difficilmente reperibili. Infine, il taglio pratico e l'organizzazione schematica facilitano l'apprendimento e il reperimento delle nozioni cercate.

È quindi con grande piacere che invito i giovani chirurghi a tenere nella propria biblioteca questo volume. Ne trarranno un utile e pratico aiuto in grado di accompagnarli nel corso della loro formazione e carriera.

Torino, Ottobre 2011

Lorenzo Capussotti
Dipartimento di Chirurgia Generale e Oncologica
Azienda Ospedaliera Ordine Mauriziano
Presidio Ospedaliero "Umberto I"
Torino

Presentazione all'edizione inglese

Più di 2 anni fa, quando il Dr. Ribes mi ha invitato a lavorare alla stesura di questo libro, ho pensato che fosse una grande idea. Ero tuttavia convinto di non essere in grado di collaborare al progetto per due ragioni: primo, non mi sentivo abbastanza competente per questo compito; in più, pensavo che non avrei mai trovato il tempo per lavorarci.

In seguito, il Dr. Ribes mi ha dato le copie di due eccellenti libri che ha scritto in collaborazione con altri, *Medical English* e *Radiological English*, con una dedica scritta a mano: "Sei la persona giusta per scrivere Surgical English." Questo mi ha fatto riconsiderare l'idea di intraprendere il progetto. Mi sono serviti più di due anni per terminare la mia parte del libro.... Ringrazio il Dr. Ribes per la sua pazienza.

Ringrazio i miei genitori per avermi "costretto" a imparare l'inglese quando andavo a scuola e per avermi veramente spinto a studiare negli USA da ragazzo nell'ambito di un programma di scambio culturale. Come nefrologo specialista, mio padre sa bene che senza un inglese di livello minimo è difficile andare oltre i limiti della propria lingua o essere coinvolto in progetti internazionali. In seguito, ho avuto il privilegio di trascorrere dei brevi periodi in diversi ospedali Europei e Statunitensi, sia come studente di medicina, sia come specializzando, sia infine come esperto chirurgo. Nel corso di queste esperienze ho avuto la possibilità di visitare ospedali sia di paesi anglofoni, come Hammersmith a Londra o Stanford Hospital in California, che di paesi non anglofoni, come il Berlin Heart Center, Il Leiden University Medical Center e il Cologne City Hospital, tra gli altri. Questa è stata una delle esperienze più utili della mia vita e mi ha aperto molte porte, sia dal punto di vista personale che professionale. Come tutti gli altri specialisti, anche i chirurghi devono studiare molto per mantenere costantemente aggiornate le proprie conoscenze. Tuttavia, al contrario di altri specialisti, abbiamo bisogno di vedere altri chirurghi lavorare e di acquisire le abilità per padroneggiare le loro tecniche chirurgiche.

Una buona competenza inglese ha un'importanza fondamentale per la comprensione della letteratura scientifica (inutile dirlo, il 90% delle pubblicazioni mediche è scritto in inglese), per capire i colleghi durante i congressi internazionali e per comunicare quando si partecipa attivamente.

Forse tutti sanno che l'inglese è la lingua scientifica per eccellenza. Ma è solo andando in un altro paese che ci si rende realmente conto di quanto sia importante saper parlare inglese. Prima di tutto, avete bisogno di una conoscenza minima dell'inglese per presentarvi e per richiedere il permesso di frequentare un ospedale o per richiedere un posto di lavoro all'estero. Inoltre avrete bisogno delle tecniche per sopravvivere all'interno di una sala operatoria: per esempio, avrete bisogno di conoscere i nomi degli strumenti chirurgici e di sapere come stabilire un contatto personale e professionale con lo staff. Indifferentemente dal fatto che andiate in un paese anglofono o no, l'inglese sarà comunque il vostro più importante strumento all'estero.

C'è realmente bisogno di un libro come questo. Crediamo sinceramente che questo libro vi fornirà le tecniche di base per sopravvivere nell'"arena chirurgica" del nuovo millennio.

Málaga, Spagna   Pedro J. Aranda

Prefazione all'edizione inglese

Scrivere un libro su un argomento vasto come l'"Inglese per chirurghi" è audace quasi come parlare della "Storia dell'Impero Romano". Tuttavia, il vasto compito di questo libro è compensato dal suo approccio semplice e dai suoi scopi reali. Se da un alto sarebbe praticamente impossibile includere tutta la terminologia utilizzata nelle varie specialità chirurgiche, bisogna però considerare che molti argomenti e modi di agire sono comuni a tutte le specialità chirurgiche e molti strumenti sono comuni alla maggior parte di esse. In più i chirurghi di tutto il mondo affrontano situazioni simili come scrivere un protocollo chirurgico, visitare i pazienti in reparto, far firmare un consenso informato. In questo libro, vi forniremo consigli su come tenere una presentazione orale in un congresso internazionale, scrivere articoli, e muoversi all'interno della sala operatoria (o OR, come viene invariabilmente chiamata negli ospedali Americani).

Data l'importanza della lingua inglese in medicina, i chirurghi di tutto il mondo dovrebbero trarre vantaggio dalla lettura di questo libro; sarà prezioso per chi desidera lavorare in un altro paese, lavorare come fellow in un ospedale diverso o semplicemente trascorrere alcune settimane in un ospedale dove si parla una lingua diversa dalla propria. Anche nei paesi dove l'inglese non è una delle lingue principali parlate dalla popolazione, la sua conoscenza vi permetterà di comunicare con le persone che vi circondano, all'interno dell'ospedale, nella maggior parte dei paesi.

Sebbene la gran parte di questo libro abbia lo scopo di aiutarvi a padroneggiare i concetti essenziali, vi sarà utile anche se possedete già un'ottima padronanza della lingua inglese. La vita professionale in un paese straniero pone di fronte a un numero infinito di sfide anche gli oratori più capaci. Sarà sempre utile avere un libro tascabile per ricordarvi di alcuni termini specifici o per fronteggiare particolari situazioni.

Potete leggere questo libro dall'inizio alla fine o saltare da un capitolo all'altro, dal momento che ogni capitolo tratta un argomento indipendente.

Speriamo che questo libro vi piaccia e che vi sia utile nella vita e nella carriera.

Ramón Ribes
Pedro J. Aranda
John Giba

Indice

Capitolo 1

Capitolo 2

Capitolo 3

Capitolo 4

Capitolo 5

Capitolo 6

Capitolo 7

Capitolo 8

Capitolo 9

Capitolo 10

Capitolo 11

Capitolo 12

Capitolo 13

Capitolo 14

Capitolo 15

Capitolo 16

Capitolo 17

Capitolo 18

Capitolo 19

Capitolo 20

Capitolo 21

Capitolo 22

Capitolo 1

Approccio metodologico all'inglese chirurgico

Per iniziare

Una profonda conoscenza della grammatica inglese è essenziale per costruire il vostro inglese chirurgico nel modo più solido. I chirurghi hanno bisogno di una conoscenza fluida dell'inglese anatomico, la cui padronanza è fondamentale per capire i vari approcci chirurgici così come i riscontri radiologici. L'anatomia è così collegata al latino e al greco che, a meno che non abbiate una certa familiarità con la terminologia latina e greca, non sarete mai in grado di parlare e scrivere in modo corretto l'inglese anatomico o chirurgico. Inoltre, i chirurghi devono sapere che i propri dettagli tecnici iperspecialistici, nella maggior parte dei casi, non sono compresi dai profani e pertanto devono essere in grado di parlarne in modo comprensibile a pazienti, medici curanti, specializzandi, infermieri, tecnici e studenti di medicina, in maniera tale che essi possano capire.

Anche la comunicazione con i pazienti e i loro parenti è di importanza fondamentale. I chirurghi hanno bisogno di comprendere i pazienti quando parlano dei loro problemi e devono essere in grado di informare i pazienti e le loro famiglie, con un linguaggio comprensibile anche ai profani, sia prima che dopo un intervento chirurgico.

Infine, è sempre più frequente operare pazienti svegli e questa situazione richiede una comunicazione scorrevole per assicurare sicurezza e comfort.

Facciamo ora un semplice esercizio. Leggete questa frase:

> ❯ Furthermore, partial resection of the suprarenal tumor could result in seeding of the operating field and hemostasis would be cumbersome without the use of BioGlue or the harmonic scalpel.

Siamo sicuri che abbiate capito la frase e siate in grado di tradurla in

R. Ribes, P. J. Aranda, J. Giba, *Inglese per chirurghi*,
© Springer-Verlag Italia 2012

italiano immediatamente; sfortunatamente la traduzione letterale è non solo inutile, ma anche deleteria ai fini della scorrevolezza del vostro inglese chirurgico. Questo è il primo punto chiave: capire non è la stessa cosa di tradurre.

Se provate a leggere il paragrafo ad alta voce in inglese, vi appariranno le prime difficoltà.

Se si aprisse una discussione su questa frase e il pubblico si aspettasse di sentire la vostra opinione, potreste iniziare ad agitarvi.

Controllate le parole che non siete in grado di pronunciare facilmente e cercatele sul dizionario.

Chiedete a un collega che parla inglese di leggervi la frase ad alta voce; provate a scriverla, probabilmente incontrerete delle difficoltà nello scrivere alcune parole.

Controllate le parole che non riuscite a scrivere correttamente e cercatele nuovamente sul dizionario.

Infine, provate a intavolare una discussione sull'argomento.

Notate quanti problemi sono nati da una sola frase in inglese chirurgico. I nostri suggerimenti, una volta valutato il reale livello del vostro inglese chirurgico, sono:

- non deprimetevi se il vostro livello è inferiore alle vostre aspettative;
- continuate con questo tipo di esercizio con paragrafi progressivamente più lunghi, a partire da quelli inerenti la vostra area di specialità;
- organizzate delle sedute di inglese chirurgico nel vostro istituto. Un incontro alla settimana potrebbe essere un buon punto di partenza e vi permetterà di restare in contatto con i vostri colleghi. Vi sentirete molto più sicuri nel parlare con i colleghi che hanno un livello di inglese inferiore al vostro piuttosto che parlare con il vostro insegnante madrelingua, così come vi sentirete meglio parlando con chirurghi non madrelingua piuttosto che con colleghi madrelingua inglese. In questi incontri, potrete provare a esporre presentazioni e lezioni, in modo che, quando dovrete farlo a un meeting internazionale, non sarà la prima volta.

Potete utilizzare questo esercizio per valutare il livello del vostro inglese scientifico:

Le seguenti frasi sono corrette?

1. The carotid artery must be dissected from the jugular vein.
   - ERRATO

In questo caso "dissected" fa riferimento a due strutture differenti, perciò è necessario dire: "dissected free from"

> The carotid artery must be dissected free from the jugular vein.

2. The flexor digitorum long tendon is rarely involved.
   - ERRATO
La frase corretta è:
> The flexor digitorum longus tendon is rarely involved.
Ricontrollate sempre lo *spelling* della terminologia Latino/Greca.

3. A 57-years-old patient with severe abdominal pain.
   - ERRATO
La frase corretta è:
> A 57-year-old patient with severe abdominal pain.
In questo caso l'espressione "57-year-old" si comporta come un aggettivo e gli aggettivi che precedono i nomi non possono essere scritti al plurale.

4. There was not biopsy of the lesion.
   - ERRATO
La frase corretta è:
> There was no biopsy of the lesion.
Anche se tecnicamente non è scorretto dire "there was not a biopsy of the lesion" o "there were not any biopsies of the lesion," queste frasi sono poco eleganti e nessuna persona madrelingua le direbbe. Altre alternative corrette includono "a biopsy was not taken" e "the lesion was not biopsied."

5. An 87-year-old patient with arrithmya.
   - ERRATO
Arrhythmia è una delle parole dell'inglese scientifico delle quali si sbaglia l'ortografia più spesso. Potete evitare questo errore ricorrente controllando la parola *rhythm* (premesso che sia scritta correttamente!), contenuta in *arrhythmia*.

6. Cosa significa "heart burn"?
Familiarmente, si riferisce all'insieme dei sintomi del reflusso gastroesofageo.

7. Cosa capireste se una strumentista vi dicesse: "Dance with me"?
Vi sta chiedendo di allacciare il suo camice sterile.

8. I due termini "Harvard students" e "Harvard alumni" sono sinonimi?
NO. Il primo termine si riferisce agli attuali studenti, il secondo agli ex studenti.

9. In che modo chiedereste a un paziente di eseguire una manovra di Valsalva?

❯ Bear down as if you were having a bowel movement.

10. I termini "home calls" e "in-house calls" sono sinonimi?

NO. Hanno significati opposti. In "home calls", se tutto va bene, potrete dormire a casa; in "in-house calls" dovrete restare in ospedale per tutta la durata del turno.

Questa serie di domande è rivolta a coloro che ritengono che l'inglese chirurgico non sia degno di un approfondimento. D'altro canto, la maggior parte dei chirurghi che non hanno mai lavorato in un ospedale dove si parla inglese tende a sottovalutare le difficoltà dell'inglese chirurgico pensando che, una volta imparato l'inglese, non si faccia fatica a parlarlo in un ambiente chirurgico. Al contrario, coloro che hanno vissuto sulla propria pelle situazioni imbarazzanti lavorando all'estero, non si azzarderebbero a dire che l'inglese in generale o l'inglese chirurgico siano semplici.

Capitolo 2

La grammatica chirurgica

Introduzione

I primi capitoli di un libro sono probabilmente i meno letti dai lettori in generale e dai chirurghi in particolare, ma è nostra opinione che proprio nei primi capitoli siano contenute le informazioni più importanti di un libro. È infatti nei primi capitoli che sono poste le basi e, saltando le parti fondamentali, molti lettori non ottimizzano la lettura di un manuale.

Questo capitolo è essenziale, poiché, a meno che non abbiate una conoscenza approfondita della grammatica inglese, sarete assolutamente incapaci di parlare inglese come ci si aspetterebbe da un chirurgo preparato. Per il livello di inglese appropriato per voi, non è assolutamente sufficiente essere soltanto capiti: dovrete parlare in modo scorrevole e la vostra proprietà di linguaggio vi dovrà permettere di comunicare con i vostri colleghi indipendentemente dalla loro nazionalità.

Come vedrete, questa sezione di grammatica utilizza come esempi frasi che sono adatte alle necessità di un chirurgo così, mentre ripassate ad esempio le forme passive, ripasserete frasi comuni nell'inglese chirurgico quotidiano, come per esempio "the CT scan had already been performed when the surgeon arrived at the CT unit".

Potremmo dire, sintetizzando, che abbiamo sostituito le classiche frasi dei vecchi manuali di inglese come "My tailor is rich" con espressioni quali "The first year surgery resident is on call today". Senza un certo grado di conoscenza della grammatica non è possibile parlare correttamente, così come senza una certa conoscenza di anatomia non sarebbe possibile creare un buon campo operatorio. La tendenza a saltare sia la grammatica che l'anatomia, considerate da molti come semplici materie preliminari, ha avuto effetti deleteri sull'apprendimento sia dell'inglese che della chirurgia.

R. Ribes, P. J. Aranda, J. Giba, *Inglese per chirurghi*,
© Springer-Verlag Italia 2012

Tempi

Parlando del presente

Present Continuous

Il *present continuous* indica un'azione che si sta compiendo nel momento stesso in cui si parla.
Questo tempo è formato dal presente semplice del verbo to be (am/are/is) + il gerundio del verbo (Infinito (senza to) + ing).

La frase negativa si forma aggiungendo not tra il verbo to be e il gerundio.
Esempio: She is not working today = She's not working today = She isn't working today.

F O R M A	Simple present del verbo *to be* + gerundio del verbo: *am/are/is…-ing*.

Studiate questo esempio:

❭ It is 7.30 in the morning. Dr. Hudson is in his new car on his way to the Ginecology Department. Dunque, "he is *driving* to the Ginecology Department" significa che sta guidando adesso, nel momento in cui stiamo parlando.

U S I	Per parlare di: Qualcosa che sta accadendo nel momento in cui stiamo parlando (cioè, ora): ❭ Dr. Hudson *is walking* to the operating room. ❭ Dr. Smith and his colleagues are *performing* an enteroclysis. Qualcosa che sta accadendo in un momento vicino a quello in cui stiamo parlando, ma non necessariamente contemporaneamente alla conversazione: ❭ Jim and John, general surgery residents, *are having* a sandwich in

the cafeteria. John says "I *am writing* an interesting article on chordomas. I'll let you have a look at it when I'm finished".

Come potete notare, John non sta scrivendo l'articolo nel preciso momento in cui sta parlando, ma vuol dire che ha iniziato a scriverlo, ma non l'ha ancora finito. È a metà del processo di scrittura.

Qualcosa che sta accadendo in un periodo limitato vicino al presente (ad esempio oggi, questa mattina, questa stagione, quest'anno...):
> Our junior neurosurgery residents *are working* hard this term.

Situazioni in evoluzione:
> Clinically speaking, the patient's condition *is getting* better.

Situazioni temporanee:
> I *am living* with other residents until I can buy my own apartment.
> I *am doing* a rotation in the surgery division until the end of May.

Usi speciali: il present continuous con significato di futuro.
Nei prossimi esempi si parla di cose già organizzate.

Per parlare di qualcosa che avete organizzato di fare nel prossimo futuro (impegni personali):
> We *are stenting* a renal artery on Monday.
> I *am having* dinner with a cardiothoracic surgeon from the United States tomorrow.

Possiamo anche usare la forma *going to* in queste frasi, ma è meno naturale quando si parla di impegni personali.
Non utilizziamo il simple present o *will* per gli impegni personali.

Simple Present

Il simple present mostra un'azione che si ripete al presente, ma non necessariamente mentre ha luogo la conversazione.

F O R M A	Il simple present ha le seguenti forme:

Il simple present ha le seguenti forme:

Affermativa: la stessa dell'infinto (senza to) (ricordate di aggiungere –s o –es alla terza persona singolare).

Negativa
> I/we/you/they do not (don't) + infinto (senza to)
> He/she/it doesn't + infinto (senza to)

Interrogativa
> Do I/we/you/they + infinto (senza to)?
> Doesn't he/she/it...?

Studiate questo esempio:

> Dr. Allan is the chairman of the Traumatology Department. He is at an International course in Greece at this moment.

Quindi: non sta dirigendo il Dipartimento di Traumatologia in questo momento (poiché è in Grecia), ma lo dirige abitualmente.

U S I	Per parlare di qualcosa che succede sempre ripetutamente o qualcosa che è vero in generale.

Per parlare di qualcosa che succede sempre ripetutamente o qualcosa che è vero in generale. Non è importante se l'azione sta avendo luogo al momento della conversazione:

> I do pediatric surgery.

> Nurses take care of patients after the implantation of the pacemaker.

> For colon surgery, pre-intervention preparation serves to cleanse the bowel.

Per dire quanto spesso facciamo qualcosa:
> I *begin* to see patients at 8.30 every morning.
> Dr. Taylor *does* laparoscopic surgery two evenings a week.
> How often *do you go* to an International surgical course? Once a year.

U S I	Il simple present è usato spesso con avverbi di frequenza *come* *always*, *often*, *sometimes*, *rarely*, *never*, *every week* e *twice a year*:

> The heart surgery chairman *always* works very hard.
> We have a pathology conference *every week*.

Per una situazione permanente (una situazione che resta uguale per un lungo periodo):

> I *work* as consultant in the breast cancer program of our hospital. I have been working there for 10 years.

Alcuni verbi sono utilizzati solo nei tempi semplici. Questi sono i verbi di pensiero o attività mentale, sentimento, possesso, percezione e i verbi per riferire. Spesso con questi verbi si utilizza *can* invece del tempo:

> I *can understand* now why X-ray machine is in such a bad condition.
> I *can see* now the solution to the diagnostic problem.

Il simple present può essere utilizzato con significato di futuro. Lo usiamo per parlare di orari, programmi, ecc.:

> What time *does* the arthroscopic knee surgery conference *start?* It *starts* at 9.30.

Parlando del futuro

Am/is/are + Going to + infinito

U S I	Per esprimere quello che abbiamo già deciso di fare o quello che intendiamo fare in futuro (non utilizzate *will* in questo caso):

> *I am going* to attend the 20th International Congress of Angiology and Vascular Surgery next month.
> There is a hands-on minimally invasive course in Boston next fall. *Are you going to* attend it?

Per dire quello che qualcuno ha organizzato di fare (impegni personali), ma ricordate che si preferisce utilizzare il present continuous, poiché suona più naturale.

> What time *are you going to meet* the vice chairman?
> What time are *you going to* begin the ooferectomy?

U S I	Per dire quello che riteniamo succederà (fare previsioni): ❯ The patient is agitated. I think we *are not going* to be able to do the operation under local anesthesia alone. ❯ "Oh, the patient's chest X-ray looks terrible. I think he *is going to* die soon", the radiologist said. Se vogliamo dire quello che qualcuno intendeva fare in passato, ma che non ha fatto, usiamo *was/ were going to*: ❯ He *was going to* do a radical resection of the tumour but finally changed his mind and did a more limited one. Per parlare di previsioni passate utilizziamo *was/ were going to*: ❯ The resident had the feeling that the patient *was going to* suffer a reaction to the antibiotic.

Simple Future (Will)

F O R M A	*Will* + infinito (senza to), ma anche *shall* può essere usato con I o We (will è più comune di shall, ma solo shall è utilizzato nelle domande per fare offerte e dare suggerimenti): ❯ *Shall* we go to the Thorachoscopy Symposium next week? You/he/she/it/they *will* (*'ll*) + infinito (senza to). Negativo: shall not = *shan't*, will not = *won't*.

U S I	Utilizziamo *will* quando decidiamo di fare qualcosa nel momento in cui stiamo parlando (ricordate che in questo caso non potete usare il simple present): ❯ Have you finished the report? ❯ No, I haven't had time to do it. ❯ Ok, don't worry, I *will* do it. Quando offriamo, concordiamo, rifiutiamo o promettiamo di fare qualcosa, o quando chiediamo a qualcuno di fare qualcosa: ❯ That case looks difficult for you. Do not worry, I *will* help you out. ❯ Can I have the book about brain tumour that I lent you back? Of course. I *will* give it back to you tomorrow.

<table>
<tr>
<td>U
S
I</td>
<td>

> Don't ask to perform the appendectomy by yourself. The consultant *won't* allow you to.
> I promise I *will* send you a copy of the latest article on intra-operative ultrasound as soon as I get it.
> *Will* you help me out with this amputation, please?

Non usate *will* per dire quello che qualcuno ha già deciso di fare o organizzato di fare (ricordate che in questa situazione useremo *going to* o il *present continuous*).

Per predire un evento o una situazione futuri:
> The specialty of General Surgery *will* be very different in a hundred year's time.
> Twenty years from now, heart surgeons won't need to perform thoracotomy.
Ricordate che se c'è qualcosa nella situazione presente che ci indica cosa succederà in futuro (prossimo futuro) si utilizza *going to* invece di *will*.

Con espressioni tipo: *probably, I am sure, I bet, I think, I suppose, I guess*:
> I *will probably* attend the European Congress.
> You should listen to Dr. Helms's conference. *I am sure* you *will* love it.
> I *bet* the patient *will* recover satisfactorily after the bypass.
> I *guess* I *will* see you at the next annual meeting.

</td>
</tr>
</table>

Future Continuous

<table>
<tr>
<td>F
O
R
M
A</td>
<td>

La forma del future continuous è: *will be* + gerundio.

Per dire che staremo facendo qualcosa in un dato momento in futuro:
> This time tomorrow morning I *will be performing* a CABG.

</td>
</tr>
</table>

U S I	Per parlare di cose che sono già programmate o decise (simile al present continuous con significato di futuro): ❯ We can't meet this evening. I *will be stenting* the aneurysmin in the patient we talked about. Per chiedere dei programmi di altre persone, soprattutto quando vogliamo qualcosa o vogliamo che qualcuno faccia qualcosa (forma interrogativa): ❯ *Will* you *be attending* the congress this year?

Future Perfect

F O R M A	La forma del future perfect è: *will have* + participio passato del verbo.

U S I	Per dire che qualcosa sarà già avvenuta prima di un dato momento nel futuro: ❯ I think the resident *will have arrived* by the time we begin the osteosynthesis. ❯ Next spring I *will have been working* in the Oral and Maxillofacial Department of this institution for 25 years.

Parlando del passato

Simple Past

F O R M A	Il simple past ha queste forme: Affermativa ❯ Il passato dei verbi regolari è formato aggiungendo –*ed* o -*d* all'infinito. ❯ Il passato dei verbi irregolari ha una sua forma propria. Negativa ❯ Did not = didn't + infinito (senza to).

U S I	Interrogativa ❯ *Did I/ did you/...*+ infinito (senza to). Per parlare di azioni o situazioni del passato (che si sono già concluse): ❯ I really *enjoyed* the trauma resident's party very much. ❯ When I *worked* as a visiting resident in Madrid, I *performed* 100 vasectomies. Per dire che una cosa è successa dopo un'altra: ❯ Yesterday we *had* a terrible duty. We *did* three embolectomies and then we performed an emergency mitral valve repair. Per chiedere o dire quando o a quale ora è successo qualcosa: ❯ When *were* you last on call? ❯ I arrived 5 min ago. Per raccontare una storia e parlare di fatti e azioni che non sono connessi al presente (eventi storici): ❯ Christian Barnard performed the first human-to-human heart transplantation.

Past Continuous

F O R M A	La forma del past continuous è: *was/were* + gerundio del verbo.

U S I	Per dire che qualcuno stava facendo qualcosa in un certo momento. L'azione o situazione era già cominciata prima di adesso, ma non era ancora finita: ❯ This time last year, I *was writing* the case report that I plan to publish next year in the *World Journal of Surgery*. Notate che il past continuous non ci dice se un'azione fosse finita o meno. Forse lo era, forse no. Per descrivere una scena: ❯ A lot of patients *were waiting* in the corridor to have their chest X-ray done.

Present Perfect

F O R M A	La forma del present perfect è: *Have/has* + participio passato del verbo.

U S I	Per parlare del risultato attuale di un'azione passata. • Per parlare di un avvenimento. • Per parlare di un evento recente. In quest'ultima situazione, potete utilizzare il present perfect con le seguenti preposizioni: *Just* (cioè poco tempo fa), per dire che qualcosa è appena accaduta: ❯ Dr. Ho *has just arrived* at the hospital. He is our new pediatric surgeon. *Already*, per dire qualcosa che è successo prima di quanto previsto: ❯ The second year resident *has already finished* her presentation. Ricordate che per parlare di un evento recente possiamo utilizzare il simple past. Per parlare di un periodo che dura fino al presente (un periodo di tempo non finito): • usiamo le espressioni: *today, this morning, this evening, this week...* • spesso usiamo *ever* e *never*. Per parlare di qualcosa che stiamo aspettando. In questa situazione utilizziamo *yet* per mostrare che chi parla sta aspettando che qualcosa succeda, ma solo nelle domande e nelle frasi negative: ❯ Dr. Helms *has not arrived yet*. Per parlare di qualcosa che non avete mai fatto o di qualcosa che non avete fatto in un periodo di tempo che dura fino al presente: ❯ I *have not performed* a mastectomy since I was a resident.. Per parlare di quanto abbiamo fatto, di quante cose abbiamo fatto o di quante volte abbiamo fatto qualcosa:

U **S** **I**	❯ I *have reported* that intervention twice because the first report was lost. ❯ Dr. Yimou *has performed* twenty vertebroplasties this week. Per parlare di situazioni che sono esistite per un lungo periodo, specialmente se utilizziamo *always*. In questi casi, la situazione sussiste tuttora: ❯ We *have already had* an excellent internal medicine department. ❯ Dr. Olmedo *has always been* a very talented urologist. Inoltre, utilizziamo il present perfect con queste espressioni: Superlativo; *It is the most...*: ❯ This is the most interesting case that *I have ever seen.* La *prima, (seconda, terza...)* volta: ❯ This is the *first time* that I have seen a CT of an inferior vena cava leiomyosarcoma.

Present Perfect Continuous

Illustra un'azione che è iniziata nel passato e continua fino al momento presente.

F **O** **R** **M** **A**	La forma del present perfect continuous è: *have/has been* + gerundio del verbo.

U **S** **I**	Per parlare di un'azione che è iniziata nel passato ed è finita di recente o in questo momento: ❯ You look tired. *Have you been working* all night? ❯ No, I *have been writing* an article on breast implants. Per chiedere o dire per quanto a lungo sia andata avanti una cosa. In questo caso, l'azione o situazione è iniziata nel passato ed è ancora in corso o è appena finita: ❯ Dr. Sancho and Dr. Martos *have been working* together from the beginning of this project.

| U
S
I | Utilizziamo le seguenti preposizioni:

• *How long...?* (per chiedere quanto a lungo):
> *How long have you been working* as personal assistant to Dr. Miller?

• *For, since* (per dire quanto a lungo):
> I *have been working for* 10 years.
> I *have been working* very hard *since* I got this grant.

• *For* (per dire quanto a lungo come periodo di tempo):
> I *have been doing* flap correction *for* 3 years.

Non usate *for* nelle espressioni con *all*: "I have been working as a plastic surgeon all my career" (non "for all my career").

• *Since* (per dire quando è iniziato un periodo):
> I *have been teaching* laparoscopy *since* 1994.

Nel present perfect continuous la cosa importante è l'azione stessa e non importa se sia conclusa o meno: l'azione può essere conclusa (appena finita) o no (ancora in corso).
Nel present perfect è importante il risultato dell'azione e non l'azione stessa. L'azione è del tutto conclusa. |

Past Perfect

Illustra un'azione che è iniziata nel passato prima di un'altra azione passata. È il passato del present perfect.

| F
O
R
M
A | La forma del past perfect è: *had* + participio passato del verbo. |

| U
S
I | Per dire che qualcosa era già successo prima che succedesse qualcos'altro:
> When I arrived at the operating room, the traumatologist had already begun the external fixation of the shoulder. |

Past Perfect Continuous

Illustra un'azione che è iniziata nel passato ed è continuata fino a un certo momento passato. È il passato del present perfect continuous.

F O R M A	La forma del past perfect continuous è: *had been* + gerundio del verbo.

U S I	Per dire quanto a lungo qualcosa stava già succedendo prima che succedesse qualcos'altro: 〉 She *had been working* as a urologist for 40 years before she was awarded the Foley Prize.

Congiuntivo

Immaginate questa situazione:
〉 The surgeon says to the radiologist, "Why don't you do a CT Scan on the patient with acute abdominal pain?"
〉 The surgeon proposes (that) the radiologist do a CT Scan on the patient with abdominal pain.

F O R M A	Il congiuntivo si forma sempre con la forma base del verbo (l'infinito senza to): 〉 I suggest (that) you work harder. 〉 She recommended (that) he give up smoking while dictating. 〉 He insisted (that) she perform an ultrasound examination on the patient as soon as possible. 〉 He demanded (that) the nurse treat him more politely. Notate che il congiuntivo del verbo to be è di solito passivo. 〉 He insisted (that) the surgical report be dictated immediately.

<table>
<tr><td>U
S
I</td><td>

Potete usare il congiuntivo dopo i seguenti verbi:

> *Propose*
> *Suggest*
> *Reccomend*
> *Insist*
> *Demand*

Potete usare il congiuntivo per il passato, presente o futuro:

> He *suggested* (that) the resident change the dressing of the wound.
> He *recommends* (that) his patient give up smoking.

Talvolta si può utilizzare Should al posto del congiuntivo, specialmente nell'Inglese Britannico.

> The doctor recommended that I should have an MRI examination; he suspects that my meniscus is torn.

</td></tr>
</table>

Wish, If Only, Would

Wish

<table>
<tr><td>F
O
R
M
A</td><td>

- *Wish* + simple past. Per dire che ci dispiace qualcosa del presente (cioè che qualcosa non è come vorremmo che fosse):
> I wish I were not on call tomorrow (but I am on call tomorrow)

- *Wish* + past perfect. Per dire che ci dispiace qualcosa che è successo o non è successo nel passato:
> I wish he hadn't treated the patient's family so badly (but he treated the patient's family badly)

- *Wish* + would + infinito senza to quando vogliamo che qualcosa succeda o cambi o che qualcuno faccia qualcosa:
> I wish you wouldn't dictate so slowly (notare che chi parla si sta lamentando della situazione presente o del modo in cui le persone fanno le cose).

</td></tr>
</table>

If Only

If only può essere usato esattamente come *wish*. Ha lo stesso significato di *wish*, ma è più teatrale.

F O R M A	• *If only* + past simple (esprime rimpianto nel presente): ❯ *If only* I *were not* on call. • *If only* + past perfect (esprime rimpianto nel passato): ❯ *If only* he *hadn't treated* the patient's family so badly. Dopo wish e if only usiamo were (con I, he, she, it) invece di was e di solito non usiamo would, anche se a volte è possibile, o would have. Quando ci riferiamo al presente o al futuro, wish e if only sono seguiti da un tempo passato e quando ci riferiamo al passato, sono seguiti da un past perfect.

Would

F O R M A	*Would* è usato: • Come un verbo modale in offerte, inviti e richieste (cioè per chiedere a qualcuno di fare qualcosa): ❯ *Would* you help me write an article on hepatic cholangiocarcinoma? (Richiesta). ❯ *Would* you like to come to the residents' party tonight?(Offerta e invito). ❯ Dopo *wish* (vedi Wish). ❯ Nelle frasi con *if* (vedi Condizionali). • A volte come il passato di will (nei discorsi riferiti): ❯ Dr. Smith: "I will do your bladder resection next week". ❯ Patient: "The Doctor said that he would do my bladder resection next week". • Quando ricordate cose che succedevano spesso (simile a used to): ❯ When we were residents, we used to prepare the clinical cases together. ❯ When we were residents, we would prepare the clinical cases together.

Verbi modali

F O R M A	• I verbi modali hanno sempre la stessa forma.
	• La terza persona singolare non finisce con –*s*, non ci sono forme in –*ing* o –*ed*.
	• Dopo un verbo modale usiamo l'infinito senza *to* (cioè, la forma base del verbo).

I verbi modali in inglese sono questi:
> *Can* (il passato è *could*)
> *Could* (anche con significato proprio)
> *May* (il passato è *might*)
> *Might* (anche con significato proprio)
> *Will*
> *Would*
> *Shall*
> *Should*
> *Ought to*
> *Must*
> *Need*
> *Dare*

Usiamo i verbi modali per parlare di:
• Abilità
• Necessità
• Possibilità
• Certezza
• Permesso
• Obbligo

Esprimere abilità

Per esprimere abilità possiamo usare:

> *Can* (solo al tempo presente)
> *Could* (solo al tempo passato)
> *Be able to* (in tutti i tempi)

Abilità nel presente

Can (più usato) o *am/is/are able to* (meno usato):

> Dr. Williams *can do* a bypass on an extremely difficult mesenteric artery stenosis.
> Dr. Douglas *is able to* dilate esophageal stenoses in children.
> *Can* you speak medical English? Yes, I *can*.
> *Are you able to* speak medical English? Yes, I *am*.

Abilità nel passato

Could (passato di can) o *was/were able to*

<table>
<tr>
<td>U
S
I</td>
<td>

Usiamo could per dire che qualcuno ha una generale abilità a fare qualcosa:
> When I was a resident, I could speak German.

Usiamo was/were able to per dire che qualcuno è riuscito a fare qualcosa in una determinata situazione (abilità specifica di fare qualcosa), anche se, con i verbi di percezione, possiamo utilizzare could
> When I was a resident, I was able to publish seven articles.
> We *could* see that the LAD was completely blocked.

Managed to può sostituire *was able to* (soprattutto quando si parla di qualcosa particolarmente difficile):
> When I was a resident, I managed to publish seven articles.

Usiamo *could have* per dire che avevamo la capacità di fare qualcosa, ma non l'abbiamo fatta:
> He could have been a surgeon but he became a radiologist instead.

A volte usiamo *could* per parlare di abilità in una situazione ipotetica (in questo caso *could* equivale a *would be able to*):
> I couldn't do your job; I'm not clever enough.

Usiamo *will be able to* per parlare di abilità con significato futuro:
> If you keep on studying surgical English, then you will be able to write articles for The Annals of Surgery very soon.

</td>
</tr>
</table>

Esprimere necessità

Necessità significa che non si può evitare di fare qualcosa.
Per dire che è necessario fare qualcosa, possiamo usare *must* o *have to*.

> Necessità nel presente: *must, have/has to*
> Necessità nel passato: *had to*
> Necessità nel futuro: *must, will have to*

Notate che per esprimere necessità nel passato non usiamo *must*.
Ci sono alcune differenze tra *must* e *have to*:

<table>
<tr><td>U
S
I</td><td>

• Usiamo *must* quando chi parla sta esprimendo sentimenti personali o autorità, dicendo quello che ritiene sia necessario:
> Your chest X-rays film shows severe emphysema. You must give up smoking.
• Usiamo *have* to quando chi parla non sta esprimendo sentimenti personali o autorità, ma sta solo esponendo fatti o esprimendo l'autorità di un'altra persona (autorità esterna), spesso una legge o una regola:
> All surgery residents have to learn how to dictatate the different types of surgical reports in their first year of residency.

Se vogliamo dire che è necessario evitare di fare qualcosa, usiamo *mustn't* (cioè, not allowed to):
> You mustn't eat anything before the operation.
</td></tr>
</table>

Esprimere l'assenza di necessità

Per dire che non c'è necessità, possiamo usare le forme negative di *need* o *have to*:
> Non c'è necessità nel presente: *needn't* o *don't/doesn't have to*
> Non c'era necessità nel passato: *didn't need, didn't have to*
> Non ci sarà necessità nel futuro: *won't have to*
Notate che "there is no necessity to do something" è totalmente diverso da "there is a necessity not to do something".

In conclusione, usiamo *mustn't* quando non siamo autorizzati a fare qualcosa o quando non c'è bisogno di farlo e usiamo la forma negativa di *have to o needn't* quando non c'è bisogno di fare qualcosa, ma possiamo farla se vogliamo:

> The urologist says I *mustn't* get overtired before the procedure but I *needn't* stay in bed.

> The urologist says I *mustn't* get overtired before the procedure but I *don't have to* stay in bed.

Esprimere possibilità

Per esprimere possibilità possiamo usare: *can, could, may, o might* (dal grado maggiore a minore di certezza: *can, may, might, could*).
Notate inoltre che *can* può essere usato per l'abilità (o capacità) di fare qualcosa; *may* per il permesso o l'autorizzazione a farlo.
Parlando di possibilità, *can* è usato in senso generale e *may* è usato in un caso particolare:

> Patients with defective heart valves *can* develop endocarditis.

> This patients *may* develop endocarditis.

Possibilità nel presente

Per dire che qualcosa è possibile, usiamo *can, may, might, could*; tutti esprimono possibilità, ma l'utilizzo di might e could indica un grado di probabilità leggermente più scarso:

> Patients undergoing Billroth II stomach resection *can* get postoperative pneumonia.

> They *may* develop anastomosistis.

> The anastomosis suture *could* leak.

> They *might* develop thrombosis of the mesenteric vessels.

Possibilità nel passato

Per dire che qualcosa era possibile nel passato usiamo *may have, might have, could have*:

> The lesion might have been detected on the screen if the field had been cleaner.

Could have è inoltre usato per dire che qualcosa era una possibilità o un'opportunità, ma non è successo:

> You were lucky to be treated with an emergency operation, otherwise you could have died.

I couldn't have done something (cioè, non sarei stato in grado di farlo se avessi voluto o provato a farlo):

> She couldn't have selectively excised that lung metastasis anyway, because it was extremely small.

Possibilità nel futuro

Per parlare di possibili azioni o fatti futuri usiamo *may, might, could* (soprattutto nei suggerimenti):

> I don't know where to do my last six months of residency. I *may/might* go to the States.
> We *could* meet later in the hospital to practice mattress sutures, couldn't we?

Quando parliamo di possibili piani futuri possiamo inoltre usare la forma continua *may/might/could be* + *forma in -ing*:

> I *could be going* to the next AATS meeting.

Esprimere certezza

Per dire che siamo sicuri che qualcosa è vero, usiamo *must*:

> You have been operating all night. You *must* be very tired (i.e., in all probability you are tired).

Per dire che pensiamo che qualcosa sia impossibile usiamo *can't*:

> According to his clinical situation and clinical studies, this diagnosis *can't* be right (i.e., it is impossible that this diagnosis be right or I am sure that this diagnosis is not right).

Per situazioni passate usiamo *must have* e *can't have*. Possiamo inoltre usare *couldn't have* invece di *can't have*:

> Considering the situation, the patient's family *couldn't have* asked for more.

Ricordate che per esprimere certezza possiamo anche usare *will*:

> The minimally invasive mitral valve plasty protocol *will* vary from institution to institution.

Esprimere permesso

Per parlare di permessi possiamo usare *can, may* (più formale di can) o *be allowed to* (utilizzato di solito nelle frasi negative per esprimere proibizione).

Permesso nel presente

Can, may o *am/is/are allowed to*:
> You *can* smoke if you like.
> You *are allowed to* smoke.
> You *may* attend the Congress.

Permesso nel passato

Was/were allowed to:
> *Were you allowed to* go into the OT without surgical scrubs?

Permesso nel futuro

May, can, o *be allowed to*:
> May I leave the hospital when I finish this operation?
> You can take a break after you finish this operation, but you can't leave the hospital.
> I will be allowed to leave the hospital when my duty is finished.

Per chiedere un permesso possiamo usare *can, may, could o might* (da meno a più formale), ma non *be allowed to*:

> Hi Hannah, *can* I borrow your digital camera? (if you are asking for a friend's digital camera).
> Dr. Chang, *may* I borrow your digital camera? (if you are talking to an acquaintance).
> Could I use your digital camera, Dr. Coltrane? (if you are talking to a colleague you do not know at all).
> Dr. Ho, *may* I borrow your digital camera? (if you are talking to a colleague you do not know at all).
> *Might* I use your digital camera, Dr. Escaned? (if you are asking for the chairman's digital camera).

Esprimere obbligo morale o dare consigli

Obbligo morale vuol dire che qualcosa è la cosa giusta da fare.
Quando vogliamo dire che quello che pensiamo è una buona cosa da fare, o la cosa giusta da fare, usiamo *should* o *ought to* (un po' più forte di *should*).

Should o *ought to* possono essere usati per dare consigli:

> You *ought to* sleep.
> You *should* work out.
> You *ought to* give up smoking.
> *Ought* he *to* see a doctor? Yes, I think he ought to.
> *Should* he see a doctor? Yes, I think he *should*.

Condizionali

Le frasi al condizionale si compongono di due parti:
1. Frase con *if*.
2. Frase principale.

Nella frase "If I were you, I would go to the annual meeting of maxillofacial residents", *If I were you* è la frase con if e *I would go to the annual meeting of maxillofacial residents* è la frase principale.

La frase con *if* può essere prima o dopo la frase principale. Spesso mettiamo una virgola se la frase con *if* è la prima.

Tipi principali di frasi al condizionale

Tipo 0

Per parlare di cose che sono sempre vere (verità generali).
- *If* + simple present + simple present:
> *If* you perform a full laparotomy, the approach to the gallbladder is extremely easy.
> *If* you see free air in the abdomen, the patient is perforated.
> *If* you drink too much alcohol, you get a sore head.
> *If* you take drugs habitually, you become addicted.

Notate che gli esempi si riferiscono a cose che sono generalmente vere. Non fanno alcun riferimento al futuro; rappresentano un semplice dato di fatto presente. Questa è la forma base (o classica) del condizionale di tipo 0.
Esistono alcune possibili variazioni di questa forma. Nella frase con *if* e nella frase principale possiamo usare il present continuous, il present perfect simple o il present perfect continuous invece del present simple. Nella frase principale possiamo anche usare l'imperativo invece del present simple:

> Residents only get certificate *if* they *have attended* the course regularly.

La forma tipo 0 può essere riassunta così:
> *If* + present form + forma presente o imperativo.

Le forme presenti includono il present simple, il present continuous, il present perfect simple e il present perfect continuous.

Tipo 1

Per parlare di situazioni future che chi parla ritiene probabili (chi parla pensa a una reale possibilità nel futuro):

- If + simple present + future simple (*will*):
> *If* I find something new about the laser treatment of varicose veins, I will tell you.
> *If* we analyze different incisions, we will be able to approach the same anatomic target from different perspectives.

Questi esempi si riferiscono a fatti futuri, che sono possibili ed è abbastanza probabile che si verifichino. Questa è la forma base (o classica) del condizionale di tipo 1.
Esistono alcune possibili variazioni di questa forma. Nella frase con *if* possiamo usare il present continuous, il present perfect o il present perfect continuous invece del present simple. Nella frase principale possiamo usare il future continuous, il future perfect simple o il future perfect continuous invece del present simple. Si possono anche usare verbi modali come *can, may* o *might*.
La forma di tipo 1 può dunque essere riassunta in:

- *If* + forma presente + forma futura.

Le forme future includono il future simple, il future continuous, il future perfect simple e il future perfect continuous.

Tipo 2

Per parlare di situazioni future che chi parla ritiene possibili, ma non probabili (chi parla immagina una possibile situazione futura) o per parlare di situazioni irreali al presente.

- *If* + simple past + condizionale (*would*).
> Peter, *if* you *studied* harder, you *would* be better prepared for doing your PhD in thoracic surgery.

Le seguenti frasi ci dicono che Peter non sta studiando abbastanza.

> *If* I *were* you, *I would go* to the Annual Meeting of the American Academy of Orthopaedic Surgeons.
> *If* I *were* a resident again, *I would* go to Harvard Medical School for a whole year to complete my training period (but I am not a resident and do not plan on being one again).

Esistono alcune possibili variazioni di questa forma. Nella frase con *if* possiamo usare il past continuous invece del past simple. Nella frase principale possiamo usare *could*, o *might* invece di *would*.

La forma di tipo 2 può dunque essere trasformata in:
> *If* + past simple o continuous + *would/could/might*.

Tipo 3

Per parlare di situazioni passate che non si sono verificate (azioni impossibili nel passato).

- *If* + past perfect + perfect conditional (*would have*):

> *If* I *had known* the patient's symptoms, I probably would not have missed the small pancreatic lesion on the CT scan.

Come potete vedere, stiamo parlando del passato. La situazione reale è che non sapevo dei sintomi del paziente, quindi non ho notato la piccola lesione pancreatica.

Questa è la forma base (o classica) del condizionale di tipo 3. Esistono alcune possibili variazioni di questa forma. Nella frase con *if* possiamo usare il past perfect continuous invece del past perfect simple. Nella frase principale possiamo usare la forma continua del perfect conditional invece del perfect conditional simple. Si possono anche usare *would probably*, *could* o *might* invece di *would* (quando non siamo sicuri di qualcosa).

Condizionali misti:
Talvolta possiamo mischiare i condizionali di tipo 2 e 3 per parlare dei risultati attuali di azioni passate o di ipotetici effetti passati di ipotetiche condizioni attuali.
> *If* we *had operated*, the patient *would be* alive.
> *If* I *were* you, I *would have* referred her to Dr Zehr.

In case

"The heart surgeon wears two pairs of latex gloves during an intervention *in case* one of them tears." *In case one of them tears,* poichè è possibile che uno di essi si rompa durante l'intervento (nel futuro).

Notate che non usiamo *will* dopo *in case*. Utilizziamo un tempo presente dopo *in case* quando parliamo del futuro.

In case non è la stessa cosa di *if*. Confrontate queste frasi:
> We'll buy some more food and drink *if* the new residents come to our department's party. (Perhaps the new residents will come to our party. If they come, we will buy some more food and drink; if they don't come, we won't.)
> We will buy some food and drink *in case* the new residents come to our department's party. (Perhaps the new residents will come to our department's party. We will buy some more food and drink whether they come or not.)

Possiamo anche usare *in case* per dire il motivo per cui qualcuno ha fatto qualcosa nel passato:
> He rang the bell again *in case* the nurse hadn't heard it the first time. (Because it was possible that the nurse hadn't heard it the first time).

In case of (= if there is):
> *In case of* fire, leave the building immediately.

Unless

"Don't take the pills *unless* you are extremely anxious". (Don't take these pills except if you are extremely anxious). Questa frase significa che puoi prendere le pillole solo se sei estremamente ansioso.
 Utilizziamo *unless* per definire un'eccezione a qualcosa che diciamo. Nel precedente esempio l'eccezione è che siate estremamente ansiosi.

Spesso usiamo *unless* negli avvertimenti:

> *Unless* you send the application form today, you won't be able to attend the next National Congress of Gynecology.

È anche possibile usare *if* in una frase negativa al posto di *unless*:

> Don't take those pills *if* you aren't extremely anxious.
> *If you don't send* the application form today, you won't be able to attend the next Congress of Gynecology.

As long as, Provided (that), Providing (that)

Le seguenti espressioni significano "ma solo se":
> You can use my new pen to sign your report *as long as* you write carefully (i.e., *but only if* you write carefully).
> Going by car to the hospital is convenient *provided (that)* you have somewhere to park (i.e., *but only if* you have somewhere to park).
> *Providing (that)* she studies the clinical cases, she will deliver a brilliant presentation.

Forme passive

Studiate questi esempi:
> The first sentinel node biopsy was performed at our hospital in 1980 (passive sentence).
> Someone performed the first sentinel node biopsy at our hospital in 1980 (active sentence).

Entrambe le frasi sono corrette e hanno il medesimo significato. Ci sono due modi di dire la stessa cosa, ma nella frase passiva cerchiamo di rendere l'oggetto della frase attiva ("the first sentinel node biopsy") più importante, mettendolo all'inizio. Quindi, preferiamo usare il passivo quando non è importante chi o cosa abbia compiuto l'azione. Nel precedente esempio, non è così importante (o non è noto) chi abbia eseguito la prima biopsia di un linfonodo sentinella.

Frase attiva:
> Fleming (soggetto) discovered (verbo attivo) penicillin (oggetto) in 1950.

Frase passiva:
> Penicillin (soggetto) was discovered (verbo passivo) by Fleming (agente) in 1950.

La forma passiva si ottiene mettendo il verbo *to be* nello stesso tempo del verbo attivo e aggiungendo il participio passato del verbo attivo:
> Discovered (verbo attivo) – Was discovered (be + participio passato del verbo attivo).

L'oggetto del verbo attivo diventa il soggetto di una verbo passivo ("penicillin"): il soggetto di un verbo attivo diventa l'agente del verbo passivo ("Fleming"). Possiamo omettere l'agente se non è importante citarlo o se non lo conosciamo. Se vogliamo citarlo, lo metteremo alla fine della frase, preceduto dalla preposizione *by* ("...by Fleming").

Alcune frasi hanno due oggetti, indiretto e diretto. In queste frasi, il soggetto passivo può essere sia l'oggetto diretto che l'oggetto indiretto della frase attiva:

> The doctor gave the patient a new treatment.

Ci sono due possibilità:

> A new treatment was given to the patient.
> The patient was given a new treatment.

Forme passive dei tempi presenti e passati

Simple Present

Attivo:
> The surgeons review the most interesting cases in the clinical session every day.

Passivo:
> The most interesting cases are reviewed in the clinical session every day.

Simple Past

Attivo:
> The nurse checked the renal function of the patient before the CT examination.

Passivo:
> The renal function of the patient was checked before the CT examination.

Present Continuous

Attivo:
> Dr. Golightly is resecting a tumor right now.

Passivo:
> A tumor is being resected right now.

Past Continuous

Attivo:
> They were carrying the injured person to the operating room.

Passivo:
> The injured person was being carried to the operating room.

Present Perfect

Attivo:
> The plastic surgeon has performed ten blepharoplasties this morning.

Passivo:
> Ten blepharoplasties have been performed this morning.

Past Perfect

Attivo:
> They had sent the CT films before the operation started.

Passivo:
> The CT films had been sent before the operation started.

Nelle frasi del tipo "la gente dice/considera/sa/pensa/crede/si aspetta/capisce...che...", come "Doctors consider that AIDS is a fatal disease", abbiamo due possibili forme passive:

> AIDS is considered a fatal disease.
> It is considered that AIDS is a fatal disease.

Comunque, la prima forma è la più comune e suona più naturale.

Have/Get Something Done

F O R M A	*Have/Get* + oggetto + participio passato.

U S I	Get è un po' più informale di have ed è spesso utilizzato nell'inglese parlato informale: > You should get your laser machine tested. > You should have your laser machine tested.

Quando vogliamo dire che non vogliamo fare qualcosa o che non possiamo farla noi stessi e facciamo in modo che qualcun altro lo faccia per noi, utilizziamo l'espressione *have something done*:

> Dr. Flick has his Porsche washed every Friday.
> The patient had all his body hair removed in order to prevent infections after the operation.
> I'm going to have my eyes tested next week.

Talvolta l'espressione *have something done ha un significato diverso:*
> John had his knee injured playing football. MRI showed a meniscal tear.

È ovvio che non vuol dire che John abbia fatto sì che qualcuno gli rompesse il ginocchio. Con questo significato, utilizziamo *have something done* per dire che qualcosa (spesso qualcosa di spiacevole) è successo a qualcuno.

Supposed to

Supposed to può essere utilizzato nei seguenti modi:

- Può essere usato come *said to*:
> The chairperson *is supposed to* be the one who runs the department.

- Può essere usato per dire cosa è stato programmato o organizzato (e questo è spesso diverso da ciò che succede in realtà):
> The fourth-year resident is *supposed to* perform this operation.

- Per dire cosa non è concesso o non è consigliabile:
> She was not *supposed to* be on call yesterday.

Discorsi indiretti

Immaginate di voler riferire a qualcuno ciò che ha detto un paziente. Potete ripetere le parole del paziente oppure usare il discorso riportato. Il verbo per riferire (*said* negli esempi seguenti) può precedere o seguire la frase riportata, ma di solito la precede. Quando il verbo per riferire viene prima, possiamo usare *that* per introdurre la frase riportata o ometterlo (quest'ultima opzione è meno formale). Quando il verbo per riferire segue, non possiamo usare *that* per introdurre la frase riportata. Si possono riferire affermazioni e pensieri, domande, ordini e richieste.

Riferire nel presente

Quando il verbo del riferire è al tempo presente, non è necessario cambiare il tempo del verbo:

"I'll help you guys with this cataract," he says.
> He says (that) he will help us with this cataract.
"The vertebroplasty will take place this morning," he says.
> He says (that) the vertebroplasty will take place this morning.

Riferire nel passato

Quando il verbo del riferire è al tempo passato, il verbo nel discorso diretto di solito cambia nei seguenti modi:
- Il simple present diventa simple past.
- Il present continuous diventa past continuous.
- Il simple past diventa past perfect.
- Il past continuous diventa past perfect continuous.
- Il present perfect diventa past perfect.
- Il present perfect continuous diventa past perfect continuous.
- Il past perfect resta tale.
- Il futuro diventa condizionale.
- Il future continuous diventa conditional continuous.
- Il future perfect diventa conditional perfect.
- Il condizionale resta tale.
- Le forme presenti dei verbi modali restano tali.
- Le forme passate dei verbi modali restano tali.

Anche i pronomi, gli aggettivi e gli avverbi cambiano. Di seguito alcuni esempi:
- La prima persona singolare diventa terza persona singolare.
- La seconda persona singolare diventa prima persona singolare.
- La prima persona plurale diventa terza persona plurale.
- La seconda persona plurale diventa prima persona plurale.
- La terza persona singolare rimane terza persona singolare.
- *Now* diventa *then.*
- *Today* diventa *that day.*
- *Tomorrow* diventa *the day after.*
- *Yesterday* diventa *the day before.*
- *This* diventa *that.*
- *Here* diventa *there.*
- *Ago* diventa *before.*

Non è sempre necessario cambiare il verbo quando si utilizza il discorso indiretto. Se state riferendo qualcosa e pensate che sia ancora vero, non serve cambiare il tempo del verbo, tuttavia volendo è possibile farlo:

> The treatment of choice for severe bleeding after the operation is the administration of fresh frozen plasma.
> He said (that) the treatment of choice for severe bleeding after the operation is the administration of fresh frozen plasma.

Or

> He said (that) the treatment of choice for severe bleeding after the operation was fresh frozen plasma.

Riferire domande

Yes/No questions

Utilizziamo *whether* o *if*:

"Do you smoke or drink any alcohol?"
> The doctor asked if I smoked or drank any alcohol.

"Have you ever had hives after intravenous contrast injections?"
> The doctor asked me whether I had ever had hives after intravenous contrast injections.

"Are you taking any pills or medicines?"
> The doctor asked me if I was taking any pills or medicines.

Domande con Wh...

Utilizziamo lo stesso avverbio interrogativo che nella domanda diretta:

"What do you think about doing the operation laparoscopically?"
> The patient asked me what I thought about doing the operation laparoscopically.

"Why do you think you need to operate?"
> The patient asked me why I thought we needed to operate.

"When will I be able to be discharged?"
> The patient asked when she would be able to be discharged.

"How often do you have headaches?"
> The doctor asked how often I had headaches.

Domande riferite

Le domande riferite hanno queste caratteristiche:

- L'ordine delle parole è diverso da quello della domanda originaria.
- Il verbo segue il soggetto come in una frase comune.
- Il verbo ausiliario *do* non è utilizzato.
- Non vi è alcun punto interrogativo.
- Il verbo cambia nello stesso modo del discorso diretto.

Studiate i seguenti esempi:
"How old are you?"
> The doctor asked me how old I was.
"Do you smoke?"
> The doctor asked me if I smoked.

Riferire ordini e richieste

F O R M A	*Tell* (pronome) + oggetto (indiretto) + infinito. "Take the pills before meals." > The doctor *told* me to take the pills before meals. "You mustn't smoke." > The doctor *told* me not to smoke. "Could you please have a look at this brain scan and let me know what you think?" > The neurosurgeon asked the radiologist to look at the brain scan and let her know what he thought. "Will you help me with this?" > He asked her to help him.

Riferire suggerimenti e consigli

Suggerimenti e consigli vengono riferiti nei seguenti modi:

> | F | • Suggerimenti: |
> |---|---|
> | O | "Why don't we operate on that patient this evening?" |
> | R | ❯ The surgeon suggested operating on that patient this evening. |
> | M | |
> | A | • Consigli: |
> | | "You had better stay in bed." |
> | | ❯ The doctor advised me to stay in bed. |

Domande

Nelle frasi con *to be*, *to have* (nelle forme ausiliarie), e con i verbi modali, di solito creiamo le frase cambiando l'ordine delle parole:

> | F | • Affermativo |
> |---|---|
> | O | ❯ You are an eye surgeon. |
> | R | Interrogativo: Are you an eye surgeon? |
> | M | |
> | A | • Negativo |
> | | ❯ You are not an eye surgeon. |
> | | Interrogativo: Aren't you an eye surgeon? |

Nelle domande al simple present utilizziamo *do/does*:
> His stomach hurts after having a nasogastric probe for 3 days in a row.
> *Does* his stomach hurt after having a nasogastric probe for 3 days in a row?

Nelle domande al simple past utilizziamo *did:*
> The nurse arrived on time.
> *Did* the nurse arrive on time?

Se *who, what* o *which* sono il soggetto della frase, non utilizziamo *do*:
> Someone paged Dr. Heijmen.
> *Who* paged Dr. Heijmen?

Se *who, what* o *which* sono l'oggetto della frase, utilizziamo *did*:
> Dr. Heijmen paged someone
> *Who* did Dr. Heijmen page?

Quando facciamo una domanda a qualcuno e cominciamo la frase con
Do you know... o *Could you tell me...* il resto della frase mantiene l'ordine delle parole della frase affermativa:

❯ Where is the reading room?
ma
❯ *Do you know* where the reading room is?

❯ Where is the library?
ma
❯ *Could you tell me* where the library is?

Anche le domande riferite conservano l'ordine delle parole della frase
affermativa:
❯ Dr. Wilson asked: How are you?
ma
❯ Dr. Wilson asked me how I was.

Le domande in cui *be, do, can, have* e *might* sono verbi ausiliari
ammettono risposte brevi:
❯ *Do* you smoke? Yes, I do.
❯ *Did* you smoke? No, I didn't.
❯ *Can* you walk? Yes, I can.

Usiamo i verbi ausiliari anche con *so* (affermativo) e *neither* o *nor*
(negative) cambiando l'ordine delle parole:
❯ I am feeling tired. *So* am I.
❯ I can't remember the name of the disease. *Neither* can I.

Quando siamo in disaccordo con delle dichiarazioni positive o negati-
ve, usiamo i verbi ausiliari:
❯ I think we should wait to do the operation. I don't.
❯ I won't be going to the congress. I will.

Spesso usiamo *so* o *not* per fornire delle risposte brevi a delle doman-
de semplici:
❯ Is he going to pass the boards? I think *so*.
❯ Will you be on call tomorrow? I guess *not*.
❯ Will you be off call the day after tomorrow? I hope *so*.
❯ Has the chairperson been invited to the party? I'm afraid *so*.

Tag questions

Usiamo una tag question affermativa con una frase negativa e viceversa:
> The first year resident isn't feeling very well today, is he?
> You are working late at the lab, aren't you?

Dopo *let's* la tag question è *shall we?*
> Let's read a couple of articles, *shall we?*

Dopo l'imperativo, la tag question è *will you?*
> Turn down the cautery, *will you?*

Infinito/ -ing

Verbo + -ing

Alcuni verbi sono sempre seguiti da un gerundio quando sono seguiti da un altro verbo. Altri possono essere seguiti da un gerundio o un infinito con un cambiamento minimo o nullo del proprio significato, e altri ancora possono essere seguiti da un gerundio o da un infinito con un grosso cambiamento di significato.

> *Finish*: *I've finished translating* the article into English.
> *Enjoy*: I *enjoy talking* to patients while I'm doing operation under local anesthesia.
> *Mind*: I *don't mind being* told what to do.
> *Suggest*: Dr. Svenson *suggested going* to the ER and trying to operate on the aneurysm we couldn't stent.
> *Dislike*: She *dislikes going* out late after a night on-call.
> *Imagine*: *I can't imagine you operating.* You told me you hate blood.
> *Admit*: The resident *admitted forgetting* to report Mrs. Smith's mammogram.
> *Consider*: Have you *considered finishing* your residency in the *United States?*

Altri verbi che seguono questo modello sono *avoid, deny, involve, practice, miss, postpone* e *risk*.

Anche le seguenti espressioni utilizzano *–ing*:
> *Give up*: Are you going to *give up smoking*?
> *Keep on*: She *kept on interrupting* me while I was speaking.
> *Go on*: *Go on studying*, the exam will be next month.

Quando parliamo di azioni concluse possiamo anche usare il verbo *to have*:
> The resident *admitted forgetting* to write Mrs. Smith's discharge report.

o
> The resident *admitted having forgotten* to write Mrs. Smith's discharge report.

Con alcuni di questi verbi (*admit, deny, regret* e *suggest*) si può anche usare la struttura "*that...*":
> The resident *admitted forgetting* to visit Dr. Smith's patient that day.

o
> The resident *admitted that he had forgotten* to visit Dr. Smith's patient that day.

Verbo + infinito

Quando sono seguiti da un altro verbo, i seguenti verbi hanno la struttura verbo + infinito:
> *Agree*: The patient *agreed to give up* smoking.
> *Refuse*: The patient *refused to give up* smoking.
> *Promise*: I *promised to give up* smoking.
> *Threaten*: Dr. Font *threatened to close* the Vascular Department.
> *Offer*: The unions *offered to negotiate*.
> *Decide*: Dr. Knight's patients *decided to leave* the waiting room.

Altri verbi che seguono questa struttura sono: *attempt, manage, fail, plan, arrange, afford, forget, learn, dare, tend, appear, seem, pretend, need* e *intend*.

Dopo i verbi *want, ask, expect, help, would like* e *would prefer* si possono avere due possibili strutture:

> Verbo + infinito: I asked to see Dr. Knight, the surgeon who operated on my patient.

> Verbo + oggetto + infinito: I *asked Dr. Knight to inform* me about my patient.

Would like è un modo elegante per dire *want*:

> *Would you like to be* the chairman of the hepatic transplantation division?

Dopo i verbi *tell, order, remind, warn, force, invite, enable, teach, persuade* e *get* si può avere solo una possibile struttura:
> Verbo + oggetto + infinito: *Remind me to send* that grant application before 10 a.m. tomorrow.

Dopo questi verbi si possono avere due forme diverse:
Advise
> I *wouldn't advise doing* an internship in that Urology Department.
> I *wouldn't advise you to do* an internship in that Urology Department.

Allow
> They *don't allow smoking* in the lunchroom.
> They *don't allow you to smoke* in the lunchroom.

Permit
> They *don't permit eating* in the surgery reading room.
> They *don't permit you to eat* in the surgery reading room.

Quando usate *make* e *let* dovreste utilizzare la struttura: verbo + forma base (infinito senza *to*) anziché verbo + infinito:
> Blood *makes me feel* dizzy (you cannot say: Blood makes me to feel…)
> Dr. Knight *wouldn't let me practice on* his patient.

Ma nella forma passiva, c'è bisogno di usare *to*:
> When I was a resident, I was made to learn all kinds of sutures that I will never use.

Dopo le seguenti espressioni, potete usare sia *–ing* che l'infinito: *like, hate, love, can't stand* e *can't bear*:
> She *can't stand being* alone while she is performing a hip replacement.
> She *can't stand to be* alone while she is performing a hip replacement.

> The patient *began to improve* after the percutaneous drainage of his collection.
> The patient *began improving* after the percutaneous drainage of his collection.

Dopo questi verbi, potete usare *–ing* ma non l'infinito: *dislike, enjoy* e *mind*:
> I *enjoy being* alone (non: I enjoy to be alone).

Would like, un modo educato di dire *I want*, è seguito dall'infinito:
> *Would you like to be* the chairman of the neuroimaging division?

Being, start e *continue* possono essere seguiti sia da *–ing* che dall'infinito:
> The patient *began to improve* after the administration of diuretics.
> The patient *began improving* after the administration of diuretics.

Con alcuni verbi, come *remember* e *try*, l'utilizzo di *–ing* o dell'infinito hanno significato differente:

Remember (ci si ricorda di fare qualcosa prima di farla; ci si ricorda di aver fatto qualcosa dopo averla fatta)
> *I did not remember to place* – the tip of the cannula in the IVC before starting the cardiopulmonary bypass. (I forgot to place the cannula properly.)
> *I distinctly remember placing* – the tip of the cannula in the IVC before starting cardiopulmonary bypass.

Try (try to do= tentare di fare; try doing= applicare una tecnica)
> *The* interventional radiologist *tried to occlude* the bleeding vessel.
> He *tried using* coils; when that didn't work, he *tried adding* gelfoam pledgets.

Verbo + preposizione + -ing

Quando un verbo è preceduto da una preposizione, esso termina in *–ing*:
> Are you interested *in working* for our hospital?
> What are the advantages *of developing* new surgical techniques?
> She's not very good *at learning* languages.

Potete usare –ing con before e after:

> Discharge Mr. Brown *before operating* on the aneurism.
> What did you do *after finishing* your residency?

Potete usare *by + -ing* per spiegare come sia successo qualcosa:

> You can improve your medical English *by reading* scientific articles.

Potete usare –ing dopo *without*:

> Jim left the hospital *without realizing* he had left his keys in his locker.

Attenzione all'utilizzo di *to* perchè può essere parte di un infinito oppure una preposizione:

> I'm looking forward *to see* you again (questa frase NON è esatta)
> I'm looking forward *to seeing* you again.
> I'm looking forward *to the next European Congress*.

Ripassate le seguenti espressioni verbo + preposizione:

> *Succeed in* finding a job.
> *Feel like* going out tonight?
> *Think about* operating on that patient.
> *Dream of* being a radiologist.
> *Disapprove of* smoking.
> *Look forward to* hearing from you.
> *Insist on* inviting me to the chair the session.
> *Apologize for* keeping Dr. Ho waiting.
> *Accuse (someone) of* telling lies.
> *Suspected of* having AIDS.
> *Stop (someone) from* leaving the ward.
> *Thank (someone) for* being helpful.
> *Forgive (someone) for* not writing to me.
> *Warn (someone) against* carrying on smoking.

Queste sono alcune espressioni seguite da –ing:

> I don't feel *like going out* tonight.
> It's no use *trying to persuade* her.
> There's no point *in waiting for* him.
> It's not worth *taking* a taxi. The hospital is only a short walk from here.
> It's worth *looking at* that radiograph *again*.
> I am having difficulty *performing* this anastomosis.
> I am having trouble *performing* this anastomosis.

Sostantivi numerabili/non numerabili

Sostantivi numerabili

I sostantivi numerabili sono oggetti che possiamo contare. Possiamo utilizzarli al plurale.

Prima di un sostantivo numerabile al singolare potete utilizzare *a/an*:
> We will put a cast on your foot.
> Dr. Calleja is looking for an anaesthetist.

Ricordate di usare *a/an* per le professioni:
> I am *a* cardiovascular surgeon.

Prima del plurale dei sostantivi numerabili in genere si usa *some*:
> I've read *some* good articles on spiral chest CT lately.

Non utilizzate *some* quando fate discorsi generici:
> Generally speaking, I like plastic surgery books.

Dovete utilizzare *some* quando intendete alcuni, ma non tutti:
> Some doctors carry a stethoscope but otorhinolaryngologists don't.

Sostantivi non numerabili

I sostantivi non numerabili sono oggetti che non possiamo contare. Non hanno una forma plurale, di conseguenza quando vengono utilizzati come soggetto di una frase usano sempre un verbo singolare.

Prima di un sostantivo non numerabile, non si possono utilizzare *a/an*; in questo caso, bisogna utilizzare *the, some, any, much, this, his,* ecc... o lasciare il sostantivo non numerabile senza l'articolo:
> The chairman gave me *an* advice (errato).
> The chairman gave me *some* advice.

Molti sostantivi possono essere utilizzati come numerabili o non numerabili. Generalmente c'è una differenza nel loro significato:
> I had many experiences on my rotation at the *children's hospital* (numerabile).

> I need experience to become a good surgeon (non numerabile).

Alcuni nomi sono non numerabili in inglese ma spesso numerabili in altre lingue: *advice, baggage, behaviour, bread, chaos, furniture, information, luggage, news, permission, progress, scenery, traffic, travel, trouble* e *weather.*

Articoli: *a/an* e *the*

Chi parla usa *a/an* quando è la prima volta che parla di qualcosa, ma una volta che l'ascoltatore sa di cosa l'oratore stia parlando, si usa *the*:
> This morning I did *an* osteosynthesis and *a* closed reduction of the radius. *The* closed reduction did not take long.

Usiamo *the* quando è chiaro di quale cosa o persona stiamo parlando:
> Can you turn off *the* light?
> Where is *the* Skin Cancer Division, please?

Come norma generale, diciamo:
> The police.
> The bank.
> The post office ("Post Office" in British English).
> The fire department.
> The doctor.
> The hospital.
> The dentist.

Diciamo *the sea, the ground, the city* e *the country.*

Non utilizziamo *the* con il nome dei pasti:
> What did you have for lunch/breakfast/dinner?

Utilizziamo *a* quando c'è un aggettivo prima di un nome:
> Thank you. It was *a* delicious dinner.

Utilizziamo *the* per parlare di un pasto specifico:
> The chief had a bit too much to drink at *the* dinner after the congress.

Utilizziamo *the* per gli strumenti musicali:
> Can you play *the* piano?

Utilizziamo *the* con gli aggettivi assoluti (aggettivi utilizzati come sostantivi). Il significato è sempre plurale. Per esempio:
> The rich.
> The old.
> The blind.
> The sick.
> The disabled.
> The injured.
> The poor.
> The young.
> The deaf.
> The dead.
> The unemployed.
> The homeless.

Usiamo *the* con i termini che esprimono nazionalità (i quali iniziano sempre con la maiuscola):
> *The* British, *the* Dutch, *the* Spanish.

Non utilizziamo *the* prima di un nome quando ci riferiamo a qualcosa di generico:
> I love doctors (non *the* doctors).

Con le parole *school, college, prison, jail, church* utilizziamo *the* quando ci riferiamo agli edifici, altrimenti lasciamo i sostantivi senza articolo. Diciamo *go to bed, go to work* e *go home*: in questi casi non utilizziamo *the*.

Usiamo *the* con i nomi geografici seguendo queste regole:
I continenti non usano *the:*
> Our new resident comes from Asia.

Gli stati/le nazioni non usano *the*:
> The patient that underwent a liver quadrangular resection came from Sweden.
(Eccetto per i nomi di nazioni che includono parole quali: *Republic, Kingdom, States*,... Ad esempio: *The* United States of America, *The* United Kingdom, *The* Netherlands).

Come regola generale, le città non usano *the*:
> The next Ginecology Congress will be held in Malaga.

Non si usa *the* con il nome di una singola isola, ma si usa con gli arcipelaghi:
> Dr. Leon comes from Sicily and her husband from *the* Canary Islands.

Non si usa *the* con i laghi; si usa invece con gli oceani, i mari, i fiumi e i canali:
> Lake Windermere is beautiful.
> *The* Panama Canal links *the* Atlantic Ocean to *the* Pacific Ocean.

Usiamo *the* con edifici, università, ecc. seguendo queste regole:
Non si usa *the* con strade, vie, viali e piazze:
> The hospital is located at the corner of 3rd Street and 15th Avenue.

Non si usa *the* con gli aeroporti:
> The plane arrived at JFK airport.

Usiamo *the* prima di edifici noti al pubblico:
> *The* White House, *the* Empire State Building, *the* Louvre Museum, *the* Prado Museum.

Usiamo *the* prima di nomi che includono *of*:
> *The* Tower of London, *the* Great Wall of China.

Non si usa *the* con le università:
> I studied at Harvard. Ma possiamo usarlo in caso di termini composti come "*the* Autonomous University of Barcelona".

Ordine delle parole

L'ordine degli aggettivi è trattato nella sezione aggettivi, nel paragrafo "Ordine degli aggettivi".

Il verbo e l'oggetto del verbo generalmente vanno insieme e non sono separati dagli avverbi:
> I studied surgery because I like *saving lives* very much (*not* I like very much saving lives).

Di solito diciamo il luogo prima del tempo:
> She has been practicing colorectal surgery in *London* since April.

Alcuni avverbi vengono messi al centro della frase:
Se il verbo è una parola, mettiamo l'avverbio prima del verbo:
> I performed his carotid endarterectomy and *also spoke* to his family.

Mettiamo l'avverbio dopo *to be*:
> You are *always* on time.

Mettiamo l'avverbio dopo la prima parte di un verbo composto:
> Are you *definitely attending* the musculoskeletal surgery course?

Nelle frasi negative, mettiamo probably prima della negazione:
> I *probably* won't see you at the congress.

Anche *all* e *both* seguono queste regole sulle posizioni nella frase:
> Jack and Tom are both able to run a transplant program. (Or: Both Jack and Tom are able to run a transplant program.)
> We all felt sick after the meal. (Or: All of us felt sick after the meal.)

Proposizioni relative

Una proposizione è una parte di un periodo. Una proposizione relativa ci dice a quale persona o cosa (o a quale tipo di persona o cosa) faccia riferimento chi parla.

Una proposizione relativa (ad esempio, *who is on call?*) inizia con un pronome relativo (ad esempio, *who, that, which, whose*).
Una proposizione relativa segue un nome (ad esempio, *the doctor, the nurse*).

La maggior parte delle proposizioni relative sono non incidentali e alcune di esse sono incidentali.

Proposizioni relative non incidentali

> *The book on vascular access (that) you lent to me is very interesting.*

La proposizione relativa è fondamentale per il significato del periodo.

Non si usano virgole per separare la proposizione relativa dal resto del periodo.

Spesso si usa *that* invece di *who* o *which*, soprattutto nel discorso parlato.

Se il pronome relativo è l'oggetto (diretto) del periodo, può essere omesso.

Se il pronome relativo è il soggetto del periodo, non può essere omesso.

Proposizioni relative incidentali

> The first vertebroplasty in Australia, which took place at our hospital, was a complete success.

La proposizione relativa non è fondamentale per il significato del periodo, ma fornisce informazioni addizionali.

Generalmente si usano virgole per separare la proposizione relativa dal resto del periodo.

That non può essere usato al posto di *who* o *which*.

Il pronome relativo non può essere omesso.

Pronomi relativi

I pronomi relativi sono utilizzati per persone e cose.

- Per le persone:
> Soggetto: *who, that.*
> Oggetto: *who, that, whom.*
> Possessivo: *whose.*

- Per le cose:
> Soggetto: *which, that.*
> Oggetto: *which, that.*
> Possessivo: *whose.*

Who è usato solo per le persone. Può essere il soggetto o l'oggetto di una proposizione relativa:
> The patient *who* was admitted in a shock situation is getting better. Can we perform the cranial MRI now?

Which è usato solo per le cose. Come *who*, può essere il soggetto o l'oggetto di una proposizione relativa:

❯ The materials which are used for laparoscopic surgery are very expensive.

That è spesso usato al posto di who o which, soprattutto nel discorso parlato.

Whom è usato solo per le persone. È grammaticalmente corretto come oggetto di una proposizione dopo il verbo della proposizione relativa, tuttavia è molto formale e non viene usato spesso nell'inglese parlato. Usiamo *whom* invece di *who* quando *who* è l'oggetto della proposizione relativa o quando c'è una preposizione dopo il verbo della proposizione relativa:

❯ The resident *who* I am going to the congress with is very nice.
❯ The resident *with whom* I am going to the congress is a very nice and intelligent person.
❯ The patient *who* I saw in the Cardiovascular Surgery Department yesterday has been diagnosed with Leriche's syndrome.
❯ The patient *whom* I saw in the Cardiovascular Surgery Department yesterday has been diagnosed with Leriche's syndrome.

Whose è il pronome relativo possessivo. Si può usare sia per le persone che per le cose. Non può essere omesso:

❯ Nurses *whose* wages are low should be paid more.

Possiamo invece omettere *who, which* o *that*:
Quando sono l'oggetto di una proposizione relativa:

❯ The article on the spleen *that* you wrote is great.
❯ The article on splenic laceration you wrote is great.

Quando è l'oggetto di una preposizione. Ricordate che, in una proposizione relativa, di solito mettiamo una preposizione nello stesso posto della proposizione principale (cioè dopo il verbo):

❯ The congress *that* we are going to next week is very expensive.
❯ The congress we are going to next week is very expensive.

Preposizioni in frasi relative

Possiamo usare una preposizione in una frase relativa con *who, which* o *that*, o senza un pronome.
Nelle frasi relative mettiamo una preposizione nella stessa posizione

della proposizione principale (dopo il verbo). Di solito non la mettiamo prima del pronome relativo. Questo è il normale ordine nell'inglese parlato informale:

> This is a problem *which* we can do very little *about.*
> The nurse (*who*) I spoke *to* earlier isn't here now.

Nell'inglese scritto o più formale, possiamo mettere una preposizione all'inizio di una proposizione relativa, ma se mettiamo una preposizione all'inizio, possiamo solo usare *which* o *whom*; non possiamo usare *that* o *who* dopo una preposizione:

> This is a problem *about which* we can do very little.
> The nurse *to whom* I spoke earlier isn't here now.

Preposizioni relative senza pronome (casi speciali)

Infinito che introduce una proposizione

Possiamo usare l'infinito invece di un pronome relativo e di un verbo dopo:
> *The first, the second,... and the next.*
> *The only.*
> Superlativi.

Per esempio:
> Roentgen was the *first* man to use X-rays.
> Joe was the only surgeon willing *to operate* on that patient.

Forme in –ing e –ed che introducono una frase

Possiamo usare la forma in *–ing* invece di un pronome relativo e di un verbo attivo:
> Residents *wanting to train abroad* should have a good level of English.

Possiamo usare una forma in *–ed* invece di un pronome relativo e di un verbo passivo:

❯ The man *injured in the accident* was taken to the CT room.

Le forme in *–ing* e in *–ed* possono sostituire un verbo al tempo presente o passato.

Why, when e where

Possiamo usare *why, when e where* in una proposizione relativa non incidentale.
❯ This is the hospital where I did my residency.

Possiamo omettere *why* o *when*. Possiamo anche omettere *where*, ma in questo caso, dobbiamo utilizzare una preposizione.
❯ This is the hospital I did my residency in.

Possiamo formare proposizioni relative incidentali con *when* e *where*:
❯ The clinical history, *where* everything about a patient is written, is a very important document.

Non possiamo omettere *when* e *where* in una proposizione relativa incidentale.

Aggettivi

Un aggettivo descrive un nome, ovvero aggiunge delle informazioni su di esso.
In inglese, gli aggettivi precedono i nomi (*old hospital*) e hanno la stessa forma sia al singolare che al plurale (*new hospital, new hospitals*), sia al maschile che al femminile.

Gli aggettivi possono essere utilizzati con alcuni verbi come *be, get, seem, appear, look* (con il significato di *seem*), *feel, sound, tast*e...:
❯ He has been ill since Friday, so he couldn't report that bone age scan.
❯ The patient was getting worse.
❯ The trans-urethral-resection (TUR) seemed easy, but it wasn't.
❯ The kidney appeared normal.
❯ You look rather tired. Have you had your RBC checked?

> She felt sick, so she was unable to operate.
> Food in hospitals tastes horrible.

Come potete vedere, in questi esempi non c'è alcun nome dopo l'aggettivo.

Ordine degli aggettivi

Esistono aggettivi di fatto e aggettivi di opinione. Gli aggettivi di fatto (*large, new, white,...*) forniscono un'informazione oggettiva riguardo qualcosa (dimensioni, età, colore,...). Gli aggettivi di opinione invece (*nice, beautiful, intelligent,...*) ci dicono cosa qualcuno pensi di qualcosa.

Generalmente gli aggettivi di opinione precedono quelli di fatto:
> An *intelligent* (*opinione*) *young* (*fatto*) surgeon visited me this morning.
> Dr. King has a *nice* (*opinione*), *red* (*fatto*) Porsche.

A volte vi sono due o più aggettivi di fatto che descrivono un nome e di solito li mettiamo in quest'ordine:
1. Dimensioni/lunghezza.
2. Forma/larghezza.
3. Età.
4. Colore.
5. Nazionalità.
6. Materiale.

Ad esempio:
> A *tall, young* nurse.
> A *small, round* lesion.
> A *black latex, leaded* pair of gloves.
> A *large, new, white latex, leaded* pair of gloves.
> An *old* American patient.
> A *tall, young* Italian resident.
> A *small, square, old, blue* iron monitor.

Comparazione regolare di aggettivi

La forma usata per il comparativo dipende dal numero di sillabe nell'aggettivo.

Aggettivi monosillabi
Gli aggettivi monosillabi (ad esempio, *fat, thin, tall*) sono usati con espressioni del tipo:
> Less... than (inferiorità).
> As... as (uguaglianza).
> *-er*... than (superiorità).

Per esempio:
> Calls are *less hard than* a few years ago.
> Eating in the hospital is *as cheap as* eating at the Medical School.
> Ultrasound examinations are difficult nowadays because people tend to be *fatter than* in the past.

Aggettivi bisillabi
Gli aggettivi bisillabi (ad esempio, *easy, dirty, clever*) sono usati con espressioni del tipo:
> Less... than (inferiorità).
> As... as (uguaglianza).
> *-er*/more... than (superiorità).

Preferiamo *–er* per gli aggettivi che finiscono in *–y* (*easy, funny, pretty*) e altri aggettivi (quali, *quiet, simple, narrow, clever*). Per gli altri aggettivi bisillabi usiamo *more*.
Per esempio:
> The surgical problem is *less simple than* you think.
> My arm is *as swollen as* it was yesterday.
> The board exam was easier *than* we expected.
> His illness was *more* serious *than* we first suspected.

Aggettivi di tre o più sillabe
Gli aggettivi di tre o più sillabe (ad esempio, *difficult, expensive, comfortable*) sono usati con espressioni del tipo:
> Less... than (inferiorità).
> As... as (uguaglianza).
> More... than (superiorità).

Per esempio:

> Studying medicine in Spain is *less* expensive *than* in the States.
> The small hospital was *as* comfortable *as* a hotel.
> Studying the case was *more* interesting *than* I had thought.

Prima dell'aggettivo comparativo possiamo usare:

> A (little) bit.
> A little.
> Much.
> A lot.
> Far.

Per esempio:

> I am going to try something *much* simpler to solve the problem.
> The patient is a *little* better today.
> The little boy is a *bit* worse today.

A volte è possibile usare due comparativi insieme (quando parliamo di qualcosa in cambiamento continuo):

> It is becoming *more* and *more* difficult to find a job in an academic hospital.

Inoltre diciamo *twice as... as, three times as... as*:

> Going to the European Congress of Plastic Surgery is *twice as* expensive *as* going the French one.

Il superlativo

La forma usata per il superlativo dipende dal numero di sillabe nell'aggettivo:

Aggettivi monosillabi

Gli aggettivi monosillabi sono usati con espressioni del tipo:

> The... -*est*.
> The least.

Per esempio:

> The number of radiologists in your country is the *highest* in the world.

Aggettivi bisillabi

Gli aggettivi bisillabi sono usati con espressioni del tipo:
> The... -*est*/the most.
> The least.

Per esempio:
> Barium enema is one of the *commonest* tests in clinical practice.
> Barium enema is one of the *most common* tests in clinical practice.

Aggettivi di tre o più sillabe

> The most.
> The least.

Per esempio:
> Common sense and patience are *the most* important qualities for a surgeon.
> This is *the least* difficult brain tumour resection I have performed in years.

Aggettivi irregolari

> Good, better, the best.
> Bad, worse, the worst.
> Far, farther/further, the farthest/furthest.

Per esempio:
> Although I have attended several microsurgery refresher courses, my anastomotic skills are *worse* now than during my first year of residence.

Comparativi con *the*

Usiamo *the* + comparativo per parlare di un cambiamento in qualcosa che causa un cambiamento in qualcos'altro:
> The cleaner the field, the better image we have.
> The more you practice with knots, the easier it gets.
> The greater the surgeon's skill, the lower the risk of complications.

As

Due fatti che accadono in contemporanea o nello stesso periodo:
> The resident listened carefully *as* Dr. Fraser explained to the patient the different diagnostic possibilities.
> I began to enjoy the residency more *as* I got used to being on call.

Un fatto che accade durante un altro:
> The patient died *as* the CT Scan was being performed.

Notate che usiamo *as* solo se due azioni accadono contemporaneamente. Se un'azione segue un'altra non utilizziamo *as*, ma usiamo *when*:
> When the injured person came to the emergency room, I decided to call the surgeon.

Con il significato di *because*:
> *As* I was feeling sick, I decided to go to the doctor.

Like e As

Like

Like è una preposizione, quindi può essere seguita da un nome, pronome o forma in –ing.

Vuol dire "simile a " o "la stessa cosa di". La usiamo quando confrontiamo cose:
> This comfortable head coil is *like* a velvet hat.
> What does he do? He is an ophthalmologist, *like* me.

As

As + soggetto + verbo.
> Don't change the dose of antibiotics. Leave everything *as* it is.
> He should have been treated *as* I showed you.

As può avere il significato di *what*, come nei seguenti esempi:
> The resident did *as* he was told.

As può avere il significato di *in the manner,* come nei seguenti esempi:
> He made the diagnosis just with the chest X-ray, *as* I expected.
> *As* you know, we are sending an article to the *European Journal of Vascular Surgery* next week.
> *As* I thought, the patient was under the influence of alcohol.

As può anche essere una preposizione e può essere usato con un nome, ma ha un significato diverso da *like*.

As + nome è usato per dire come è (stato) qualcosa in realtà (soprattutto quando parliamo del lavoro di qualcuno o di come usiamo qualcosa):
> Before becoming a plastic surgeon I worked *as* a general practitioner in a small village.

As if, as though sono usati per dire come qualcosa o qualcuno sembra, suona, appare... o per dire come qualcuno fa qualcosa:
> The doctor treated me *as if* I were his son.
> John sounds *as though* he has got a cold.

Espressioni con *as*:
> *Such as= for example.*
> *As usual* (Dr Gonzalez was late as usual).

So e Such

So e *such* rafforzano il significato di un aggettivo.

Usiamo *so* con un aggettivo senza un nome o con un avverbio:
> The first-year resident is *so clever*.
> The weather has been *so beautiful* lately.
> The traumatologist injected lidocaine *so carefully* that the patient did not notice it.

Usiamo *such* con un nome aggettivato:
> She is *such* a *clever resident*.
> We've been having *such beautiful weather* lately. (Notate che weather non è numerabile, di conseguenza non serve un articolo indefinito).

So e *Such* vengono spesso utilizzati con *that* per mostrare un nesso causale.

> The resident was *so* tired *that* she could hardly keep her eyes open during the session.
> It was *such* a complex case *that* we had to bring in an outside consultant.

Preposizioni

At/On/In time

Usiamo *at* con gli orari:
> *At* 7 o'clock.
> *At* midnight.
> *At* breakfast time.

Di solito omettiamo *at* quando chiediamo (*at*) *what time:*
> *What time* are you operating this evening?

Usiamo *at* anche in queste espressioni:
> *At* night.
> *At* the moment.
> *At* the same time.
> *At* the beginning of.
> *At* the end of.

Ad esempio:
> I don't like to be on call *at night.*
> Dr. Artaiz is operating *at the moment.*

Usiamo *in* per lunghi periodi:
> *In* June.
> *In* summer.
> *In* 1977.

Diciamo inoltre *in the morning, in the afternoon, in the evening:*
> I'll visit the patients *in the morning.*

Usiamo *on* con giorni e date:
> *On* October 9th.
> *On* Monday.

❯ *On* Saturday mornings.
❯ *On* the weekend (ma diciamo "*at* the weekend" in inglese Britannico).

Non usiamo *at/in/on* prima di *last e next:*
❯ I'll be on call *next* Saturday.
❯ They bought a new scanner *last* year.

Usiamo *in* prima di un periodo di tempo (cioè, un tempo nel futuro):
❯ Our resident went to Boston to do a rotation on minimally invasive surgery. He'll be back *in* a year.
❯ I predict she'll need another bypass *in* 5 years (i.e., 5 years from now).

For, During e While

Usiamo *for* per dire quanto tempo richiede una cosa:
❯ I've worked as a surgeon at this hospital *for* 10 years.

Non possiamo usare *during* in questo modo:
❯ It rained *for* 5 days (non *during* 5 days).

Usiamo *during* + nome per dire quando succede qualcosa (non per quanto tempo):
❯ The resident fell asleep *during* the morning conference.

Usiamo *while* + soggetto + verbo:
❯ The resident fell asleep *while* he was attending the morning conference.

By e Until

By + un tempo definito (cioè, non più tardi di; non si può usare *until* con questo significato).
❯ I mailed the article on carotid dissection today, so they would receive it *by* Tuesday.

Until può essere usato per dire quanto a lungo dura una situazione:
> Let's wait *until* the patient gets better.

Quando si parla del passato, si può usare *by the time*:
> *By the time* they got to the hotel the congress had already started.

In/At/On

Usiamo *in* come nei seguenti esempi:
> *In* a room.
> *In* a building.
> *In* a town/*in* a country: "Dr. Concha works *in* Malaga".
> *In* the water/ocean/river.
> *In* a row.
> *In* the hospital.

Usiamo *at* come nei seguenti esempi:
> *At* the bus stop.
> *At* the door/window.
> *At* the top/bottom.
> *At* the airport.
> *At* work.
> *At* sea.
> *At* an event: "I saw Dr. Jules *at* the resident's party".

Usiamo *on* come nei seguenti esempi:
> *On* the ceiling.
> *On* the floor.
> *On* the wall.
> *On* a page.
> *On* your nose.
> *On* a farm.

In o At?

- Diciamo *in the corner of a room*, ma *at the corner of a street*.

- Diciamo *in* o *at college/school*. Usate *at* quando state parlando della scuola come di un posto o quando ne dite il nome:
> Thomas will be *in* college for three more days.
> He studied medicine *at* Harvard Medical School.

- *Arrive*. Diciamo:

> *Arrive in* a country or town: "Dr. Jimenez *arrived in* Boston yesterday".
> *Arrive at* other places: "Dr. Jimenez *arrived at* the airport a few minutes ago".

Ma omettiamo *in* e *at*:
> *Arrived home*: "Dr. Jimenez *arrived home* late after sending the article to *Circulation*".

"Prophylaxis *against* infection", non "prophylaxis *on* infection"!

Inglese Americano vs. Inglese Britannico

Le differenze tra queste due varietà di inglese sono molto più di un semplice "accento diverso". Numerose differenze possono essere riscontrate nello spelling, nel vocabolario e nella grammatica. Nel Capitolo XII c'è un testo scritto in Inglese Britannico che mostra chiaramente alcune particolarità di questa varietà di inglese. La maggior parte dei giornali scientifici accettano entrambi gli stili, a patto che siano utilizzati coerentemente all'interno dell'articolo. Probabilmente è saggio utilizzare un "Inglese Britannico" per articoli inviati a giornali Britannici e un "Inglese Americano" per articoli inviati a giornali Americani, anche se attualmente i reviewers per i giornali scritti in inglese possono essere originari di qualsiasi parte del mondo.

Ci sono molte differenze nel modo di compitare le parole in Inglese Britannico e Americano, soprattutto nella parole mediche derivanti dal latino.

British	American
OU →	**O**
Colour	Color
Tumoury	Tumor
Behaviour	Behavior
RE →	**ER**
Centre	Center
Metre	Meter
Calibre	Caliber
AE →	**E**
Anaemia	Anemia
Anaesthesia	Anesthesia
Caecum	Cecum
Aetiology	Etiology
Haematoma	Hematoma
Paediatric	Pediatric
OE →	**E**
Coeliac	Celiac
Diarrhoea	Diarrhea
Oedema	Edema
Oesophagus	Esophagus
Oestrogen	Estrogen
Foetus	Fetus
S →	**Z**
But note that Z is becoming more common in British English	
Analyse	Analyze
Catheterise	Catheterize
Criticise	Criticize
Organisation	Organization
Visualisation	Visualization
LL→	**L**
Bevelled	Beveled
Traveller	Traveler
Labelling	Labeling
L→	**LL**
Enrolment	Enrollment
Fulfil	Fulfill
Skilful	Skillful

Miscellaneous

Analogue	Analog
Programme (*for congresses, concerts, etc.,* *but computer program*)	Program (*all types*)
Practise (*verb—the noun is spelled practice*)	Practice (*verb and noun*)
PH→	**F**
Sulphur	Sulfur
Sulphonamide	Sulfonamide
Compound medical words tend to be hyphenated	*Compound medical words tend to be written without hyphens*
Hepatico-duodenostomy	Hepaticoduodenostomy
Sterno-pericardial	Sternopericardial

Ci sono molte differenze nel vocabolario. Esse tendono ad essere più frequenti nel linguaggio di tutti i giorni piuttosto che nel vocabolario dei termini medici. Molte parole sono conosciute sia in America che in Inghilterra, ma alcune sono più comuni di altre in ciascun paese. Ecco alcuni esempi.

Abiti

British	American
Mackintosh (mac)	Raincoat
Tights	Leotards/panty hose
Trousers	Pants
Nightdress	Nightgown
Dinner jacket	Tuxedo
Polo neck	Turtleneck
Vest	Undershirt
Knickers	Panties
Handbag	Purse

Acconciature e unghie

British	American
Sideboards	Sideburns
Nail varnish	Nail polish
Fringe	Bangs

Fate attenzione ad alcune parole della strada che non dovreste pronunciare, ma che potreste sentire: hanno un doppio significato....

British	American
Slut	Tramp
Tramp	Homeless person
Arse	Ass
Ass	Donkey

Vacanze e vita in casa

British	American
Rucksack	Backpack
Fortnight	Two weeks
Father Christmas	Santa Claus or Santa
Queue (to queue up)	Line (to stand in line)
Flat	Apartment
Ground floor	First floor
Garden	Yard
To let	To rent
Post code	Zip code
Lift	Elevator
Tap	Faucet
The box, the telly (TV)	The tube (TV)
To hoover	To vacuum
Toilet, loo	Bathroom, restroom, lavatory
Bin	Garbage bag
Duvet	Comforter
Blind	Shade
Clothes peg	Clothes pin
Wardrobe	Closet
Couch	Sofa
Fridge	Refrigerator
Hand basin	Sink

Cose per bambini

British	American
Nappy	Diaper
Dummy	Pacifier
Cot	Crib
Pushchair	Stroller
Mum	Mom

Salute e lavoro

British	American
Public limited company (plc)	Incorporated company (inc.)
Reception	Lobby, front desk
To sack	To fire
A rise	A raise
Chemist	Drug store, pharmacy
Surgery	Examination room
Anesthetist (*technician who administers anesthesia*)	Anesthetist (*physician specialized in anesthesiology*)
Anesthesiologist (*physician specialized in anesthesiology*)	
Operating theater	Operating room

Vita metropolitana

British	American
Trolley	Cart
Car boot sale	Garage sale
Shopping centre	(Shopping) mall
Ironmonger's	Hardware store
Current account	Checking account
Fishmonger's	Fish store
VAT (value added tax)	Sales tax
Town centre	Downtown

Altro

British	American
Tippex	White out
Rubber	Eraser
Parcel	Package
Full stop	Period
Form, year	Grade
Brackets	Parentheses
Autumn	Fall
Crisps	Chips
Chips	French fries

La lista va avanti all'infinto, potete trovare interi libri sull'argomento; le differenze grammaticali sono poche e poco importanti. Anche la pronuncia è molto differente, ma questo va al di là degli obiettivi di questo libro.

Capitolo 3

Letteratura scientifica chirurgica: scrivere un articolo

Questo capitolo non vuole essere una "Guida per gli Autori" come quelle che si trovano su ogni rivista. Il nostro consiglio più importante è: *non scrivete l'articolo nella vostra lingua per poi tradurlo in inglese, ma scrivetelo direttamente in inglese.*

(Questo consiglio è valido per i chirurghi con un inglese di buon livello. Se non si tratta del vostro caso, tenete presente che anche se la maggior parte delle persone hanno serie difficoltà a pensare e scrivere nella loro lingua, i risultati di un articolo ben tradotto sono di solito migliori di quelli di un articolo scritto male, anche se è stato corretto).

Errori comuni: un esempio reale

Questa è la prima bozza di un articolo scritto da uno specializzando di chirurgia non madrelingua inglese:

"A young fireman, 47 years old, came to emergency assistance in our Hospital because of left thoracic pain and unknown fever. During the staying in Internal Medicine the evolution was unlucky, with high fever. One echocardiography taken a few days after the incoming showed an aortic regurgitation and the 7th day in the Hospital patient suffered a severe cardiac failure. A. urinae is isolated in four blood-cultures and S. aureus was founded in urine culture.

Disnea and fever were increasing so it was decided to do an urgent aortic replacement. When the patient arrived to surgery he was in respiratory and hemodinamic failure. Killip IV. Transthoracic Echocardiography revealed the aortic regurgitation because of big vegetations on coronary valve without ring affectation or another complication, and systolic function was conserved. Urinary sound was complicated, creating a false way, so the urologist was required to place a suprapubic sound. Aortic valve is substituted for an ATS prosthesis without incidences. 69 min CPB and 49 min aortic clamped. In the immediately post-surgery the patient requires plama and blood transfusions. During ICU staying patient was still in septic shock but in good hemodinamic evolution. Euroscore: 8. Fever 38° during 2 days with peak curve and after that light fever. Bilateral lung edema is important, and the left one is needed to be evacuated. Neurological symptoms are not patent but sleepiness. Post-extubated echocardiography showed rigth function of prosthetic aortic valve. Antibiotics treatments are justified with the literature and cultures: Penicillin G 4 x 106/4 h, Levofloxacine 500 mg/12 h and Gentamicine 60 mg sc/12 h. After 8 days in Intensive Care Unit patient is moved to Internal Medicine area were is going up."

Questi sono alcuni dei molti errori presenti in questo breve paragrafo:
 "Unknown fever": l'autore intende dire "fever of unknown origin," ma "fever" dovrebbe essere sufficiente perché nella letteratura medica "fever" significa temperatura corporea continua o ricorrente maggiore di 37,5°C misurata dalla bocca della durata di 2 o più settimane, della quale non è stato possibile stabilire la causa dopo accurate indagini mediche. Quindi la frase dovrebbe essere la seguente: "because of left-sided chest pain and fever."
"During the staying" dovrebbe essere sostituito con "during the stay."
"Unlucky" dovrebbe essere sostituito con "unfortunate," o meglio ancora la frase "the evolution was unlucky" dovrebbe essere sostituita da una constatazione emotivamente più neutrale come "his condition worsened."
"One echocardiography ..." non è abbastanza preciso (ne sono state eseguite più di una?). Per inciso, il termine corretto sarebbe "echocardiogram". Si dovrebbe precisare il grado di insufficienza aortica. La frase "the patient suffered a severe cardiac failure" andrebbe sostituita con "the patient developed severe heart failure."
Nella frase "A. urinae is isolated in four blood cultures and S. Aureus was founded in ...." vi è una discordanza temporale: presente e passato contemporaneamente nella stessa frase. La parola "founded" significa "set up" e l'autore intende dire "found."
Siamo sicuri che possiate trovare molti altri errori in questo breve passaggio. Anche se il contributo scientifico fosse stato rilevante per il giornale, l'articolo sarebbe stato rifiutato senza esitazioni. Comunque, anche se il livello dell'inglese è scadente, scrivere la bozza direttamente in inglese è sempre un buon esercizio. Una volta messa giù la vostra idea, è essenziale ricorrere a un aiuto prima di inviare l'articolo.

Lavoro preliminare

Quando volete scrivere di un argomento, innanzitutto dovete fare una ricerca bibliografica. Potete fare riferimento all'*Index Medicus*® (http://www.ncbi.nlm.nih.gov/entrez/ query.fcgi?db=PubMed) per cercare gli articoli. Una volta trovati, leggeteli attentamente e sottolineate quelle frasi o paragrafi che pensate di poter citare nel vostro articolo.

Consigliamo di non scrivere l'articolo in italiano e poi tradurlo in inglese, ma di scriverlo direttamente in inglese. Per fare ciò, scegliete tra la vostra bibliografia o all'interno della rivista nella quale vorreste pubblicare il vostro lavoro, l'articolo che ritenete più simile al tipo di studio di cui volete scrivere.

Ovviamente dovrete seguire le istruzioni della rivista alla quale volete mandare l'articolo; tuttavia, qui utilizzeremo una forma standard che potrebbe essere adeguata alla maggior parte delle riviste. In ogni sezione forniremo alcuni esempi per mostrarvi come estrarre alcune espressioni dagli altri articoli.

Intestazione dell'articolo

Titolo

Il titolo dell'articolo dovrebbe essere breve, ma informativo. Riflettete molto bene sul titolo del vostro articolo.

Abstract

Insieme a ogni articolo si deve inviare un *abstract* di 150-200 parole (a seconda della rivista). Ricordate che l'*abstract* è un riassunto, non un'introduzione all'articolo e dovrebbe rispondere alla domanda: "Cosa dovrebbe apprendere il lettore da questo articolo?".

La maggior parte delle riviste richiede che l'*abstract* sia diviso in quattro paragrafi con i seguenti titoli: Obiettivo, Materiali e Metodi, Risultati e Conclusioni.

Obiettivo

Definite gli scopi dello studio o dell'indagine, l'ipotesi che viene testata
o la procedura che viene valutata.
Notate che molto spesso potrete costruire la frase iniziando con un
infinito:

> › *To evaluate* the impact of preoperative antibiotics on prosthesis
> infection after knee replacement.
> › *To present* our experience with limited mastectomy in early breast
> cancer.
> › *To study* the long-term evolution of ovarian cancer.
> › *To assess* perioperative results of thoracoabdominal aneurysm
> resection.
> › *To compare* radical excision versus functional prostate resection in
> prostate cancer.
> › *To determine* the prevalence of stenoses in dysfunctional autoge-
> nous hemodialysis fistulas and of patency following angioplasty
> and to identify predictors of this patency.
> › *To develop* a predictive model for functional status after lung resec-
> tion for lung cancer.
> › *To investigate* the prognostic value of FDG-PET uptake parameters
> in patients who undergo an R0 resection for carcinoma of the lung.
> › *To ascertain* recent trends in imaging workload among the various
> medical specialties.
> › *To describe* the clinical presentation, sonographic diagnosis, and
> radiological treatment of uterine AVMs.
> › *To assess* the usefulness of three-dimensional (3D) gadolinium-
> enhanced MR urethrography and virtual MR urethroscopy in the
> evaluation of urethral pathologies.
> › *To establish ..., To perform ..., To study ..., To design ..., To analy-
> ze ..., To test..., To define ..., To illustrate ...*

Potete inoltre iniziare con: "The aim/purpose/objective/goal of this study
was to..."

> › *The aim of this study was to* report the medium-term results after
> femoropopliteal bypass using PTFE conduits in diabetic patients.

> *The purpose of this study was to* compare the feasibility of non-complicated cholecystectomy using two different laparoscopic approaches.

> *The goal of this study was to* ascertain the safety of endoscopic saphenous vein harvest in obese patients.

> *The objective of this study was to* determine whether multislice CT is as sensitive as conventional cardiac catheterization in the diagnosis of coronary artery disease.

Potete fornire alcune informazioni introduttive e poi descrivere quello che avete fatto:

- Autoimmune pancreatitis is a new clinical entity which frequently mimics pancreatic carcinoma, resulting in unnecessary radical surgery of the pancreas. The purpose of this study was to describe the radiologic findings of autoimmune pancreatitis.

- Myocardial fibrosis is known to occur in patients with hypertrophic cardiomyopathy (HCM) and to be associated with myocardial dysfunction. This study was designed to clarify the relation between myocardial fibrosis demonstrated by gadolinium-enhanced magnetic resonance imaging (Gd-MRI) and procollagen peptides or cytokines.

- Posterior fossa tumors have traditionally been treated with open surgery alone.

- The objective of this study was to evaluate whether preoperative radiotherapy improves long-term prognosis.

- We hypothesized that ...

- We compared ...

- We investigated ...

Materiali e metodi

Definite brevemente cosa è stato fatto e quali materiali sono stati usati, incluso il numero dei soggetti. Includete, inoltre, i metodi utilizzati per analizzare i dati e controllare i bias.

- N patients with...were included.
- N patients with...were excluded.
- N patients known to have/suspected of having...
- ...was performed in N of patients with...
- N patients underwent...
- Quantitative/qualitative analyses were performed by...
- Patients were followed clinically for... months/years.
- We examined the effects of inhaled nitric oxide on blood pressure, heart rate, and renal function after 10 min' inhalation in 14 healthy young volunteers.

Risultati

Fornite i reperti dello studio, inclusi gli indicatori di significatività statistica. Includete numeri reali e percentuali:

- A total of 24 patients were included; 15 (62.5%) presented with bowel obstructions, 4 (16.5%) with perforations, and 5 (21%) with septicemia. Thirteen tumors (54%) were located in the descending colon and 11 (46%) in the transverse or ascending portions. Thirty-day mortality for perforated patients was double that of those presenting with obstruction (11 (46%) vs 5 (21%)), $p < 0.05$; perforated patients were more prone to present with metastatic liver disease (n = 4 (16.5%) vs n = 0 (0%), ns).

- A total of 62 patients were included in the MP group and 63 in the RP group. Age was 37.73 ± 7.28 in MP patients vs 35.33 ± 7.63 in RP patients (ns). Gender, etiology, functional class, and the rest of the preoperative variables were comparable between groups. Operative mortality was 6.45% (4 patients) in MP vs 1.58% (1 patient) in RP (ns).

- Twelve patients had acute myocardial infarction (AMI) and nine had acute myocarditis (AM). Patients with AMI were older (67.3 vs 55.4, $p < 0.05$) but the survival rate after left ventricular assist device implantation (LVAD) was similar at 30 days.

Conclusioni

Riassumete in una o due frasi le conclusioni raggiunte in base ai risultati. Questa parte dovrebbe enfatizzare gli aspetti o le osservazioni dello studio che sono nuovi e importanti:

- Multi-detector row CT is an effective tool for depicting orthopedic hardware complications.
- Radical mastectomy for T1N1M1 breast tumors is associated with longer post-operative stay and worse quality of life, but also with a decreased number of reinterventions.
- Contrast-enhanced color Doppler imaging demonstrated an overall accuracy of 100% for the detection of crossing vessels at the obstructed UPJ. This technique showed comparable results to CT and MRI and therefore provides accurate information for the detection of vessels crossing at the obstructed UPJ.
- In our setting, intra- and early post-operative morbidity and mortality rates are similar for RP and MP patients, although a learning curve was noted in the first RP cases. Although follow-up is still limited and homograft-related morbidity exists in the RP group, our overall 5-year major complication rate supports the use of the pulmonary autograft for aortic valve replacement in patients 20–50 years old.
- The study data demonstrate ..., Preliminary findings indicate ..., Results suggest...

Parole chiave

Dopo l'abstract, dovreste fornire e identificare da tre a dieci parole chiave o brevi frasi che aiutino nella classificazione dell'articolo e possano essere pubblicate con l'abstract. Questi termini dovrebbero provenire dalla lista del *Medical Subject Headings* dell'*Index Medicus* (http://www.nlm.nih.gov/mesh/meshhome.html).

Testo principale

Il testo di articoli osservazionali e sperimentali è di solito (ma non necessariamente) diviso in sezioni con i titoli *Introduction, Methods, Results* e *Discussion*. Gli articoli più lunghi possono richiedere dei sottotitoli in alcune sezioni (soprattutto nei risultati e nella discussione) per chiarire il loro contenuto. Altri tipi di articoli, quali Case Reports, Reviews ed Editorials, generalmente richiedono formati differenti. Dovrete consultare le singole riviste per ulteriori indicazioni.

Non usate abbreviazioni. Quando le usate, le abbreviazioni del termine dovrebbero essere scritte la prima volta per esteso, per esempio Magnetic Resonance Imaging (MRI).

Introduzione

Il testo dovrebbe iniziare con un'introduzione che specifichi la natura e lo scopo dello studio e che citi la bibliografia più importante. Fornite solo le informazioni preliminari che ritenete necessarie per capire perché l'argomento sia importante e le citazioni bibliografiche che spieghino al lettore perché avete intrapreso questo studio. Non fate un'analisi estensiva della letteratura. Il paragrafo finale dovrebbe definire chiaramente l'ipotesi e lo scopo dello studio. La brevità e l'appropriatezza sono importanti.

Materiali e metodi

Dopo l'introduzione, dovrebbero essere esposti i dettagli delle procedure cliniche e tecniche.

Descrivete chiaramente la vostra selezione di soggetti sperimentali o osservazionali (pazienti o animali di laboratorio, inclusi i controlli) e definitene età, sesso e altre caratteristiche importanti. Poiché la rilevanza di alcune variabili come età, sesso e razza rispetto all'oggetto di studio non è sempre chiara, gli autori dovrebbero giustificarle chiaramente quando sono incluse nei risultati di uno studio. Il principio chiave dovrebbe essere la chiarezza sui metodi e sulle ragioni per le quali uno studio è stato condotto in un determinato modo. Ad esempio, gli autori dovrebbero spiegare perché sono stati inclusi solo soggetti di alcune età, o perché le donne sono state escluse. Dovreste evitare termini come "race", che mancano di un preciso significato biologico e usare invece concetti come "ethnicity" o "ethnic group". Dovreste inoltre specificare attentamente cosa vogliono dire i descrittori e come sono stati raccolti i dati (ad esempio, quali termini sono stati usati nei moduli di raccolta dati, se i dati erano riferiti dai pazienti o da altri, ecc.).

- Our study population was selected from...
- N patients underwent...
- N consecutive patients...
- N patients with proven...
- Patients were followed clinically.
- N patients with... were examined before and during...
- N patients with known or suspected... were prospectively enrolled in this study.
- More than N patients presenting with... were examined with... over a period of N months.
- N patients were prospectively enrolled between... (date) and... (date).
- N patients (N men, N women; age range N-N years; mean N.N years)
- In total, 140 patients, aged 50-70 years (mean 60 years), all with severe acute pancreatitis fulfilling Ranson's criteria, were included in the study.
- Patients undergoing elective coronary arteriography for evaluation of chest pain were considered eligible if angiography documented...

Definite metodi, apparecchiature (nome commerciale, nome e indirizzo del produttore tra parentesi) e procedure in dettaglio sufficiente a permettere ad altri di riprodurre il vostro studio. Identificate in modo preciso tutti i farmaci e composti utilizzati, includendone il nome generico, la dose e la modalità di somministrazione.

- After the administration of 200 Units of heparin directly into the atrium, the aorta was cannulated with a standard tip cannula (Stocker 345 model) and extracorporeal circulation was started...
- The prostatic resection was performed using the Da Vinci Robotic System (Intuitive, USA).

- Aortic valve replacement was performed using the St. Jude Medical Regent Valve (St. Paul, Minnesota, USA).
- After baseline PET investigation, 40 mg of fluvastatin (Cranoc, Astra) was administered once daily.
- Dynamic PET measurements were performed with a whole-body scanner (CTI/ ECAT 951R/31; Siemens/CTI). After a transmission scan for attenuation correction, 20 mCi of 13N-labeled ammonia was administered as a bolus over 30 s by an infusion pump. The dynamic PET data acquisition consisted of varying frame durations (12 x 10 s, 6 x 30 s, and 3 x 300 s). For the stress study, adenosine was infused at a dose of 0.14 mg + kg 1 + min 1 over 5 min. 13N-labeled ammonia was administered in a similar fashion as in the baseline study during the third minute of the adenosine infusion.

È fondamentale che indichiate in quale modo sono stati valutati i risultati: in base agli esiti clinici, mediante questionari sulla qualità di vita, mediante ecografie o TC eseguite ogni X mesi, così come è necessario che il lettore conosca gli endpoint primari dello studio (nella maggior parte dei casi la mortalità) o gli eventi intermedi (reinterventi, riospedalizzazione ecc.).

La natura retrospettiva o prospettica del vostro studio dovrebbe essere chiara.

- Entry/inclusion criteria included...
- These criteria had to be met:...
- Patients with... were not included.
- Further investigations, including... and..., were also performed.
- We retrospectively studied N patients with...
- The reviews were not blinded to the presence of...
- The following patient inclusion criteria were used: age between 16 and 50 years and closed epipheses, ACL injury of one knee that required surgical replacement with a bone-to-patellar tendon-to-bone autograft, and informed written consent with agreement to attend follow-up visits. The following exclusion criteria were used: additional ligament laxities with a grade higher than 2 (according to the European classification of frontal laxity) in the affected knee, ...
- Two skeletal radiologists (O.J., C.V.) in consensus studied the following parameters on successive MR images ...

- Both the interventional cardiologists and echocardiographers who performed the study and evaluated the results were blinded to drug administration.
- Histologic samples were evaluated in a blinded manner by one of the authors and an outside expert in rodent liver pathology.

Indicate i riferimenti bibliografici a metodi già consolidati, includendo metodi statistici che sono stati pubblicati, ma non sono ben conosciuti; descrivete metodi nuovi o modificati in modo sostanziale e spiegate i motivi per l'utilizzo di queste tecniche e le loro eventuali limitazioni. Identificate chiaramente tutti i farmaci e composti utilizzati includendone il nome generico, la dose e la modalità di somministrazione. Non usate il nome commerciale di un farmaco tranne nel caso in cui sia importante.

- The imaging protocol included...
- To assess objectively the severity of acute pancreatitis, all patients were scored using the Balthazar criteria (10).
- The stereotactic device used for breast biopsy has been described elsewhere (12); it consists of a ...
- Gut permeability was measured in isolated intestinal segments as described previously (2).

Statistica

Descrivete i metodi statistici con sufficiente dettaglio per permettere a un lettore esperto, che abbia accesso ai dati originali, di verificare i risultati riportati. Inserite una descrizione generale dei metodi nella sezione *Methods*. Quando i dati sono riassunti nella sezione *Results*, specificate i metodi statistici utilizzati per analizzarli:

- The statistical significance of differences was calculated with Fisher's exact test.
- The probability of... was calculated using the Kaplan-Meier method.

- To test for statistical significance,...
- Statistical analyses were performed with... and... tests.
- The levels of significance are indicated by p-values.
- Interobserver agreement was quantified by using K statistics.
- All p-values less than 0.05 were considered significant statistical indicators.
- Univariate and multivariate Cox proportional hazards regression models were used.
- The V2 test was used for group comparison. Descriptive values of variables are expressed as means and percentages.
- We adjusted RRs for age (5-year categories) and used the Mantel extension test to test for linear trends. To adjust for other risk factors, we used multiple logistic regression.

Fornite dettagli sulla randomizzazione:

- They were selected consecutively by one physician between February 1999 and June 2000.
- This study was conducted prospectively during a period of 30 months from March 1998 to August 2000. We enrolled 29 consecutive patients who had...

Specificate ogni programma di software di uso generale utilizzato:

- All statistical analyses were performed with SAS software (SAS Institute, Cary, N.C.).
- The statistical analyses were performed using a software package (SPSS for Windows, release 8.0; SPSS, Chicago, Ill).

Risultati

Presentate i vostri risultati in sequenza logica nel testo, insieme a tabelle e illustrazioni. Non ripetete nel testo tutti i dati delle tabelle o illustrazioni; sottolineate o enfatizzate solo le osservazioni importanti. Evitate l'uso non tecnico di termini propriamente statistici quali "random" (che implica l'utilizzo di un metodo per la randomizzazione), "normale", "significativo", "correlazioni" e "campione". Definite i termini statistici, le abbreviazioni e la maggior parte dei simboli:

- Statistically significant differences were shown for both X and X.
- Significant correlation was found between X and X.
- Results are expressed as means ± SD.
- All the abnormalities in our patient population were identified on the prospective clinical interpretation.
- The abnormalities were correctly characterized in 12 patients and incorrectly in...
- The preoperative and operative characteristics of these patients are listed in Table X.
- The results of the US-guided ASD-closure are shown in Table X.
- Table 1 summarizes the clinical findings.

Riportate ogni complicanza:

- Two minor complications were encountered. After the second procedure, one patient had a slight hemoptysis that did not require treatment and one patient had chest pain for about 2 h after a puncture in the supraclavicular region. Pneumothorax was never encountered.
- Among the 11,101 patients, there were 373 in-hospital deaths (3.4%), 204 intraoperative/postoperative CVAs (1.8%), 353 patients with postoperative bleeding events (3.2%) and 142 patients with sternal wound infections (1.3%).

Indicate il numero di osservazioni e riportate il numero di casi persi (ad esempio, chi ha abbandonato un trial clinico):

- The final study cohort consisted of...
- Of the 961 patients included in this study, 69 were reported to have died (including 3 deaths identified through the NDI), and 789 patients were interviewed. For 81 surviving patients, information was obtained from another source. Twenty-two patients (2.3%) could not be contacted and were not included in the analyses because information on nonfatal events was not available.

Discussione

In questa sezione, fate ampio uso dei sottotitoli. Enfatizzate gli aspetti nuovi e importanti dello studio e le conclusioni che ne conseguono. Non ripetete in dettaglio i dati o altro materiale fornito in *Introduction* o in *Results*. Includete in *Discussion* le implicazioni dei risultati e le loro limitazioni, incluse le implicazioni per la ricerca futura. Correlate le osservazioni ad altri studi importanti.

Collegate le conclusioni con gli obiettivi dello studio, ma evitate affermazioni non attinenti e conclusioni non completamente supportate dai dati. In particolare, evitate di fare commenti su costi e vantaggi economici a meno che non abbiate incluso dati e analisi dei costi. Evitate di fare riferimento a lavori che non sono stati completati. Se necessario, formulate nuove ipotesi, ma indicatele chiaramente come tali. Quando appropriato, possono essere incluse raccomandazioni.

- In conclusion...
- In summary...
- This study demonstrates that...
- This study found that...
- This study highlights...
- Another finding of our study is...
- One limitation of our study was...
- Other methodological limitations of this study...
- Our results support...
- Further research is needed to elucidate...
- However, the limited case number warrants a more comprehensive study to confirm these findings and to assess the comparative predictive value of relative lung volume versus LHR.
- Some follow-up is probably appropriate for these patients.. Further research should be undertaken to randomly compare all the surgical options and evaluate their results in the long term.

Ringraziamenti

Elencate tutti i collaboratori che non soddisfano i criteri per essere autori, ad esempio una persona che abbia fornito assistenza puramente tecnica, assistenza nello scrivere, o un capo-reparto che abbia concesso solo un generico supporto. Dovrebbero anche essere riconosciuti i contributi economici e materiali.

 Le persone che hanno contribuito materialmente all'articolo, ma i cui contributi non soddisfano i criteri per essere autori, possono essere elencate in un paragrafo dal titolo "clinical investigators" oppure "participating investigators" e i loro ruoli e contributi dovrebbero essere descritti (ad esempio, "served as scientific advisors", "critically reviewed the study proposal", "collected data" o "provided and cared for study patients").

Poiché i lettori potrebbero dedurre la loro approvazione dai dati e dalle conclusioni, tutti dovranno aver fornito il permesso scritto per essere ringraziati.

- The authors express their gratitude to... for their excellent technical support.
- The authors thank Wei J. Chen, M.D., Sc.D,. Institute of Epidemiology, College of Public Health, National Taiwan University, Taipei, for the analysis of the statistics and his help in the evaluation of the data. The authors also thank Pan C. Yang, D, Ph.D., Department of Internal Medicine, and Keh S. Tsai, M.D., Ph.D., Department of Laboratory Medicine, National Taiwan University, medical College and Hospital, Taipei, for the inspiration and discussion of the research idea of this study. We also thank Ling C. Shen for her assistance in preparing the manuscript.

Riferimenti bibliografici

I riferimenti bibliografici dovrebbero essere numerati consecutivamente nell'ordine con cui vengono citati la prima volta nel testo. Identificate i riferimenti bibliografici nel testo, nelle tabelle e nelle didascalie con numeri arabi tra parentesi (alcune riviste richiedono numeri arabi scritti in apice). I riferimenti bibliografici citati solo nelle tabelle o nelle didascalie dovrebbero essere numerati secondo la sequenza stabilita dalla prima citazione nel testo di quella particolare tabella o figura.

- Clinically, resting thallium-201(^{201}Tl) single-photon emission computed tomography (SPECT) has been widely used to evaluate myocardial viability in patients with chronic coronary arterial disease and acute myocardial infarction [8-16].
- In addition, we have documented a number of other parameters previously shown to exhibit diurnal variation, including an assessment of sympathetic activity, as well as inflammatory markers recently shown to relate to endothelial function [14].

Usate lo stile degli esempi di seguito, che sono basati sui formati usati dalla National Library of Medicine (NLM) nell'*Index Medicus*. I nomi delle riviste dovrebbero essere abbreviati secondo lo stile usato nell'*Index Medicus*. Consultate la *List of Journals Indexed in Index Medicus*, pubblicata ogni anno dalla biblioteca come volume separato e come lista nel numero di gennaio dell'*Index Medicus*. La lista può anche essere ottenuta attraverso il sito internet della biblioteca (http://www.nlm.nih.gov).

Evitate di citare abstract. I riferimenti ad articoli accettati, ma non ancora pubblicati, dovrebbero essere indicati come "*in press*" o "*forthcoming*"; gli autori dovrebbero ottenere il permesso scritto di citare tali lavori e la conferma che sono stati accettati per la pubblicazione. Dati tratti da articoli inviati a riviste, ma non ancora accettati, dovrebbero essere citati nel testo come "*unpublished observations*", con il permesso scritto della fonte.

Evitate di citare una comunicazione personale a meno che non fornisca informazioni essenziali non disponibili da una fonte pubblica, nel qual caso il nome della persona e la data della comunicazione dovrebbero essere citati tra parentesi nel testo. Per gli articoli scientifici, gli autori dovrebbero ottenere l'autorizzazione scritta e la conferma dell'accuratezza dalla fonte della comunicazione personale.

Gli autori devono controllare le citazioni bibliografiche con i documenti originali.

Lo stile *Uniform Requirements* (o stile *Vancouver;* http://www.icmje.org/) si basa soprattutto sullo stile standard ANSI adottato dalla NLM per i suoi database (http://www.nlm.nih.gov/bsd/uniform_requirements.html). Di seguito sono stati aggiunti commenti quando lo stile *Vancouver* differisce dallo stile attualmente utilizzato dalla NLM.

Articoli in riviste

Articolo standard su rivista

Elencate i primi sei autori seguiti da *et al.* (si noti che NLM ora elenca fino a 25 autori; se ve ne sono più di 25, NLM elenca i primi 24, poi l'ultimo autore, infine et al.):

> ❯ Theodorou SJ, Theodorou DJ, Schweitzer ME, Kakitsubata Y, Resnick D. Magnetic resonance imaging of para-acetabular insufficiency fractures in patients with malignancy. Clin Radiol 2006 Feb;61(2):181–190

Se una rivista ha una numerazione delle pagine continua per tutto un volume (come fanno molte riviste mediche), si possono omettere il mese e il numero della rivista. (Nota: questa opzione viene usata in tutti gli esempi di *Uniform Requirements*, per omogeneità. NLM non utilizza questa opzione).

> ❯ Theodorou SJ, Theodorou DJ, Schweitzer ME, Kakitsubata Y, Resnick D. Magnetic resonance imaging of para-acetabular insufficiency fractures in patients with malignancy. Clin Radiol 2006 Feb;61(2):181–190

Organizzazione come autore

> ❯ The Evidence-based Radiology Working Group. Evidence-based radiology: a new approach to the practice of radiology. Radiology 2001;220:566–575

Nessun autore

> ❯ Cancer in South Africa (editorial). S Afr Med J 1994; 84:15

Articolo in lingua diversa dall'inglese

(Nota: NLM traduce il titolo in inglese, racchiude la traduzione tra parentesi quadre e aggiunge un indicatore linguistico abbreviato).

> ❭ Zangos S, Mack MG, Straub R, et al. [Transarterial chemoembolization (TACE) of liver metastases: a palliative therapeutic approach]. Radiologie 2001:41(1):84–90. German

Volume con supplemento

> ❭ Shen HM, Zhang QF. Risk assessment of nickel carcinogenicity and occupational lung cancer. Environ Health Perspect 1994;102 Suppl 1:275–282

Numero con supplemento

> ❭ Payne DK, Sullivan MD, Massie MJ. Women's psychological reactions to breast cancer. Semin Oncol 1996;23(1 Suppl 2):89–97

> ❭ Hamm B, Staks T, Taupitz M. SHU 555A: a new superparamagnetic iron oxide contrast agent for magnetic resonance imaging. Invest Radiol 1994;29(Suppl 2):S87–S89

Volume con parti

> ❭ Ozben T, Nacitarhan S, Tuncer N. Plasma and urine sialic acid in noninsulin dependent diabetes mellitus. Ann Clin Biochem 1995; 32 (pt 3):303-306

Numero con parti

> Poole GH, Mills SM. One hundred consecutive cases of flap lacerations of the leg in ageing patients. N Z Med J 1994; 107 (986 pt 1):377-378

Numero senza volume

> Turan I, Wredmark T, Fellander-Tsai L. Arthroscopic ankle arthrodesis in rheumathoid arthritis. Clin Orthop 1995; (320):110-114

Nessun numero o volume

> Browell DA, Lennard TW. Immunologic status of the cancer patient and the effects of blood transfusion on antitumor responses. Curr Opin Gen Surg 1993; 325-333

Pagine in numeri romani

> Fischer GA, Sikic BI. Drug resistance in clinical oncology and haematology. Introduction. Hematol Oncol Clin North Am 1995 Apr; 9(2):xi-xii

Tipologia di articolo indicata secondo necessità

> Ezensberger W, Fischer PA. Metronome in Parkinson's disease (letter). Lancet 1996; 347:1337

Articolo con ritrattazione

> Garey CE, Schwarzman AL, Rise ML, Seyfried TN. Ceruloplasmin gene defect associated with epilepsy in EL mice [retraction of Garey CE, Schwarzman AL, Rise ML, Seyfried TN. In: Nat Genet 1994; 6:426-431]. Nat Genet 1995; 11:104

Articolo ritirato

> Liou GI, Wang M, Matragoon S. Precocious IRBP gene expression during mouse development [retracted in Invest Ophthalmol Vis Sci 1994; 35:3127]. Invest Ophthalmol Vis Sci 1994; 35:108-138

Articolo con published erratum

> Hamlin JA, Kahn AM. Herniography in symptomatic patients following inguinal hernia repair [published erratum appears in West J Med 1995; 162:278]. West J Med 1995; 162:28-31

Libri e altre monografie

Autori personali

> Helms CA. Fundamentals of skeletal radiology. 1st ed. Philadelphia: W.B. Saunders Company; 1992.

(Nota: il precedente "Vancouver Style" presentava, in maniera non corretta, una virgola al posto di un punto e virgola tra il nome dell'editore e la data di pubblicazione.)

Editor(s)/curatori come autori

> Rumack CM, Wilson SR, Charboneau JW, editors. Diagnostic ultrasound. St. Louis: Mosby-Year Book; 1998.

Organizzazione come autore ed editore

> Institute of medicine (US). Looking at the future of the Medicaid program. Washington: The Institute; 1992

Capitolo di un volume

> Levine MS. Benign tumors of the esophagus. In: Gore RM, Levine MS, editors. Textbook of gastrointestinal radiology. 2nd ed. Philadelphia, PA: Saunders; 2000. pp. 387–402

Conference proceedings

> Kimura J, Shibasaki H, editors. Recent advances in clinical neuro-physiology. Proceedings of the 10th International Congress of EMG and Clinical Neurophysiology; 1995 Oct 15–19; Kyoto, Japan. Amsterdam: Elsevier; 1996

Articolo di un congresso

> Bengtsson S, Solheim BG. Enforcement of data protection, privacy and security in medical informatics. In: Lun KC, Deoulet P, Piemme TE, Rienhoff O, editors. MEDINFO 92. Proceedings of the 7th World Congress on Medical Informatics; 1002 Sep 6-10; Geneva, Switzerland. Amsterdam: North-Holland; 1992. pp. 1561-1565

Relazione scientifica o tecnica

Prodotta da un'agenzia di funding/sponsoring:
> Smith P, Golladay K. Payment for durable medical equipment billed during skilled nursing facility stays. Final report. Dallas (TX): Dept. of Health and Human Services (US) office of Evaluation and Inspections; 1994 Oct. Report No. HHSI-GOEI69200860

Prodotta dall'agenzia che l'ha eseguita:
> Field MJ, Tranquada RE, Feasley JC, editors. Health services research: work force and educational issues. Washington: National Academy Press; 1995. Contract No. AHCPR282942008. Sponsored by the Agency for Health Care Policy and Research

Tesi

> Kaplan SJ. Post-hospital home health care: the elderly's access and utilization [dissertation]. St. Louis (MO): Washington Univ.; 1995

Brevetto

> Larsen CE, Trip R, Johnson CR, inventors; Novoste Corporation, assignee. Methods for procedures related to the electrophysiology of the heart. US patent 5,529,067. 1995 Jun 25

Altro materiale edito a stampa

Articolo di giornale

> Lee G. Hospitalization tied to ozone pollution: study estimates 50,000 admissions annually. The Washington Post 1996 Jun 21; Sect. A:3(col.5)

Materiale audiovisivo

> ❯ HIV+/AIDS: the facts and the future [videocassette]. St. Louis (MO): Mosby-Year Book; 1995

Vocabolari e altra bibliografia simile

> ❯ Stedman's medical dictionary. 26th ed. Baltimore: Williams&Wilkins; 1995. Apraxia; pp. 119-120

Materiale non pubblicato

In press

(Nota: NLM preferisce "*forthcoming*" poiché non tutto il materiale verrà stampato).

> ❯ Assessment of chest pain in the emergency room: What is the role of multidetector CT? Eur J radiol. In press 2006

Materiale elettronico

Articolo di rivista in formato elettronico

> ❯ Morse SS. Factors in the emergence of infectious diseases. Emerg Infect Dis [serial online] 1995 Jan-Mar [cited 1996 Jun 5];1(1):[24 screens]. Available from: URL:http://www.cdc.gov/ncidod/ EID/eid.htm

Monografia in formato elettronico

> CDI, clinical dermatology illustrated [monograph on CD-ROM]. Reeves JRT, Maibach H. CMEA Multimedia Froup, producers. 2nd ed. Version 2.0. San Diego: CMEA; 1995

File informatico

> Hemodynamics III: the ups and downs of hemodynamics [computer program]. Version 2.2. Orlando (FL): Computerized Educational Systems; 1993

Materiale aggiuntivo

Tabelle

Tutti i dati tabulati identificati come tabelle dovrebbero avere un numero di tabella e una didascalia descrittiva. Controllate con attenzione che le tabelle siano citate in ordine sequenziale nel testo.

La presentazione di dati e informazioni forniti nelle intestazioni della tabella non dovrebbe ripetere informazioni già fornite nel testo. Spiegate nelle note in fondo alla tabella tutte le abbreviazioni non standard utilizzate nella stessa.

Se dovete utilizzare tabelle o figure da un'altra rivista, assicuratevi di ottenere il permesso e aggiungete una nota di questo tipo:

Adapted, with permission, from reference 5.

Figure

Le figure dovrebbero essere numerate consecutivamente nell'ordine in cui sono citate per la prima volta nel testo. Seguite la "sequenza" di illustrazioni simili dei vostri riferimenti bibliografici.

- Figure 1. Non-enhanced CT scan shows...
- Figure 2. Contrast-enhanced CT scan obtained at the level of...
- Figure 3. renal arteriogram shows ...

- Figure 4. Photograph of a fresh-cut specimen shows ...
- Figure 5. Photomicrograph (original magnification, _10; hematoxylin-eosin stain) of...
- Figure 6. Coronal contrast-enhanced T1-weighted MR image of ...
- Figure 7. Typical metastatic compression fracture in a 65-year-old man. (a) Sagittal T1-weighted MR image (400/11) shows ...
- Figure 8. Nasal-type extranodal NK/T-cell lymphoma involving the nasal cavity in a 42-year-old woman. Photomicrograph (original magnification,_400; hematoxylin-eosin [H-E] stain) of a nasal mucosal biopsy specimen shows intense infiltration of atypical lymphoid cells into the vascular intima and subintima (arrow). This is a typical appearance of angiocentric invasion in which the vascular lumen (V) is nearly obstructed.
- Figure 9. AFX with distortion of histopathologic architecture as a consequence of intratumoral ...
- Figure 10. CT images obtained in a 75-year-old man with gross hematuria. MIP image obtained during the compression-release excretory phase demonstrates a non-obstructing calculus (arrow) in the distal portion of the right ureter.
- Figure 11. Diagram of the surgical setting. A. Surgeon B. Assistant 1, C. Assistant 2, D. Nurse.

Consigli finali

Prima di inviare il vostro articolo, controllate l'ortografia e rileggete il testo, cercando parole eventualmente omesse o scritte due volte, così come parole che potreste aver mal utilizzato, ad esempio, scrivendo "there" invece di "their". Non inviate un articolo con errori di ortografia o di dosaggio o altre inaccuratezze mediche. E non aspettatevi che il controllo ortografico automatico del vostro computer rilevi tutti gli errori di ortografia.

Siate accurati. Controllate e ricontrollate i vostri dati e le citazioni bibliografiche. Anche quando avete la sensazione che l'articolo sia completo, lasciatelo da parte un paio di giorni e poi rileggetelo. I cambiamenti che fate al vostro articolo, dopo averlo visto in una nuova luce, spesso fanno la differenza tra un buon articolo e un grande articolo.

Una volta che pensate che tutto sia corretto, consegnate la bozza al vostro insegnante di inglese per una correzione finale informale. Non mandate la vostra prima (e nemmeno la seconda) bozza all'editor (il direttore scientifico della rivista)!

Non dimenticate infine di leggere e seguire scrupolosamente le specifiche "*Instructions for Authors*" della rivista sulla quale vorreste pubblicare il vostro articolo.

Capitolo 4

Lettere agli editor delle riviste chirurgiche

In questo capitolo, riportiamo diversi esempi di lettere inviate all'editor (direttore scientifico) di riviste chirurgiche. È nostra intenzione, infatti, fornirvi strumenti utili per comunicare in modo formale con gli editor e i reviewer delle riviste. È nostra convinzione che le lettere agli editor abbiano un ruolo importante e spesso sottovalutato nel decidere il destino di un articolo scientifico chirurgico.

Anche se non ci soffermeremo sulle lettere dagli editor, poiché sono in genere facili da comprendere, esse si dividono in lettere di accettazione "a determinate condizioni", lettere di accettazione e lettere di rifiuto.

- Lettere di accettazione "a determinate condizioni": sono abbastanza comuni, e di solito significano una gran quantità di lavoro, poiché l'articolo in genere deve essere riscritto.
- Lettere di accettazione: congratulazioni! Il vostro articolo è finalmente stato accettato e non necessita di correzioni. Queste lettere sono sfortunatamente relativamente rare e abbastanza facili da leggere. Inoltre, non richiedono risposta.
- Lettere di rifiuto: esistono molti modi educati per comunicarvi che il vostro articolo non sarà pubblicato in una determinata rivista. Queste lettere sono di immediata comprensione e, poiché non richiedono alcuna risposta, non ci soffermeremo su di esse dal punto di vista linguistico.

Abbiamo diviso le lettere agli editor in:

- Lettere di sottomissione.
- Lettere di risottomissione.
- Lettere di riconfigurazione.
- Lettere di ringraziamento per l'invito a pubblicare un articolo su una rivista.

R. Ribes, P. J. Aranda, J. Giba, *Inglese per chirurghi*,
© Springer-Verlag Italia 2012

- Lettere per chiedere informazioni sullo stato di un articolo.
- Altri tipi di lettere.

Lettere di invio

Le lettere di sottomissione (*submission letters*) sono abbastanza facili da scrivere poiché l'unico messaggio da trasmettere è il titolo dell'articolo che viene inviato insieme al nome dell'autore che terrà i contatti (*corresponding author*). Si possono usare molte lettere standard per questo scopo e riteniamo che non dobbiate investire troppo tempo su di esse poiché sono solo materiale preliminare che va inviato insieme all'articolo stesso.

Vostro indirizzo

Nome e indirizzo del destinatario   Data

Dear Dr. Massa,

Please find enclosed (*N*) copies of our manuscript entitled "..." (authors..., ..., ...), which we hereby submit for publication in the... Journal of... Also enclosed is a CD with a copy of the text file in Microsoft Word for Windows (version...).

I look forward to hearing from you.

Yours sincerely,

A.J. Merckel, M.D.

Lettere di reinvio

Le lettere di risottomissione (*resubmission letters*) devono rispondere in dettaglio ai commenti e suggerimenti espressi nelle lettere di accettazione. È in queste lettere che il corresponding author deve far sapere all'editor che sono stati fatti tutti i cambiamenti richiesti, o almeno la maggior parte di essi, e che così facendo l'articolo potrebbe essere pronto alla pubblicazione. Queste lettere possono avere un ruolo abbastanza importante nell'accettazione o rifiuto di un articolo. A volte una mancanza di dimestichezza con l'inglese può impedire al corresponding author di comunicare quali correzioni siano state fatte nel testo e le ragioni per cui altre correzioni suggerite non siano state fatte.

Vediamo questo esempio:

Dear Dr. Ho,

After a thorough revision in light of the reviewers' comments, we have decided to submit our paper "Radical mastectomy versus selective lumpectomy in breast cancer" for re-evalutation.

First of all, we would like to thank you for this second chance to present our paper for publication in your journal.

The main changes in the paper are related to your major comments:
- to improve overall image quality (including some new cases);
- to indicate what the clinical role of radical mastectomy is;
- to present our surgical strategy algorihtm in cases of axillary node involvement.

Following your advice, we have also addressed the reviewer's comments.

We hope this new revision will now be suitable for publication in your journal.

Yours sincerely,

Antonio Belafonte, M.D., and co-authors

Lettere di riconfigurazione

A volte un articolo viene accettato a condizione che la sua configu-
razione sia cambiata, ad esempio da *pictorial review* a *pictorial essay*. Le
lettere di riconfigurazione sono lettere di risottomissione e quindi tendono a essere lunghe.
Leggete questo esempio da cui abbiamo estratto e sottolineato diverse
frasi che vi possano aiutare nella corrispondenza con le riviste.

"Staged bilateral knee replacement is better than single-stage bilateral
replacement"
RE:01-1343

Dear Dr. Woods, (1)

We have reconfigured the manuscript referenced above (2) in the form
of a Review article *following your suggestion (3)* and we have made as
many changes as possible with regard to the reviewers' recommendations taking into account the *space limitation imposed by the new format of the paper (4)*.

We have tried to cover all possible clinical situations involving knee
disease while *giving priority to the most prevalent conditions (5)*. The
re-configuration of the manuscript has shortened it so drastically that
we have had to rewrite it entirely and *for this reason we do not attach
an annotated copy (6)–if you still consider this necessary we will
include one (7)*. Although tables are not common in Review articles,
we think that the inclusion of a single table on the classification of
degenerative knee disease would *"allow the reader to more easily categorize the described imaging findings" (8)* as stated by reviewer no. 2
(9) in his general remarks. The table has not been included due to the
new format of the paper but *if you take our suggestion into consideration we will be pleased to add it (10)*.

The major changes in our manuscript are:

1. *The title has been modified to* "Staged bilateral knee replacement is
   better than single-stage bilateral replacement" *following your recommendation (11)*.

2. *We have included the technical details of our surgical protocol,* although it has not been possible to expand the technical section *as suggested by reviewer no. 1 (12)* due to the space limitations.

3. *Similarly,* the description of infectious lesions and postoperative quality of life *could not be expanded as suggested by reviewer no. 2 due to the space limitations (13).*

4. *With regard to figures (14):*
   a. We have included two new figures.
   b. *Intraoperative photos have been included (15),* as suggested, in figures 4, 7, 12, and 14.
   c. *The image quality of figure 5 has been improved (16).*

5. *We have assigned distinct figures to different entities in most cases although the* limited number of figures allowed—5—made it impossible to do so in all cases.

6. *With regard to comments on figures by reviewer no. 1 (17):*
   - *Figure 4e is indeed a right not left knee MRI and its legend has been corrected.*
   - *Figure 6b shows a ghosting artifact due to poor breath-holding (18).*

We look forward to hearing from you (19)

Yours sincerely (20)

John Best, MD, and Co-authors (21)

---

1. *Dear Dr. Woods,*
   - Questa frase termina con una virgola anziché con il punto e virgola.

2. *We have reconfigured the manuscript referenced above...*
   - Il primo paragrafo deve riassumere il contenuto della vostra lettera.

3. *...following your suggestion...*
   - Questa è una delle frasi più comuni nelle lettere di risottomissione/riconfigurazione.

4. *...space limitation imposed by the new format of the paper...*
   - Le limitazioni di spazio, se il nuovo formato lo limita, devono essere prese in considerazione sia dagli autori che dai reviewer.

5. ...giving priority to the most prevalent conditions...
- Può essere un criterio per la riduzione della lunghezza dell'articolo.

6. ... for this reason we do not attach an annotated copy...
- Quando non seguite un suggerimento, dovete fornire una spiegazione.

7. ... if you still consider this necessary we will include it...
- Lasciatevi sempre la possibilità di aggiungere ulteriore materiale nelle comunicazioni future.

8. ..." allow the reader to more easily categorize the described complications"...
- Potete citare i commenti/suggerimenti dei reviewer se necessario, inserendoli tra virgolette.

9. ... as stated by reviewer no. 2...
- Questo è un modo tipico di rispondere al commento di un reviewer.

10. ... if you take our suggestion into consideration we will be pleased to add it...
- Questa frase può essere usata ogni volta che volete includere qualcosa che non è stato richiesto dai revisori.

11. The title has been modified to...following your recommendation.
- Questo è un modo tipico di rispondere al commento di un reviewer.

12. We have included the technical details of our surgical protocol as suggested by reviewer no.1...
- Questo è un modo tipico di rispondere al commento di un reviewer.

13. Similarly...could not be expanded as suggested by reviewer no.2 due to space limitations.
- Quando non seguite un suggerimento, dovete fornire una spiegazione.

14. With regard to figures:
- Oppure *regarding figures, as regards figures, as for figures* (senza la preposizione "to").

15. Intraoperative photos have been included
– Questo è un modo tipico di rispondere al commento di un reviewer.

16. The image quality of figure 3 has been improved...
– Questo è un modo tipico di rispondere al commento di un reviewer.

17. With regard to comments on figures by reviewer no. 1...
– Questo è un modo tipico di rispondere al commento di un reviewer.

18. We look forward to hearing from you,
– Ricordate che il verbo che segue il verbo "to look forward to" deve essere nella forma *–ing*.

19. Yours sincerely,
– Ricordate che se non conoscete il nome dell'editor dovreste usare invece "Yours faithfully".

20. John Best, M.D., and co-authors
– Anche se la lettera è firmata solo dal corresponding author, a volte si fa riferimento anche ai coautori.

Lettere di ringraziamento per l'invito a pubblicare un articolo su una rivista

Queste sono lettere semplici e generalmente brevi, nelle quali comunichiamo all'editor di una rivista quanto siamo lieti del suo invito e quanto apprezziamo la sua considerazione.

Vostro indirizzo

Nome e indirizzo del destinatario   Data

Dear Dr. Massa,

Thank you for the invitation to submit a manuscript on the surgical staging of focal hepatic lesions to your journal.

Please find attached our paper which details protocols, and provides a thorough review of the literature on the subject.

I look forward to hearing from you.

Yours sincerely,

A.J. Cantona, M.D.

Lettere per chiedere informazioni sullo stato di un articolo

In queste lettere, chiediamo informazioni sulla situazione del nostro articolo poiché non abbiamo ricevuto alcuna risposta dalla rivista. Sfortunatamente, nel mondo accademico "niente nuove" non vuol dire "buone nuove" e molte di queste richieste finiscono con una cortese lettera di rifiuto.

Dear Dr. Ross,

As I have not received any response regarding the manuscript "Surgical resection of cholangiocarcinoma," I am interested in obtaining some information on the status of the paper.

Please use the following e-mail address for further correspondence: sanzzap@seram.es

I look forward to hearing from you at your earliest convenience,

J. Sanz, MD, PhD.

Altri tipi di lettere

Candidarsi per un posto di lavoro

11 St Albans Road
London SW 17 5TZ

17 November 2006

Medical Staffing Officer
Brigham and Women's Hospital
18 Francis St.
Boston, MA 02115, USA

Dear Sir/Madam,

I wish to apply for the post of Consultant General Surgeon as advertised in the *European Journal of Surgery* of 22 October.

I enclose my CV and the names of two referees as requested.

Yours faithfully,

Albert Mas, M.D.

Chiedere il permesso di citare qualcuno come referenza

Platero Heredia, 19
Cordoba 14012
Spain
17 April 2006

John G. Adams M.D.
Department of Surgery
Massachusetts General Hospital
22 Beacon St
Boston, MA 02114, USA

Dear Dr. Fishman,

I am applying for a post of Consultant Surgeon at Cleveland Clinic.
I should be most grateful if you allow me to use your name as a referee.

Yours sincerely,

Guido Andreotti, M.D.

Posporre l'inizio dell'attività lavorativa

Gran Via, 113
Madrid 28004
Spain

17 November 2006

Robert H. Shaw, M.D.
Department of Surgery
Massachusetts General Hospital
22 Beacon St
Boston, MA 02114, USA

Dear Dr. Oesterle,

I would like to thank you for your letter of 11 February 2001, offering me the post of Consultant Surgeon from 12 March 2005.

I am very pleased to accept the post but unfortunately I will not be able to arrive in Boston until 25 March 2005 due to personal reasons. Would it, therefore, be possible for you to postpone the commencement of my duties to 26 March 2005?

I look forward to hearing from you.

Yours sincerely

Angela Maldini, M.D.

Riassumendo

Per riassumere, bisogna ricordare alcuni semplici dettagli formali:

- *"Dear Dr. Smith"* è il modo tipico di iniziare una lettera accademica. Ricordate che dopo il nome dell'editor dovete mettere una virgola, anziché il punto e virgola, e continuare la lettera con un nuovo paragrafo.

- Poiché la maggior parte degli articoli al giorno d'oggi viene inviata tramite internet, la classica formula *"find enclosed…"* può oggi essere sostituita da *"find attached"*.

- *"I look forward to hearing from you"* è la frase standard alla fine di ogni lettera formale e dovete ricordarvi, per evitare un errore piuttosto frequente, che *"to look forward to"* è un phrasal verb che deve essere seguito dal gerundio piuttosto che dall'infinito. Non fate l'errore di scrivere "I look forward to hear from you". Frasi simili sono *"I look forward to receiving your comments on…"*, *"Very truly yours,"*.

- *"Your consideration is appreciated"* o *"Thank you for your and the reviewer's consideration"* sono frasi standard da scrivere alla fine delle lettere agli editor.

- *"I look forward to receiving your feedback on…"* è una frase un po' più informale spesso usata nelle lettere agli editor.

- *"Yours faithfully"* viene usato quando non conoscete il nome della persona alla quale state scrivendo, mentre *"sincerely"*, *"sincerely yours"*, *"yours sincerely"* e *"very truly yours"* devono essere usati quando si indirizza la lettera a qualcuno di preciso. Quindi, se la lettera comincia con *"Dear Dr. Olsen"* dovrà concludersi con *"yours sincerely"*, mentre se la lettera è indirizzata all'editore dovrà concludersi con *"yours faithfully"*. Non dimenticate che dopo l'avverbio o il pronome dovete mettere una virgola piuttosto che un punto e poi la vostra firma sotto.

- Quando non potete seguire uno dei suggerimenti dell'editor, spiegate nella lettera di risottomissione perché non è stato possibile farlo, in modo che i reviewer non perdano tempo a cercarla nel testo. Per esempio:
  - ❯ We have included the technical details of our surgical protocol although it has not been possible to expand the technical section as suggested by reviewer no. 1 due to the space limitations.

Capitolo 5

Partecipare a un congresso internazionale di chirurgia

Introduzione

Nelle pagine seguenti, ci dedicheremo ai congressi internazionali di chirurgia. Consigliamo a chi ha un livello di inglese medio-alto di leggerle rapidamente, mentre a chi ha un livello di inglese intermedio di soffermarsi con attenzione su questa sezione, in modo da acquisire familiarità con il gergo dei congressi internazionali e con quello dei luoghi di conversazione più comuni come aeroporto, aereo, dogana, taxi, check-in dell'albergo e infine sede congressuale, luoghi che generalmente compongono l'itinerario di un chirurgo che partecipa a un congresso internazionale.

La maggior parte dei principianti non si reca da sola al suo primo congresso all'estero. All'inizio questo è un sollievo poiché non si devono affrontare le difficoltà linguistiche da soli, ma comporta un importante svantaggio: la maggior parte degli specializzandi di chirurgia non madrelingua inglese ritorna al proprio paese di origine senza aver pronunciato una sola parola di inglese. Anche se può sembrare molto innaturale, parlare inglese con i vostri colleghi è l'unico modo per parlare inglese a un congresso, poiché parlerete con vostri connazionali per oltre il 90% del tempo. Quando si è in gruppo, diventa virtualmente impossibile fare questo semplice esercizio.

Viaggiare da soli è l'unico modo per parlare inglese durante un congresso chirurgico internazionale e per i chirurghi non di madrelingua inglese può essere il solo modo per mantenere attivo il proprio inglese durante l'anno. Non perdete questa eccellente opportunità di esercitare il vostro livello di inglese colloquiale e scientifico.

R. Ribes, P. J. Aranda, J. Giba, *Inglese per chirurghi*,
© Springer-Verlag Italia 2012

Il seguente aneddoto mostra il livello di insicurezza dei giovani chirurghi non di madrelingua inglese quando partecipano ai loro primi congressi internazionali. Era il mio primo *European Congress* a Vienna. Mentre attendevo al banco della registrazione che qualcuno mi consegnasse il materiale e la borsa del congresso, qualcuno mi ha chiesto "*Have you got your badge?*". Non sapendo cosa fosse un badge, ho risposto "*no*" poiché era improbabile che avessi con me qualcosa di cui non conoscevo nemmeno il nome. Così mi dissero in modo molto autoritario: "Si metta in quella fila" e andai in modo obbediente a mettermi in coda senza avere la minima idea del motivo per il quale dovessi farlo. Quella è stata la prima volta, ma non l'ultima, in cui mi sono dovuto mettere in fila senza conoscerne minimamente il motivo. Quando si suppone che dobbiate tenere una lezione su – per esempio – "Il trattamento chirurgico dell'epatocarcinoma", e vi succede una cosa del genere, il desiderio di tornare a casa sarà l'unica certezza che vi resta.

Non lasciate che la vostra mancanza di dimestichezza con l'inglese di uso quotidiano diminuisca la vostra capacità di fare una buona o anche una grande presentazione. L'inglese colloquiale e quello scientifico sono due mondi differenti e per avere successo con il secondo, dovete avere una buona conoscenza del primo.

Questo capitolo vi fornisce trucchi e frasi utili nell'itinerario abituale di un congresso internazionale: aeroporto, aereo, dogana, taxi, check-in dell'albergo e infine, la sede congressuale stessa. Se non riuscirete a superare gli ostacoli nella conversazione nelle situazioni che precedono il congresso stesso, non sarete in grado di arrivare alla sede congressuale e, se ci arriverete, non avrete molta voglia di fare la vostra presentazione.

La maggior parte degli oratori non di madrelingua inglese si rassegna a fare il proprio discorso e "sopravvivere", dimenticando che, se non ci si diverte facendo la propria presentazione, neanche il pubblico si divertirà. Si pensa che per tenere una relazione in inglese si debba essere madrelingua inglese. Noi non siamo d'accordo con quest'idea, poiché molti oratori non amano parlare nemmeno nella propria lingua e riteniamo che divertirsi nel tenere un discorso sia molto più legato alla personalità.

Organizzazione di viaggio e albergo

Aeroporto

Andare in aeroporto

- How can I get to the airport?
- How soon should we be at the airport before take-off?

Check-in

- May I have your passport and flight tickets, please? Of course, here you are.
- Are you Mr. Macaya? Right, I am. How do you spell it? M-A-C-A-Y-A. (rehearse the spelling of your last name since if it is not an English one, you are going to be asked about its spelling many times).
- Here is your boarding pass. Your flight leaves from gate 14. Thank you.
- You are only allowed two carry-on items. You'll have to check in that larger bag.

Domande che un passeggero potrebbe fare

- I want to fly to London leaving this afternoon. Is there a direct flight? Is it via Amsterdam?
- Is it direct? Yes, it is direct/ No, it has one stopover.
- Is there a stopover? Yes, you have a stopover in Berlin.
- How long is the stopover? About 1 hour.
- Do I have to change planes? Yes, you have to change planes at...
- How much carry-on luggage am I allowed?
- What weight am I allowed?

- My luggage is overweight. How much more do I need to pay?
- Is a meal served? Yes, lunch will be served during the flight.
- What time does the plane to Boston leave?
- When does the next flight to Boston leave?
- Can I get onto the next flight?
- Can I change my flight schedule?
- What's the departure time?
- Is the plane on time?
- What's the arrival time?
- Will I be able to make my connection?
- I have misplaced my hand luggage. Where is Lost Property?
- How much is it to upgrade this ticket to first class?
- I want to change the return flight date from Atlanta to Madrid to September 28th.
- Is it possible to purchase an open ticket?
- I have missed my flight to New York. When does the next flight leave, please?
- Can I use the ticket I have, or do I need to pay for a new one?

Annuncio di cambiamenti su un volo

- Our flight to Vigo has been cancelled because of snow.
- Our flight to Chicago has been delayed; however, all connecting flights can be made.
- Flight number 0112 to Paris has been cancelled.
- Flight number 1145 has been moved to gate B15.
- Passengers for flight number 110 to London, please proceed to gate 7. Hurry up! Our flight has been called over the loudspeaker.

Al cancello d'imbarco

- We will begin boarding soon.
- We are now boarding passengers in rows 24 through 36.
- May I see your boarding card?

Arrivo

- Pick up your luggage at the terminal.
- Where can I find a luggage card?
- Where is the taxi rank?
- Where is the subway stop?
- Where is the way out?

Reclami su bagagli smarriti o danneggiati

- My luggage is missing.
- One of my bags seems to be missing.
- My luggage is damaged.
- One of my suitcases has been lost.

Ufficio di cambio

- Where is the Exchange Office?
- What is the rate for the Dollar?
- Could you change 1,000 Euros into Dollars?

Controlli di dogana e immigrazione

- May I see your passport, please?
- Do you have your visa?
- What is your nationality?
- What is the purpose of your journey? The purpose of my journey is...
- How long do you plan on staying?
- Empty your pockets and put your wallet, keys, mobile phone and coins on this tray.

- Remove any metallic objects you are carrying and put them on this tray.
- Open your laptop.
- Take your shoes off. Put them in this tray too.
- Do you have anything to declare? No, I don't have anything to declare.
- Do you have anything to declare? No, I only have personal effects.
- Do you have anything to declare? Yes, I am a doctor and I'm carrying some surgical instruments.
- Do you have anything to declare? Yes, I have bought six bottles of whisky and four cartons of cigarettes in the duty-free shop.
- How much currency are you bringing into the country? I haven't got any foreign currency.
- Open your bag, please.
- I need to examine the contents of your bag.
- May I close my bag? Sure.
- Please place your suitcases on the table.
- What do you have in these parcels? Some presents for my wife and kid.
- How much duty do I have to pay?
- Where is the Exchange Office?

Durante il volo

Durante un volo normalmente si hanno poche occasioni di conversazione. Se siete a vostro agio con l'inglese, vi renderete conto di come la dimestichezza con la lingua possa influire in modo positivo sul vostro umore. Altrimenti, se vi serve un cuscino e non siete in grado di chiederlo, la vostra autostima si ridurrà, il collo vi farà male e non oserete chiedere nient'altro per tutto il resto del volo.

Durante il mio primo volo per gli Stati Uniti non sapevo come chiedere un cuscino e cercavo di convincermi che in realtà non mi servisse. Quando poi ho guardato finalmente sulla guida, l'ho chiesto e la hostess mi ha portato il cuscino, mi sono addormentato felice e comodo.

Non lasciate che la mancanza di dimestichezza con la lingua vi rovini un volo altrimenti perfetto.

- Is there an aisle/window seat free? (I asked for one at the check-in and they told me I should ask onboard just in case there had been a cancellation).
- Excuse me, you are in my seat. Oh! Sorry, I didn't notice.
- Fasten your seat belt, please.
- Your life-jacket is under your seat.
- Smoking is not allowed during the flight.
- Please would you bring me a blanket/pillow?
- Is there a business class seat free?
- Can I upgrade to first class on board?
- Would you like a cup of tea/coffee/a glass of soda? A glass of soda, please.
- What would you prefer, chicken or beef/fish or meat? Beef/fish please.
- Is there a vegetarian menu?
- Stewardess, I'm feeling bad. Do you have anything for flight-sickness? Could you bring me another sick-bag, please?
- Stewardess, I have a headache. Do you have an aspirin?
- Stewardess, this gentleman is disturbing me.

In taxi (anche chiamato Cab negli Stati Uniti)

Immaginate di prendere un taxi nella vostra città. Quante frasi scambiereste in condizioni normali, o anche in condizioni non convenzionali? Vi assicuro che con meno di due dozzine di frasi sareste in grado di risolvere oltre il 90% delle possibili situazioni.

Chiedere dove prendere un taxi

- Where is the nearest taxi rank?
- Where can I get a taxi?

Istruzioni di base

- Hi, take me downtown/to the Sheraton Hotel, please.
- Please, would you take me to the airport?
- It is rush hour; I don't go to the airport.
- Sorry, I am not on duty.
- It will cost you double fare to leave the city.
- I need to go to the Convention Center.
- Which way do you want me to take you, via Fifth or Seventh Avenue? Either one would be OK.
- Is there any surcharge to the airport?

Riguardo la velocità del taxi

- To downtown as quick as you can.
- Are you in a hurry? Yes, I'm in a hurry.
- I'm late; please hurry up!
- Slow down!
- Do you have to drive so fast? There is no need to hurry. I am not in a rush at all.

Chiedere di fermarsi e aspettare

- Stop at number 112, please.
- Which side of the street?
- Do you want me to drop you at the door?
- Pull over; I'll be back in a minute.
- Please, wait here a minute.
- Stop here.

Riguardo la temperatura sul taxi

- Would you please wind your window up? It's a bit cold.
- Could you turn the heat up/down/on/off?
- Could you turn the air conditioning on/off?
- Is the air conditioning/heating on?

Pagamento

- How much is it?
- How much do I owe you?
- Is the tip included?
- Do you have change for a twenty/fifty (dollar bill)? Sorry, I don't (have any change).
- Keep the change.
- Would you give me a receipt?
- I need a receipt, please.
- I think that is too expensive.
- They have never charged me this before. Give me a receipt, please. I think I'll make a complaint.
- Can I pay by credit card? Sure, swipe your card here.

In albergo

Registrazione

- May I help you?
- Hello, I have reserved a room under the name of Dr. Pichard.
- For how many people? Two, my wife and me.
- Do you need my ID?
- Do you need my credit card?
- How long will you be staying? We are staying for a week.
- You will have to wait until your room is ready.

- Here is your key.
- Enjoy your stay. Thank you.
- Is there anybody who can help me with my bags?
- Do you need a bellhop? Yes, please.
- I'll have someone bring your luggage up.

Preferenze

- Can you double-check that we have a double room with a view of the beach/city…?
- I would like a room at the front/at the rear.
- I would like the quietest room you have.
- I would like a non-smoking room.
- I would like a suite.
- How many beds? I want a double bed/a single bed.
- I asked for two single beds.
- I'd like a king-sized bed.
- I'd like a queen-sized bed.
- We will need a crib for the baby.
- Are all your rooms en suite? Yes, all of our rooms have a bath or shower.
- Is breakfast included?
- Does the hotel have parking? (British English: "car park").
- Do you have a parking lot/structure nearby? (British English: "car park").

Soggiorno

- Can you give me a wake-up call at seven each morning?
- There is no hot water. Would you please send someone to fix it?
- The TV is not working properly. Would you please send someone to fix it?
- The bathtub has no plug. Would you please send someone up with one?

- The people in the room next to mine are making a racket. Would you please tell them to keep it down?
- I want to change my room. It's too noisy.
- What time does breakfast start?
- How can I get to the city center?
- Can we change Euros into Dollars?
- Could you recommend a good restaurant near to the hotel?
- Could you recommend a good restaurant?
- Would you give me the number for room service?
- I will have a cheese omelette, a ham sandwich and an orange juice.
- Are there vending machines available?
- Do you have a fax machine available?
- Do you serve meals?
- Is there a pool/restaurant...?
- How do I get room service?
- Is there wireless/Internet connection?
- The sink is clogged.
- The toilet is running.
- The toilet is leaking.
- My toilet overflowed!
- The toilet doesn't flush.
- The bath is leaking.
- My bathroom is flooded.
- The bath faucets (British English: "taps") drip day and night.
- The water is rust-colored.
- The pipes are always banging.
- The water is too hot.
- The water is never hot enough.
- I don't have any hot water.

Checking out

- How much is it?
- Do you accept credit cards?
- Can I pay in Dollars/Euros?
- I'd like a receipt please.
- What time is checkout? Checkout is at 11 a.m.
- I would like to check out.
- Is there a penalty for late checkout?

- Please, would you have my luggage brought down?
- Would you please call me a taxi?
- How far is the nearest bus stop/subway station?

Lamentele

- Excuse me; there is a mistake on the receipt.
- I have had only one breakfast.
- I thought breakfast was included.
- I have been in a single room.
- Have you got a complaints book?
- Please would you give me my car keys?
- Is there anybody here who can help me with my luggage?

Esempio di congresso

Informazioni generali

Rivediamo alcune informazioni generali sul programma di un congresso, concentrandoci sui termini che potrebbero non essere conosciuti dai principianti.

Lingua

La lingua ufficiale del corso sarà l'Inglese.

Abbigliamento

L'abito formale è richiesto per la cerimonia d'apertura e per la cena sociale. Un abbigliamento informale è accettabile per tutti gli altri eventi e occasioni (anche se è utilizzato di solito durante le lezioni).

Esposizioni commerciali

I partecipanti avranno la possibilità di esaminare dei campioni delle case produttrici di prodotti farmaceutici, diagnostici e chirurgici; gli editori nel loro stand potranno ricevere aggiornamenti sulle informazioni relative a nuovi prodotti.

Anche se la maggior parte dei partecipanti non parla con gli informatori scientifici per via dell'inglese incerto, simili conversazioni sono un'opportunità per esercitarsi nell'inglese chirurgico e, allo stesso tempo, ricevere informazioni aggiornate su apparecchiature e strumenti abitualmente utilizzati nella pratica clinica quotidiana.

Interessi commerciali

Per evitare preconcetti commerciali, I relatori devono segnalare eventuali rapporti con l'industria. Per quanto riguarda le relazioni commerciali con le imprese, esistono tre tipi di relatori:

1. Relatori (congiunti/partner e organizzatori) che non hanno rapporti significativi con ditte.
2. Relatori che hanno dichiarato di aver ricevuto qualcosa "di valore" da una compagnia i cui prodotti sono correlati al contenuto delle loro presentazioni.
3. Relatori che non hanno fornito informazioni sui loro rapporti con le ditte.

Organizzazione

- Russel J. Curtin, M.D., Staff Surgeon, Division of Bariatric Surgery, Beth Israel Deaconess Medical center, Boston, Ma

Con il termine *"Guest faculty"* si indicano quei relatori che non provengono dall'Istituto organizzatore del congresso stesso.

- Fergus B . Schwartz, Professor of Radiology and Otolaryngology, Head and Neck Surgery, New York School of Medicine; New York University Medical Center, New York, NY

How to reach...

Arrivo con l'aereo

- The International Airport is situated about 25 kilometers outside the city. To reach the city center you can use the...
- City airport train. Every half-hour. Non-stop. 18 minutes from the airport direct to downtown and from downtown direct to the airport. Fare: single EUR 10; return EUR 18.
- Regional railway, line 6. Travel time: 36 minutes. Frequency: every 30 minutes. Fare: Single EUR 12; Return EUR 20. Get off at "Charles Square". From there use the underground line "U7" to "Park Street".
- Bus. International Airport to...Charles Square. Travel time: 25 minutes. Fare: EUR 8.
- Taxi. There is a taxi rank to the south of the arrival hall. A taxi to the city center costs around EUR 45 (depending on traffic).

Arrivo con il treno

- For detailed information about the timetable you can call...
- At the railway station you can use the underground to reach the city.
- Congress venue (where the course is to be held, e.g., hotel, university, convention center...):
  Continental Hotel
  32 Park Street, 23089...
  Phone:.../Fax:...
  E-mail: continentalhotel@hhs.com
- To reach the venue from the city center (Charles Square) take the U1 underground line (green). Leave the train at Park Street and take the exit marked Continental Hotel. Travelling time: approximately 10 minutes.

Argomenti finanziari

- The common European currency is the Euro.

Tempo

- The weather in... December is usually cold with occasional snow. The daytime temperatures normally range from - 5° to +5°C.

Registrazione

Generalmente i partecipanti si iscrivono ai congressi in anticipo e non è pertanto necessario iscriversi al banco delle registrazioni. Tuttavia, nel caso in cui vi doveste iscrivere direttamente al congresso, vi suggeriamo alcune delle frasi più usate in tale occasione:

Chirurgo:	May I have a registration form, please?
Addetto al congresso:	Do you want me to fill it out (UK fill it in) for you?
	Are you a surgeon?
	Are you an ESC member?
	Are you attending the full course?
Specializzando in chirurgia:	No. I'm a surgery resident.
Addetto al congresso:	Can I see your chairpersons's confirmation letter?
Specializzando/tecnico:	I was told it was faxed last week. Would you check that, please?
Chirurgo:	I'll pay by cash/credit card. Charge it to my credit card. Would you make out an invoice?
Addetto al congresso:	Do you need an invoice? Do you want me to draw up an invoice?
Chirurgo:	Where should I get my badge?
Addetto al congresso:	Join that line.

Costi di registrazione e scadenze:

	Until 1 September 2005	Until 13 November 2006	After 13 November 2006
Full fee member	€230.-	€330.-	€450.-
Full fee non-member	€420.-	€540.-	€650.-
Resident member*	€150.-	€190.-	€260.-
Resident non-member*	€250.-	€310.-	€440.-
Radiographer*	€100.-	€140.-	€180.-
Hospital administrator*	€100.-	€140.-	€180.-
Single-day ticket	On-site only	On-site only	€240.-
Single half-day ticket	On-site only	On-site only	€80.-
(Tuesday only)			
Weekend ticket	On-site only	On-site only	€360.-
(Saturday 07:00 to Sunday 18:00)			
Industry day ticket	On-site only	On-site only	€90.-
Student**	On-site only	On-site only	Free of charge!
Radiographer			€120.-
Full fee member			€180.-
Full fee non-member			€300.-

Programma del congresso

L'idea fondamentale è che, quando partecipate a un congresso internazionale, dovete immaginare in anticipo quelle situazioni che si verificheranno inevitabilmente e così potrete ridurre al minimo le situazioni imbarazzanti che vi coglierebbero impreparati. Se solo avessi cercato (a casa!) il significato della parola "badge", non sarei stato colto di sorpresa al mio primo congresso all'estero. Sono poche le parole, le frasi fatte e le sedi che devono essere conosciute nell'ambiente dei corsi chirurgici e possiamo assicurarvi che conoscerle prima vi darà la sicurezza necessaria a rendere la vostra partecipazione al congresso un successo personale.

Il primo consiglio è: *leggete attentamente il programma del congresso e controllate sul dizionario o chiedete a colleghi più esperti il significato di parole e concetti che non conoscete. Poiché il programma è disponibile prima dell'inizio del congresso, leggetelo a casa; non avrete bisogno di leggere il programma scientifico in sede di congresso.*

"*Adjourn*" è uno di quei termini tipici dei programmi con cui uno diventa familiare una volta che la sessione diventa "*adjourned*". Anche se molti potrebbero pensare che la maggior parte dei termini saranno integrati e resi comprensibili dal contesto, la nostra intenzione è quella di analizzare quei termini "neutri" che potrebbero impedirvi di ottimizzare il vostro tempo al congresso.

Nella Tabella 5.1 è riportato un esempio di programma di congresso.

Il programma del congresso può contenere i seguenti elementi:

1. *Satellite symposia (singular symposium)*: eventi scientifici sponsorizzati da case farmaceutiche nel corso dei quali vengono presentati alla comunità chirurgica nuovi farmaci, tecniche o device.
2. *Plenary sessions*: questi eventi hanno luogo generalmente a mezzogiorno e radunano tutti i partecipanti intorno ai membri più eminenti della comunità chirurgica.
3. *Cases of the day*: Una serie di casi chirurgici riguardanti diversi settori della chirurgia. I partecipanti possono presentare i loro approcci chirurgici.
4. *Categorical courses*: Si discute un argomento chirurgico importante focalizzando l'attenzione sulle esigenze dei chirurghi generali.
5. *Refresher courses*: Un tema concreto viene esaminato attentamente da esperti del settore.
6. "*... meets*" *sessions*: Lo scopo di queste sessioni è quello di creare legami più stretti tra i partecipanti al congresso provenienti da paesi diversi. Esistono sessioni dedicate alle comunità chirurgiche di questi paesi per mostrare ai partecipanti il congresso l'eccellenza chirurgica raggiunta.
7. *Special focus session*: lo scopo è quello di discutere un argomento nuovo, presentato in modo tale da promuovere il dibattito tra esperti e pubblico.
8. "*How to do it*" *sessions*: Chirurghi esperti descrivono il loro approccio a una patologia, mostrando la loro tecnica passo per passo, spesso con l'aiuto di filmati video di casi reali.
9. *Scientific session*: La Commissione Scientifica seleziona, da tutti gli abstract presentati, i lavori di ricerca clinica e di base più rilevanti e invita gli autori a fare una presentazione sui materiali e metodi e sulle

conclusioni (generalmente non più lunga di 10-15 min). Solitamente è concessa una serie di domande.

10. *Adjourn:* break o intervallo alla fine di una sessione.

Tabella 5.1 Programma del congresso

	8:30	10:30	12:15	14:00	16:00
Dec 4	Special focus session Categorical courses Refresher courses	State-of-the-art Scientific sessions Workshops Satellite symposium	Opening ceremony Inauguration lecture	Scientific sessions Satellite symposium	Special focus session Categorical courses Refresher courses Adjourn
Dec 5	Special focus session Categorical courses Refresher courses	... meets Italy Workshops	Honorary lecture	Scientific sessions Workshops	Special focus sessions Categorical courses Refresher courses Adjourn
Dec 6	Special focus session Categorical courses Refresher courses	... meets Hungary Workshops Satellite symposium	Honorary lecture	Image interpretation session	Special focus sessions Categorical courses Refresher courses Adjourn
Dec 7	Special focus session Categorical courses Refresher courses	State-of-theart Workshops Scientific sessions	Honorary lecture	... meets Japan Scientific sessions	Special focus sessions Categorical courses Refresher courses Adjourn
Dec 8	Special focus session Categorical courses Refresher courses	Workshops Scientific sessions	Closing ceremony		

Capitolo 6

Presentare una comunicazione orale in inglese

Introduzione

I congressi chirurgici internazionali rappresentano un mondo a parte. In questo universo gli invitati e gli oratori provengono da paesi diversi con differenti culture e pertanto hanno abitudini che si diversificano sia in termini di comportamento sia nel modo di comunicare durante le presentazioni. Tuttavia, la maggioranza degli oratori mette da parte, almeno parzialmente, la propria identità culturale e cerca di adeguarsi allo stile dei congressi medici internazionali. La standardizzazione fa parte della globalizzazione cui stiamo tutti assistendo.

La lingua più parlata al mondo non è il cinese, l'inglese o lo spagnolo, ma il nuovo fenomeno di "inglese stentato". Questa lingua nasce dal tentativo di semplificare l'inglese stesso, al fine di renderlo il più naturale e comprensibile possibile, limando espressioni colloquiali, dialettali, o ancora ogni altra fonte di confusione linguistica.

In questo nuovo universo, i professionisti della sanità si trovano a dover fare uno sforzo cosciente per adattarsi a queste regole esplicite e implicite. Alcune di queste regole saranno discusse nei prossimi paragrafi.

Con la lettura di questo capitolo, non solo sarete in grado di migliorare le vostre presentazioni e sentirvi a vostro agio durante la comunicazione, ma potrete anche essere in grado di trasmettere il vostro messaggio e, magari, il tutto potrà essere piacevole anche per voi, nonostante dobbiate parlare durante il cosiddetto "graveyard slot" (ovvero la prima presentazione dopo pranzo, quando la maggior parte dell'uditorio sarà affetta da sonnolenza post-prandiale e molto probabilmente non udirete altri rumori che il russare generale).

R. Ribes, P. J. Aranda, J. Giba, *Inglese per chirurghi*,
© Springer-Verlag Italia 2012

Cosa fare e cosa non fare

Il tempo e la tempistica sono fattori strettamente correlati alla cultura e alle abitudini. Infatti, un inizio dei lavori alle otto del mattino in America Latina potrebbe sembrare troppo "precoce", mentre sarebbe interpretato come un orario perfettamente adeguato nel Nord Europa o negli Stati Uniti. Inoltre, il giorno è diviso in modo diverso nelle varie parti del mondo… e nel nostro universo chirurgico. Pertanto durante un congresso medico internazionale il giorno viene diviso secondo la seguente tabella di marcia:

- Mattina: dall'inizio fino alle 12.
- Pomeriggio: dalle 12.01 alle 17.00 o 18.00.
- Sera: dalle 18 a mezzanotte.
- Ricordatevi di seguire questi consigli nel salutare:
- *Good morning*: dall'inizio fino alle 12.
- *Good afternoon*: dalle 12.01 in poi, anche se il vostro metabolismo è lungi dal sentirsi "nella fascia pomeridiana" nonostante sia passata la vostra ora abituale di pranzo e vi urla *"good morning"*.
- *Good evening*: dalle 18 in poi. Se doveste fare una presentazione, un discorso o un brindisi alle 22, fate attenzione a non esordire mai con *"good night"*; tale espressione dovrebbe, infatti, essere usata solo nell'augurare buona notte prima di andare a dormire e non dovrebbe pertanto essere utilizzata in pubbliche occasioni.

Quando si fa una presentazione, c'è sempre un limite di tempo. So bene, anche per esperienza personale, quanto sia difficile condensare in soli 20 minuti le nostre conoscenze sull'argomento al quale abbiamo dedicato il nostro lavoro negli ultimi anni. Per superare questo limite, ci sono alcune tattiche come ad esempio parlare alla massima velocità con cui la lingua riesce a muoversi, concludere il discorso in soli 5 minuti, e spendere i rimanenti 15 a fissare l'uditorio. I medici americani, inglesi e australiani sono spesso oratori molto fluenti (lo sappiamo, lo sappiamo… stanno parlando nella loro lingua). Tuttavia, ricordatevi che mostrare e commentare cinque diapositive al minuto e parlare più velocemente di quanto anche un registratore digitale sia in grado di registrare può non essere il modo migliore per trasmettere il messaggio. Pertanto seguite alcune semplici regole:

- *Non parlate* troppo velocemente o troppo lentamente.
- *Non dite* "mi dispiace per questa diapositiva". Siete voi a scegliere le diapositive da presentare, eliminate quelle di cui vi scusereste.
- *Riassumete* la vostra presentazione e provate a vedere quanto tempo vi serve per rendere la vostra presentazione più chiara possibile.

Talvolta i relatori tendono a fornire troppi dati e dettagli minuziosi nelle loro presentazioni. Le introduzioni spesso sono sature di informazioni che risultano di scarsa rilevanza per un uditorio internazionale (ad esempio, il nome, la data e i codici di leggi locali, provinciali, regionali o nazionali che regolano gli standard chirurgici nel loro istituto; o anche le informazioni di base sui principali investigatori di un trial incluso l'anno di laurea e il numero di scarpe... o una storia dettagliata dell'edificio del sedicesimo secolo che ospita l'ospedale con i successivi restauri cui è stato sottoposto; ecc.). In tali situazioni, forniti tutti questi dettagli, la presentazione avrà superato la fase introduttiva, ma comunque il tempo a vostra disposizione sarà già terminato e al moderatore non resterà che esibirsi in gesti disperati verso il relatore. Ecco ancora qualche suggerimento:

- *Reggete* il puntatore laser con entrambe le mani.
Il miglior modo di evitare che il pointer tremi è quello di afferrarlo con entrambe le mani e tenerle sul leggio. Se questo non funziona, vi consigliamo di usare il mouse, almeno il vostro tremolio sarà confinato a un solo piano, anzichè avere un puntatore laser che trema nelle tre dimensioni.

- *Usate* un puntatore o il mouse del computer.
Anche se può sembrare incredibile, sono stato a una conferenza durante la quale il relatore piuttosto che usare il puntatore laser, cercava di indirizzare l'occhio attento dell'uditorio sulle immagini, utilizzando un giornale piegato. Inutile dire che l'unica persona che potesse vedere i dettagli indicati era lui stesso.

- *Strutturate* la vostra presentazione in modo da trasmettere pochi messaggi ma chiari, piuttosto che una pletora di informazioni non tutte particolarmente rilevanti che nessuno ha la possibilità di memorizzare.
- *Non leggete* le diapositive, ma cercate di spiegare alcuni concetti base nel modo più chiaro possibile.

Molti medici con un livello intermedio di inglese parlato potrebbero non
approvare quest'ultimo punto, dal momento che si potrebbero sentire
maggiormente a loro agio leggendo la presentazione. Tuttavia leggere è
la forma di comunicazione meno naturale; vi incoraggiamo, pertanto, a
presentare il vostro lavoro evitando di leggere. Anche se ciò dovesse
richiedere una preparazione più intensa, il discorso sarà più scorrevole e
il risultato – perché no? – addirittura brillante. Molti medici stranieri si
rassegnano a esprimersi in modo appena accettabile, rifiutando esplicita-
mente la possibilità di esporre una presentazione dello stesso livello che
riuscirebbero a raggiungere nella loro madre-lingua. Non rifiutate la possibilità di essere brillanti almeno quanto lo sareste nella vostra lingua;
l'unica differenza è nel numero di prove che vi serviranno per ottenere
risultati eccezionali. Prove accurate possono darvi risultati incredibili;
non arrendetevi anzitempo.

- *Non leggete* la vostra presentazione dagli appunti.
Leggere da un testo scritto è, se possibile, ancora peggio che leggere le diapositive. Ho assistito a veri disastri di relatori che tentavano, senza alcun
successo, di coordinare foglietti scritti e diapositive. Il rumore delle pagine sfogliate era insopportabile e la faccia del relatore sull'orlo di una crisi
di nervi impediva al pubblico di ascoltare la presentazione stessa.

- *Divertitevi.*
Quando fate la vostra presentazione rilassatevi; nessuno conosce più di
voi il tema specifico che state presentando. L'unico modo di far sì che la
gente apprezzi la vostra presentazione è quello di apprezzarla voi stessi.
Dovete solo comunicare, non esibirvi; essere un bravo ricercatore o un
clinico competente non è la stessa cosa che essere un comico o una
modella. Ciò tuttavia non vuol dire che possiamo permetterci di ignorare
le nostre abilità nelle presentazioni, soprattutto se volete che la maggior
parte dei vostri colleghi siano ancora svegli alla fine della relazione!

- *Cercate di superare la paura* da palcoscenico e concentratevi sulla
  comunicazione.
Deve esserci qualcuno là fuori interessato a quello che avete da dire...
che sia per lodarlo o farlo a pezzi, questo non importa.

- *Evitate* qualsiasi cosa che vi possa rendere nervosi durante la presentazione.
Un consiglio che posso sicuramente darvi è quello di togliere tutte le
chiavi, monete e altri oggetti metallici dalle vostre tasche, in modo che

non siate tentati di giocherellarci – riuscireste a produrre un suono veramente irritante che abbiamo tutti imparato a odiare.

• Mettete cellulare (UK: mobile phone; USA: cell phone) e cercapersone in modalità *silenziosa*.

L'unica cosa più imbarazzante del cellulare di qualcuno del pubblico che interrompe il vostro discorso è senza dubbio il vostro stesso cellulare che suona a metà della vostra presentazione.

• *Fate in modo* che le vostre battute possano essere capite da un pubblico internazionale.

La creatività e lo humour sono sempre apprezzati in una sala conferenze... naturalmente se sono appropriati e capiti! Sappiamo bene che l'umorismo è un fattore culturale, come il tempo, le cravatte, le preferenze alimentari, ecc. La maggior parte dei relatori americani iniziano i loro discorsi con una battuta che spesso non viene capita da gran parte dell'uditorio europeo, nemmeno dagli irlandesi o dai britannici. Un relatore britannico potrebbe farvi, quando meno ve lo aspettereste, un commento sarcastico probabilmente con lo stesso tono con cui parlerebbe del tasso di mortalità del proprio reparto, mentre un medico non anglosassone potrebbe provare a raccontare una lunga battuta in inglese basata su un gioco di parole nella sua lingua d'origine, che ovviamente non funziona in inglese, e probabilmente riguarderà religione, sport e/o sesso. Vi suggeriamo come regola generale di evitare battute su religione e sesso nei discorsi pubblici.

Frasi utili per discorsi chirurgici

Introdurre la presentazione

> Good afternoon. It is an honour to have the opportunity to speak to you about...
> Good afternoon. Thank you for your kind introduction. It is my pleasure to speak to you about an area of great interest to me.
> In the next few minutes I'll talk about...
> The topic I'll cover this afternoon is...
> In the next 20 minutes I'll show you...

> In my talk on focal hepatic lesions, I want to share with you all our experience on...
> Thank you for sticking around (informal way of addressing the last talk attendees).
> I'd like to thank Dr. Leon for his kind invitation.
> Thank you Dr. Pichard for inviting me to attend this course.
> Thank you Dr. Nieminem. It is a great honour to be here talking about...
> On behalf of my colleagues and assistants, I want to thank Dr. Palacios for his kind invitation.
> I'd like to welcome you to this course on...(to be said in the first talk of the course if you are a member of the organizing committee).
> Today, I want to talk to you about...
> Now, allow me to introduce...
> What I want to talk about this morning is...
> During the next few minutes, I'd like to draw your attention to...
> First of all, let me summarize the contents of my lecture on...
> Let's begin by looking at these 3D images of the heart...

Commentare immagini, grafici, tabelle, schemi, ecc.

> As you can see in the image on your right...
> As you will see in the next table...
> As we saw in the previous slide...
> The next image shows...
> The next image allows us to...
> In the bottom left image we can see...
> What do we have to look at here?
> What do we have to bear in mind with regard to this artefact?
> Notice how the lesion is...
> Bear in mind that this image was obtained in less than 10 seconds...
> Let's look at this schematic representation of the portal vein.
> As you can see in this CT image...
> Let us have a look at this schematic diagram of the portal vein.
> Looking at this table, you can see...
> Having a look at this bar chart, we could conclude that...
> To sum up, let's look at this diagram...
> The image on your right...

> The image at the top of the screen shows...
> Let's turn to the next slide in which the lesion, after the administration of contrast material, is more conspicious.
> Figure 3 brings out the importance of...
> As can be observed in this MR image...
> I apologize that the faint area of sclerosis in the femur *does not project well*. (When a subtle finding is difficult to see on a projected image, it is said that *it does not project well*).

Riassumere

> To sum up we can say that...
> In summary, we have discussed...
> To conclude...
> Summing up, I would say that...
> The take-home lesson of the talk is...
> To put it in a nutshell...
> To cut a long story short...
> In short,...
> To put it briefly...
> If there is one point I hope you will take away from this presentation, it is that ...Endovascular surgery of the thoracic aorta is safe and effective.
> Thoracoscopic resection of lung cancer can be done in patients in the early stage.
> This less invasive technique of total hip replacement provides a survival benefit in elderly patients.
> Cavum tumors respond better to a combination of surgery and radiotherapy than to surgery alone.
> Virtual colonoscopy is the most accurate technique for the assessment of ...

Concludere

> Thank you for your kind attention.
> Thank you all for sticking around until the very last talk of the session.
> Thank you all.
> Thank you very much for your time; you have been a most gracious audience.
> Thank you for your attention. I would be happy to entertain any questions.
> Thank you for your time. I would be happy to address any questions.
> This is all we have time for, so thank you and have a good time in London.
> Let me finish my presentation by saying that...
> We can say to conclude that...
> Let me end by wishing you a pleasant stay in our city.
> I'd be happy to answer any question you might have.
> I'd be happy to address your comments and questions.

La terribile sezione dedicata ai commenti e alle domande

Molti principianti sicuramente non esiterebbero a fare una comunicazione libera durante un congresso internazionale se non fosse seguita da una breve sezione di domande.

Il seguente aneddoto può mostrare i sentimenti di molti chirurghi non di madrelingua inglese alle prese con le loro prime presentazioni in inglese. Dopo una breve comunicazione libera, condotta a termine peraltro con discreto successo per un principiante, sul follow-up RM dell'operazione di Ross (la sostituzione della valvola aortica del paziente con la sua valvola polmonare e la sostituzione di quest'ultima con una protesi), stavo aspettando, come un coniglio che fissa un serpente, il giro di domande che inevitabilmente avrebbe seguito la mia presentazione.

Sull'orlo di una crisi di nervi, ho sentito un chirurgo inglese farmi una domanda che riuscivo a malapena a capire. Gli ho detto *"Would you please repeat your question?"* e lui, obbediente, ha ripetuto la domanda con le stesse esatte parole e il medesimo tono con cui l'aveva formulata prima. Poiché continuavo a non capire, il moderatore l'ha tradotta in un inglese più internazionale e comprensibile e sono finalmente riuscito a rispondere. Questa è stata l'unica domanda che mi hanno fatto poiché il tempo era finito e non c'era spazio per altri commenti.

Pensiamo a questo aneddoto in modo positivo considerando i seguenti punti che ci porteranno ad alcuni consigli:

1. Non scoraggiatevi. Nessuno vi ha detto che gli inizi sono facili.
2. Le domande e i commenti da parte di un madrelingua inglese tendono a essere più difficili da comprendere.
3. Ci sono diverse tipologie di interlocutori, ne dovete essere consci.
4. Non lamentatevi se l'interlocutore fa esattamente quello che gli avete chiesto.
5. I moderatori possono sempre aiutarvi.
6. Il tempo è limitato e potete sfruttare questo a vostro vantaggio.

Questi punti portano ad alcuni consigli:

1. Allora non sapevo che il peggio dovesse ancora venire. Ho passato l'intera mattina a ripensare alla scena più e più volte. "Come posso aver rovinato in questo modo tante ore di ricerca e studio?" Pensavo anche che la gente mi avrebbe riconosciuto come "quello che non aveva capito una semplice domanda".

Pensiamo per un momento a come è andata la prima volta che avete fatto qualcosa nella vostra vita, ad esempio, la prima volta che avete impugnato una racchetta da tennis o una mazza da golf. Rispetto a quello, non era così male.

2. Quando il chirurgo che chiede la parola non è di madrelingua inglese, potete tirare un sospiro di sollievo perché parlerete con qualcuno uguale a voi dal punto di vista linguistico, uno che ha speso molte ore a lottare per imparare una lingua diversa dalla sua. D'altro canto, quando parlate con un interlocutore inglese, potete trovarvi di fronte a due tipologie di soggetti:

Il *Tipo A* è un collega che non sfrutta il fatto di essere di madrelingua e riduce la sua normale velocità del discorso, in modo che possiate capire la domanda e quindi trasmettere al pubblico quello che avete da dire.

Il *Tipo B* è un collega che non fa alcuna distinzione tra relatori di madrelingua e non. Non è necessario sottolineare che ho incontrato un tipo B nella mia prima presentazione internazionale.

3. Tipi di interlocutori:
- *Tipo 1*: l'interlocutore che vuole conoscere un particolare della vostra presentazione. Questi interlocutori sono facilmente gestibili semplicemente rispondendo alle loro domande.

> What diameters do you measure in the aortic root?
> Annulus, Valsalva sinuses, and sinotubular junction.

- *Tipo 2*: l'interlocutore che vuole mostrare al pubblico la sua conoscenza approfondita dell'argomento che viene discusso. Questi interlocutori sono abbastanza facili da gestire in quanto non formulano domande, ma fanno commenti. Le risposte tendono a essere più brevi delle domande o dei commenti e il tempo, il cui passare gioca a favore del principiante se non sta parlando, scorre, non lasciando così spazio ad altre temibili domande.

> I do agree with your comments.
> We are planning to include this point in our next paper on...

- *Tipo 3*: l'interlocutore che è in forte disaccordo con voi. Questo è ovviamente il tipo di interlocutore più difficile da affrontare soprattutto per un principiante a causa delle lacune linguistiche. L'unico consiglio è difendere la vostra posizione con umiltà e non sfidare l'interlocutore.

> I will consider your suggestion on...
> This is a work in progress and we will consider including your suggestions...

4. Se io chiedessi al mio interlocutore di ripetere la domanda più lentamente e con parole differenti, sarebbe moralmente costretto a fare ciò. Purtroppo i principianti mancano di questo tipo di modestia e fingono di essere migliori di quanto realmente siano e di sapere più di quanto realmente sappiano, il che è per definizione un errore.

> I don't understand your question. Would you please reformulate your question in a different way, please?

5. Quando sentite di aver bisogno di sostegno, chiedete aiuto al moderatore.

> Dr. Ho(chairman) I'm not sure I've understood the question. Would you please formulate it in a different way?

6. Nella peggiore delle ipotesi tuttavia sarà solo un breve momento di stress. Non lasciate pertanto che un periodo così breve possa ostacolare una carriera potenzialmente di successo nella chirurgia internazionale.

Frasi che possono aiutare

Studiate queste frasi che possono aiutarvi a uscire da una situazione difficile e a ridurre al minimo la vostra paura della sezione delle domande e dei commenti:

Making your point

> ❯ Let me point out that this procedure is as safe as the standard one …
> ❯ You must bear in mind that performing this operation is more time consuming than the fully open procedure …
> ❯ If you look closely at this brain tumor, you will realize that …
> ❯ I want to draw your attention to the fact that …
> ❯ Don't forget the importance of liver protection in …
> ❯ Before I move on to my next slide …
> ❯ In view of the upcoming publication of …
> ❯ Surgically speaking …
> ❯ From a surgical point of view …
> ❯ As far as trackability is concerned …
> ❯ The bottom line of the subject is …

Dare spiegazioni

> ❯ To put it another way, this surgical approach was responsible for …
> ❯ Taking into consideration that the operation was done with the patient under conscious sedation …
> ❯ In a bit more detail, you can notice that …
> ❯ This fact can be explained taking into account that …

> Long-term follow-up was poor since the patients often did not live in the area.
> Although double phospho-soda was well tolerated by most patients ...
> In short, you may need larger balloons in elderly patients.
> What I'm saying is that endometriosis is related to ectopic growth of endometrial tissue ...
> We did not operate on the patient because her family refused an aggressive intervention.
> We performed an unenhanced CT scan because the patient suffered from renal insufficiency.
> The statistical analysis was underpowered because the number of patients was too small.

Rispondere a più domande

> There are two different questions here.
> It seems there are three questions here.
> It is my understanding that there are two questions to be addressed here.
> With regard to your second question,...
> Regarding your second question,...
> As far as your first question is concerned,...
> In answer to your first question, I should say that...
> I'll begin with your second question.
> Let me address your last question first.
> I'll address your last question first and then the rest of them.
> Would you please repeat your second question?
> I didn't understand your first question. Would you repeat it?

Essere in disaccordo

> With all due respect, I believe that there is no evidence of...
> To the best of our knowledge no article has been published on this topic.

> With all respect, I think that your point overlooks the main aspect of...
> Yours is an interesting point of view, but I'm not sure of its...
> I see it from a different point of view.
> With all respect, I don't go along with you on...
> I think that the importance of... cannot be denied.
> I strongly disagree with your comment on...
> I disagree with your point.
> I don't see a valid argument for supporting such a comment.

Sottolineare un punto

> I do believe that...
> I strongly agree with Dr. Ho's comment on...
> It is of paramount importance...
> It is a crucial fact that...
> And this fact cannot be overlooked.
> I'd like to stress the importance of...
> Don't underestimate the role of...
> The use of antibiotic prophylaxis in this case is of the utmost importance.
> With regard to..., you must always bear in mind that...
> It is well known that...

Incomprensioni

> I am not sure I understood your question...
> Sorry, I don't quite follow you.
> Would you repeat the question, please?
> Would you repeat the second part of your question, please?
> I'm afraid I still don't understand.
> Could you be a bit more specific with regard to...?
> What do you mean by...?
> Could you repeat your question? I couldn't hear you.

> Could you formulate your question in a different way?
> I'm not sure I understand your final question.

Far passare il tempo

> I am not sure I understood your question. Would you repeat it?
> I don't understand your questions. Would you formulate it in a different way?
> That's a very interesting question...
> I wonder if you could be a bit more specific about...
> I'm glad you asked that question.
> Your question is of the utmost importance, but I'm afraid it is beyond the scope of our paper...
> What aspect of the problem are you referring to by saying...

Evitare un argomento

> I'm afraid I'm not really in a position to be able to address your question yet.
> We'll come back to that in a minute, if you don't mind.
> I don't think we have enough time to discuss your comments in depth.
> It would take extremely long time to answer that.
> I will address your question in my second talk, if you don't mind.
> At my institution, we do not have experience on...
> At our department, we do not perform...
> Perhaps we could return to that at the end of the session.
> We'll probably address your question in further papers on the subject.
> I have no experience of...

Problemi tecnici

> May I have another laser pointer?
> Does anyone in the audience have a pointer?
> Video images are not running properly. In the meantime I'd like to comment on...
> My microphone is not working properly. May I have it fixed?
> My microphone is not working properly. May I use yours?
> Can you hear me?
> Can the rows at the back hear me?
> Can you guys at the back see the screen?
> Can we turn off the lights, please?

Capitolo 7

Moderare una sessione chirurgica

Introduzione

La possibilità di moderare sessioni di congressi internazionali, generalmente, si presenta una volta acquisito un adeguato livello di competenze nel corso della propria carriera accademica. Il raggiungimento di tale traguardo prevede inevitabilmente la sottomissione di numerosi articoli e che siano già state sostenute molte presentazioni; è, pertanto, plausibile che il livello di inglese scientifico posseduto dal lettore sia superiore a quello del destinatario "tipo" di questo manuale.

Perché, dunque, includiamo un capitolo su come moderare una sessione? Al contrario di quanto si possa pensare, anche i moderatori più esperti possono trovarsi di fronte a situazioni difficili o addirittura imbarazzanti da dover gestire.

Agli occhi di chi non ha mai moderato una sessione, infatti, il moderatore potrebbe apparire come la sola persona libera dall'onere di preparare una presentazione ed il cui ruolo sarebbe limitato unicamente all'impiego di frasi semplici come: "thank you Dr. Smith, for your interesting presentation" oppure "the next speaker will be Dr. Spurek who comes from . . .".

Fare il moderatore, invece, vuol dire molto di più. Innanzitutto il moderatore non deve preparare una singola presentazione, ma deve studiare attentamente tutto il materiale di recente pubblicazione sull'argomento in discussione. In più, il moderatore deve rivedere tutti gli abstract ed è tenuto a preparare interventi e domande per sopperire alla platea, qualora quest'ultima non ne avesse.

Abbiamo diviso questo capitolo in quattro paragrafi principali:
1. Tipici commenti da moderatore
2. Il moderatore dovrebbe fare domande?
3. Cosa dovrebbe dire il moderatore quando qualcosa va storto?
4. Commenti specifici di un moderatore chirurgo.

R. Ribes, P. J. Aranda, J. Giba, *Inglese per chirurghi*,
© Springer-Verlag Italia 2012

Tipici commenti da moderatore

Tutti coloro che hanno partecipato a un congresso internazionale conoscono le tipiche frasi che i moderatori usano per introdurre la sessione.
Alcune espressioni chiave sono indispensabili per garantire fluidità alla
moderazione. La buona notizia è che se si conoscono tali espressioni e,
soprattutto, se le si utilizza in modo appropriato, moderare una sessione
diventa realmente semplice. La cattiva notizia è che se, in caso contrario,
non si dovessero conoscere tali espressioni, un compito tecnicamente
semplice potrebbe trasformarsi in una situazione imbarazzante. C'è sempre una prima volta per tutto, e se questa è la prima volta che siete invitati a moderare una sessione, ripassate alcune di queste frasi e vi troverete-
te a vostro agio. Accettate un consiglio da amico: riuscirete ad apparire
spontanei solo se avrete provato e riprovato, con lungo anticipo, la vostra
"spontaneità".

Introdurre la sessione

Vi suggeriamo questi utili commenti per introdurre la sessione:

> Good morning ladies and gentlemen. My name is Dr. Vida and I
> want to welcome you all to this workshop on laparoscopic knee sur-
> gery. My co-chair is Dr. Vick, who comes from King's College.
> Good afternoon. The session on minimally invasive heart surgery is
> about to start. Please take a seat and disconnect your cellular
> phones and any other electrical devices that could interfere with the
> oral presentations. We will listen to ten 6-min lectures with a 2-min
> period for questions and comments after each one. Afterwards, pro-
> vided we are still on time, we will have a final round of questions
> and comments from the audience, speakers, and panelists.
> Good morning. We will proceed with the session on mitral valve
> replacement. As many papers have to be delivered, I encourage the
> speakers to keep an eye on the time.

Presentare gli oratori

Vi suggeriamo le seguenti frasi:

> Our first speaker is Dr. Muñoz from Xanit International Hospital in Málaga, Spain, who will present the paper: "Stent grafting of abdominal aneurysms."

I seguenti oratori sono introdotti quasi nella stessa maniera attraverso frasi quali:

> Our next lecturer is Dr. Adams. Dr. Adams comes from Brigham and Women's Hospital, Harvard Medical School, and his presentation is entitled "Nonoperative treatment of intraosseous ganglion."
> Next is Dr. Shaw from Beth Israel Deaconess Hospital, presenting "Stem cells in hepatic surgery."
> Dr. Olsen from UCSF is the next and last speaker. His presentation is: "Metastatic disease. Pathways to the heart."

Una volta che gli oratori hanno concluso la propria presentazione, si suppone che il moderatore dica qualcosa del tipo:

> Thank you, Dr. Vida, for your excellent presentation. Any questions or comments?

Il moderatore di solito commenta la presentazione, anche se a volte non lo fa:

> Thank you, Dr. Vida, for your presentation. Any questions or comments from the audience?

Vi sono alcune formule e aggettivi comuni (*nice, elegant, outstanding, excellent, interesting, clear, accurate*) spesso utilizzati per descrivere le presentazioni. Alcuni esempi nei seguenti commenti:

> Thanks, Dr. Shaw, for your accurate presentation. Does the audience have any comments?
> Thank you very much for your clear presentation on this always-controversial topic. I would like to ask a question. May I? (Although being the chairperson you are the one who gives permission, to ask the speaker is a usual formality.)

> I'd like to thank you for this excellent talk Dr. Olsen. Any questions?
> Thanks a lot for your talk, Dr. Barba. I wonder if the audience has any questions.

Aggiornare

Vi suggeriamo questi utili commenti per aggiornare la sessione:

> I think we all are a bit tired, so we'll have a short break.
> The session is adjourned until 4 p.m.
> We'll take a short break.
> We'll take a 30-minute break. Please fill out the evaluation forms.
> The session is adjourned until tomorrow morning. Enjoy your stay in Paris.

Concludere la sessione

Vi suggeriamo questi utili commenti per chiudere la sessione:

> I'd like to thank all the speakers and the audience for your interesting presentations and comments. (I'll) see you all at the congress dinner and awards ceremony.
> The session is over. I want to thank all the participants for their contribution. (I'll) see you tomorrow morning. Remember to take your attendance certificates if you have not taken them already.
> We should finish up over here. We'll resume at 10.50.

Il moderatore dovrebbe fare domande?

Secondo noi, il moderatore dovrebbe fare domande soprattutto all'inizio della sessione, quando il pubblico generalmente non fa commenti. Promuovere il dibattito è uno dei doveri del moderatore e, se nessuno tra il pubblico si sente di fare domande, il moderatore deve invitare il pubblico a partecipare:

> Are there any questions?

Nessuno alza la mano:

> Well, I have two questions for Dr. Adams. Do you think surgery alone
  is the mainstay of prostate cancer treatment or do you see a role for
  hybrid interventions with radiotherapy? And second: What, in your
  opinion, should the role of chemotherapy be in this surgical algo-
  rithm?

Una volta acceso il dibattito, il moderatore utilizzerà domande e/o commenti solo per gestire adeguatamente la tempistica e se, come spesso
accade, la sessione è in ritardo, il moderatore non è tenuto a partecipare
a meno che non sia strettamente indispensabile.
Il moderatore, inoltre, non deve dimostrare al pubblico la propria conoscenza sugli argomenti trattati, facendo troppe domande o commenti. La
sua competenza è indubbia, altrimenti non sarebbe stato messo lì.

Cosa dovrebbe dire il moderatore quando qualcosa non va bene?

In ritardo

Molti relatori, pur sapendo in anticipo di avere a disposizione una determinata quantità di tempo per la loro presentazione, spesso cercano di parlare un po' più a lungo, rubando parte del tempo destinato alle domande
e ai commenti e/o invadendo lo spazio dedicato ai relatori successivi. Un
bravo moderatore dovrebbe essere capace di fermare questa tendenza alla
prima occasione con sollecitazioni del tipo:

> Dr. Cutty, your time is almost over. You have 30 seconds to finish your
  presentation.
> Dr. Shang, you are running out of time.

Se il relatore non finisce la sua presentazione in tempo, il moderatore può
dire:

> Dr. Cutty, I'm sorry but your time is over. We must proceed to the next
  presentation. Any questions, comments?

Dopo aver presentato il prossimo relatore, frasi come queste vi aiuteranno a gestire la sessione:

> Dr. Treasure, please keep an eye on the time, we are behind schedule.
> We are running behind the schedule, so I remind all speakers you have 6 minutes to deliver your presentation.

In anticipo

Anche se raramente, può accadere che la sessione termini in anticipo. Il tempo a disposizione potrà essere utilizzato per porre domande ai relatori circa le proprie esperienze lavorative nei rispettivi centri:

> As we are a little bit ahead of schedule, I encourage the panelists and the audience to ask questions and offer comments.
> I have a question for the panelists: What percentage of the total number of aortic operation is performed on children at your institution?

Problemi tecnici

Computer che non funziona

Vi suggeriamo questi commenti:

> I am afraid there is a technical problem with the computer. In the meantime I would like to make a comment about . . .
> The computer is not working properly. While it is being fixed, I encourage the panelists to offer their always-interesting comments.

Mancanza di corrente

Vi suggeriamo questi commenti:

> The lights have gone out. We'll take a (hopefully) short break until they are repaired.

> As you see, or indeed do not see at all, the lights have gone out. The hotel staff has told us it is going to be a matter of minutes, so do not go too far; we'll resume as soon as possible.

Mancanza di audio

Vi suggeriamo questi commenti:

> Dr. Kannel, we cannot hear you. There must be a problem with your microphone.
> Perhaps you could try this microphone.
> Please would you use the microphone? The rows at the back cannot hear you.

Il relatore è insicuro

Se l'oratore dovesse usare un tono di voce troppo basso:

> Dr. Smith, would you please speak up? The audience cannot hear you.
> Dr. Alvarez, would you please speak up a bit? The people at the back cannot hear you.

Se l'oratore fosse agitato al punto di non riuscire a proseguire la sua presentazione:

> Dr. Olsen, take your time. We can proceed to the next presentation, so whenever you feel OK and ready to deliver yours, it will be a pleasure to listen to it.

Commenti specifici di un moderatore chirurgico

Poiché il moderatore deve riempire i buchi che si possono verificare durante la sessione, in caso di problemi tecnici sarà suo compito dire qualcosa per "intrattenere" il pubblico. Ciò non creerebbe alcun disagio a un madrelingua inglese, ma potrebbe rivelarsi problematico per un moderatore non inglese. In queste situazioni, c'è sempre un argomento interessante di cui parlare "nel frattempo", in particolare lo stato attuale del tema della sessione nei paesi dei relatori:

> Regarding training in laparoscopic surgery, how are things going in Italy, Dr. Toldo?
> As for as the use of ventricular assist devices, what's the deal in Japan, Dr. Hashimoto?
> How is the current situation in Germany regarding repayment policies?
> May I ask how many cerebellar tumor resections you are performing yearly at your respective institutions?
> What's going on in the States, Dr. Olsen?

Avviando una discussione sulla situazione nei diversi paesi, un moderatore con non troppa dimestichezza riesce a condividere con i relatori il peso di riempire i buchi. Questo trucco fallisce raramente e, una volta che il problema tecnico è risolto, la sessione può continuare normalmente senza aver destato nel pubblico alcun sospetto sulle competenze linguistiche del moderatore.

Oltre le più comuni espressioni che i moderatori di qualsiasi specialità devono conoscere, ci sono alcuni commenti tipici che un moderatore chirurgo non può ignorare. Questi commenti variano in base alla sottospecialità del moderatore e sono, di solito, facili da comprendere anche per relatori non madrelingua. Ad esempio, vediamo i seguenti:

> Dr. Petit, would you please use the pointer so the audience can know what lesion you are talking about?
> Dr. Wilson, would you please point out the number of patients excluded from the study?
> Dr. Negroponte, did you perform an emergency thoracotomy on the patient with active bleeding or did you carry out an elective operation?
> Dr. Maier, did you resect the tumor on an emergent basis?
> Have you had any anaphylactic reactions to this type of contrast material?
> Dr. Olsen, you presented a case of ruptured ovarian cyst, did you rule out a heterotopic pregnancy?

> Do you use 12F catheters for this purpose or do you actually dissect the artery?

> Dr. Pons, I'm afraid that the video is not running properly. Unfortunately, I must ask you to move on with your lecture for time's sake.

> Dr. Hashimoto, why didn't you use a 0.0035 stiff guidewire to cross the stenosis?

> Dr. Soares, are you currently using the harmonic scalpel in cases like this one?

> Dr. Mas, would you recommend this operation as the first-line option for this particular disease?

> Do you do encourage young surgeons to start doing this operation straight away or do you think that it should be reserved for experienced surgeons only?

> Do you perform preprocedural pelvic MRI on all patients undergoing pelvic tumor resections?

Capitolo 8

Errori frequenti nell'inglese parlato e scritto dei chirurghi

Introduzione

In questa sezione, saranno messi in luce alcuni dei più grandi ostacoli nell'ambito dell'inglese chirurgico. Vi sono molte difficoltà che possono emergere quando vi viene chiesto di presentare una lettura in inglese. Questo capitolo, pertanto, ha lo scopo di trasmettere al lettore parte dell'esperienza che abbiamo acquisito nel mondo dell'inglese in chirurgia.

Quando si prepara e si tiene una presentazione in inglese durante un congresso internazionale di chirurgia, si devono considerare una serie di problemi di base, che sono stati raggruppati in quattro differenti aree di rischio:

1. Nomi ingannatori e *false friend*;
2. Errori grammaticali frequenti;
3. Errori comuni di ortografia;
4. Errori di pronuncia frequenti.

Nomi ingannatori e *false friend*

Ogni lingua ha i suoi *false friend*. Un elenco completo dei *false friend* va oltre lo scopo di questo manuale, quindi sarà utile ricercare quei nomi inglesi difficili che hanno pronunce simili nella vostra lingua, ma con un significato completamente diverso.

Così, d' ora in poi, individuate i *false friend* nella vostra lingua e fate una lista a cominciare da quelli appartenenti alla vostra specialità.

La medicina in generale, l'anatomia e la radiologia in particolare, sono piene di nomi ingannatori. Pensate per un attimo al termine *vena*

R. Ribes, P. J. Aranda, J. Giba, *Inglese per chirurghi*,
© Springer-Verlag Italia 2012

femorale superficiale. È difficile spiegare come un trombo nella vena femorale superficiale sia in realtà nel sistema venoso profondo.

Molti chirurghi e oncologi di tutto il mondo parlano di *linfadenopatie di piccole dimensioni*. Tenendo conto che quello dimensionale è l'unico criterio per la diagnosi dei linfonodi anormali e che linfadenopatia significa, da un punto di vista etimologico, linfonodi anormali, una *linfadenopatia "normale"* (di piccole dimensioni) è tanto assurda quanto una *psicopatia normale*. Il termine linfadenomegalia sarebbe probabilmente più accurato.

Etimologicamente, *pancreas* significa *all meat* (carne), ma non c'è tessuto muscolare all'interno di questa ghiandola eso-endocrina.

Perché chiamiamo la parte più interna del gomito, mediale e leggermente prossimale alla troclea, *epicondilo mediale* e non *epitroclea*?

Etimologicamente, *azygos* significa "dispari", il che mette *hemiazygos* in una strana posizione, in quanto i numeri dispari non sono divisibili per due.

Il termine vena anonima è tanto assurdo quanto la denominazione di un bambino "innominato".

Errori grammaticali frequenti

Questi sono alcuni degli errori fatti più frequentemente dai chirurghi quando parlano inglese:

1. The patient was operated with local anesthesia.
Probabilmente è più corretto dire:
> The operation was performed under local anesthesia.
Oppure,
> We operated on the patient using local anesthesia.

2. The intact posterior cruciate ligament was isointense and presented no signs of disruption.
L'isointensità rappresenta sempre una grandezza relativa, di conseguenza la frase corretta sarebbe:
> The intact posterior cruciate ligament was isointense to cortical bone and showed no signs of disruption.

3. The cyst was 6 cm wide on the operative field.
Anche se potreste imbattervi in questa espressione, è più corretto dire:

❯ The cyst was 6 cm wide in the operative field.

4. The hospital purchased a MRI unit.
Anche se *a magnetic resonance imaging unit* … è corretto, quando usate
un acronimo non dimenticate che "m" si legge "em" che inizia con una
vocale, di conseguenza l'articolo da usare è "an" invece di "a". In
questo caso dovete scrivere:
❯ The hospital purchased an MRI unit.

5. The chairman of surgery came from an university hospital.
Anche se "university" inizia con una vocale e si può pensare che l'articolo che la deve precedere sia "an" come in "an airport"; la "u" si pronuncia come "you", che inizia con una consonante, così l'articolo che
deve essere utilizzato è "a" invece di "an". In questo caso si dovrebbe
scrivere:
❯ The chairman of surgery came from a university hospital.

6. A 22-years-old man presenting . . .
Molto spesso la prima frase della prima diapositiva di una presentazione
contiene il primo errore. Per gli oratori di livello intermedio, questo semplice errore è così evidente da non riuscire a credere che sia uno degli
errori commessi più frequentemente. È ovvio che l'aggettivo *22-year-old*
non può essere scritto al plurale e dovrebbe essere scritto:
❯ A 22-year-old man presenting . . .

7. There was not biopsy of the lesion.
Questo è un errore frequente e relativamente sottile, commesso da oratori
di livello   medio-alto. Se continuate a preferire l'uso della forma negati-
va, dovreste dire:
❯ There was not any biopsy of the lesion.
Ma la forma affermativa è:
❯ There was no biopsy of the lesion.

8. It allows to distinguish between . . .
Dovreste utilizzare una delle seguenti frasi:
❯ It allows us to distinguish between . . .
Oppure:
❯ It allows the distinction between . . .

9. Haemorrhagic tumors can cause….
Controllate il vostro articolo o presentazione alla ricerca di eventuali dis-
cordanze nell'uso dell'inglese americano o britannico.

Questo esempio mostra l'utilizzo di un'ortografia americana (*tumors*) dopo un termine inglese (*haemorrhagic*). Dovreste scegliere tra l'ortografia americana e quella inglese in base al giornale o al congresso al quale state inviando il vostro articolo.

La frase da dire dovrebbe essere:

> Haemorrhagic tumours can cause....

Oppure:

> Hemorrhagic tumors can cause....

10. Please, would you tell me where is the operating theater?

Le domande inserite all'interno di una frase sono sempre problematiche. Ogni volta che una domanda è inserita in un'altra frase interrogativa, l'ordine delle parole ne risulta modificato. Questo succede quando, cercando di essere gentili, cambiamo erroneamente *What time is it?* con *Would you please tell me what time is it?* invece di *Would you please tell me what time it is?*

> La domanda diretta *Where is the operating theater?* deve essere trasformata come segue:

> Please would you tell me where the operating theater is?

11. Most of the times hemangiomas. . .

Potete dire *many times*, ma non *most of the times*. *Most of the time* è corretto e potete usare *commonly* o *frequently* come termini equivalenti.

Dite invece:

> Most of the time hemangiomas . . .

12. I look forward to hear from you . . .

Questo è un errore molto frequente alla fine di lettere formali come quelle inviate agli editori. Si basa su un errore di grammatica: *to* può essere sia parte di un infinito che una preposizione. In questo caso, non è parte dell'infinito del verbo *hear*, ma parte del verbo con preposizione *look forward to*; è dunque una preposizione.

Questo errore può avere conseguenze irreparabili. Se state cercando di farvi pubblicare un articolo su una prestigiosa rivista, non potete commettere errori formali che potrebbero precludere la lettura del vostro altrimenti interessante articolo.

Così, invece di *look forward to hear from you*, dovreste scrivere:

> I look forward to hearing from you.

13. Best Regards.

Anche se è utilizzato in ambito di corrispondenza accademica e informale, *best regards* è un misto di due forme inglesi forti: *kind regards* e *best wishes*. A nostro parere, invece di *best regards*, che è colloquialmente accettabile, dovreste scrivere:

> *Kind regards.*

o semplicemente:

> *Regards.*

14.Are you suffering from paresthesias?
Molti medici dimenticano che i pazienti non sono colleghi (con alcune eccezioni) e utilizzano la terminologia medica che può non essere da loro compresa. Questa domanda tecnica sarebbe facilmente comprensibile nella forma:

> Do you have pins and needles?

15. A single metastases was seen in the liver.
Single e *metastases* sono termini incompatibili perché *metastases* è plurale.
Quindi la frase corretta è:

> A single metastasis was seen in the liver.

16. Multiple metastasis were seen in the brain.
Multiple e *metastasis* sono termini incompatibili perchè *metastasis* è singolare. Ogni volta che usate un termine Latino, controllate la sua forma singolare e plurale. In questo caso dovrete scrivere:

> Multiple metastases were seen in the brain.

17. An European expert on cardiac surgery chaired the session.
Sebbene *European* inizi con una vocale e si possa pensare che l'articolo che lo deve precedere è "an" come in "an airport", la frase corretta, in questo caso, sarebbe:

> A European expert on cardiac surgery chaired the session.

18. The meeting began a hour ago.
Anche se *hour* inizia con una consonante e potreste pensare che l'articolo che deve precedere sia "a" come in "a hamstring", la frase corretta, in questo caso, sarebbe:

> The meeting began an hour ago.

Le parole che iniziano con una "h" silente sono precedute da "an", come se iniziassero con una vocale.

19. The cardiac surgeon who asked for the CMR was operating a stenotic aortic valve.

Questa frase non è corretta in quanto il verbo "to operate", quando viene
utilizzato dal punto di vista chirurgico (sia per quanto riguarda i pazienti che le parti anatomiche), è sempre seguito dalla preposizione "on". La
frase corretta sarebbe stata:

> The cardiac surgeon who asked for the CMR was operating on a
  stenotic aortic valve.

20. Medial and collateral ligaments are well defined on the coronal plane.

Usiamo "in" quando parliamo di piani (coronale, assiale, sagittale...)
poiché i reperti radiologici sono contenuti all'interno delle immagini.
Quindi dovremo dire:

> Medial and collateral ligaments are well defined in the coronal plane.

21. The hospital personal are very kind.

Quando si parla di un gruppo di persone che lavorano in un istituto, la
parola corretta è "personnel", non "personal":

> The hospital personnel are very kind.

22. Page to the surgeon.

Il verbo "to page," che potrebbe essere connesso al sostantivo "page"
(paggio, un ragazzo che è addetto a sbrigare commissioni), non è un
verbo con preposizione e non richiede la preposizione "to" dopo di esso.
Quando si desidera che il chirurgo sia chiamato al cicalino, si deve dire:

> Page the surgeon.

Errori comuni di ortografia

Create il vostro elenco di parole che potreste scrivere in modo errato e
non esitate a crearvi formule mnemoniche se ciò vi può essere di aiuto.
Ecco una lista di parole spesso non scritte correttamente (con l'errore più
frequente riportato fra parentesi):

> Sagittal (misspelled: saggital)

In una parola con consonanti doppie e singole, evitate di raddoppiare la
consonante singola e viceversa. *Sagittal* è una delle parole più frequentemente sbagliate nelle diapositive che mostrano immagini (MR, CT, ed

eco) ed è tra le parole più utilizzate in radiolgia. L'etimologia di questa parola – *sagitta* – significa "freccia".

> Parallel (misspelled: parallell)

Per questo errore comune, uso una formula mnemonica abbastanza assurda (come la maggior parte delle formule mnemoniche) per ricordarmi l'ortografia: "due gambe (ll) corrono più veloci e vengono prima di una sola (l)."

> She works in the neurorradiology division

Questo è un errore frequente dei medici spagnoli e latino-americani. In inglese, neuroradiology è scritto con una "r":
She works in the neuroradiology division.

> Dura mater (misspelled: dura matter)

Etimologicamente, "mater" significa "mother" e si scrive con una sola "t." "Dura matter" è un errore frequente dovuto alla confusione tra "dura mater" e "gray/white matter." "Matter" significa sostanza e non ha niente a che fare con "mater."

> Arrhythmia (misspelled: arrythmia)

Controllate due volte l'ortografia di *arrhythmia* e accertatevi che la parola "rhythm", da cui deriva, sia incorporato in essa.

Rivedete anche le seguenti coppie di parole (con l'ortografia errata tra parentesi) e soprattutto, come già detto, createvi il vostro elenco di parole "difficili".

> Professor (misspelled: proffesor)
> Professional (misspelled: proffesional)
> Occasion (misspelled: ocassion)
> Dissection (misspelled: disection)
> Resection (misspelled: ressection)
> Gray-white matter (misspelled: gray-white mater)
> Subtraction (misspelled: substraction)
> Acquisition (misspelled: adquisition).

Errori di pronuncia frequenti

Per semplicità, ci siamo presi la libertà di utilizzare una rappresentazione approssimativa della pronuncia, invece di utilizzare i segni fonetici. Ci scusiamo con i nostri colleghi linguisti che potrebbero avere preferito una trascrizione più ortodossa.

La pronuncia è uno degli incubi più temuti in inglese. Anche se ci sono delle regole di pronuncia, esistono così tante eccezioni che è necessario conoscere la pronuncia delle parole a orecchio. Pertanto, in primo luogo, leggete ad alta voce il più possibile, perché è l'unico modo per accorgervi delle parole di cui non conoscete la pronuncia e, in secondo luogo, quando seguite un corso, oltre a concentrarvi sul contenuto della presentazione, prestate attenzione al modo in cui i chirurghi madrelingua pronunciano le parole che non conoscete.

Alcuni consigli sulla pronuncia:

- Non abbiate paura di apparire diversi o strani. I suoni inglesi sono diversi e strani. A volte un chirurgo non di madrelingua può sapere come pronunciare una parola corretta, ma prova un po' di vergogna nel farlo, soprattutto in presenza di colleghi della stessa nazionalità. Non vergognatevi di pronunciare correttamente, indipendentemente dalla nazionalità del vostro interlocutore.

- Apprezzate lo sforzo di utilizzare un diverso gruppo di muscoli della bocca. In principio, i "muscoli inglesi" possono affaticarsi, ma perseverate, è solo un segno di duro lavoro.

- Non vi preoccupate di avere un accento particolare o addirittura imbarazzante all'inizio; non importa, purché siate capiti. L'idea è quella di comunicare, di dire cosa pensate o sentite e non di esibirvi in logopedia.

- Cercate di pronunciare correttamente le parole inglesi. Col passare del tempo, quando vi sentirete relativamente più sicuri del vostro inglese, vi incoraggiamo a studiare progressivamente la fonetica inglese. Se continuerete a usare la pronuncia da principianti, il vostro inglese suonerà come l'italiano parlato con l'inconfondibile accento degli americani o degli inglesi.

- Esercitatevi con frasi standard sia di inglese chirurgico che di conversazione. Dire cose come *"Do you know what I mean?"* or *"Would you do me a favor?"* e *"Who's on call today?"* o *"Please would you window (and level) this image?"* vi fornirà degli strumenti estremamente utili per sentirvi più sicuri.

Avere un vostro *lieve* accento nazionale in lingua inglese non è un problema grave, a patto che la presentazione trasmetta il messaggio corretto. Tuttavia, per quanto riguarda la pronuncia, ci sono molte parole difficili che non possono essere propriamente definite *false friend* e richiedono un po' più di attenzione.

In inglese ci sono parole che si scrivono in modo diverso, ma vengono pronunciate in modo molto simile. Vediamo questo esempio:

- *Ileum*: la porzione distale dell'intestino tenue, estesa dal digiuno al cieco.
- *Ilium*: la parte più alta e ampia delle tre componenti dell'anca.

Immaginate quanto sarebbe surreale per i nostri chirurghi confondere l'intestino con l'osso dell'anca. Potreste anche dire che potrebbe andare peggio: in fondo, le due strutture anatomiche sono più o meno nella stessa area!

Vediamo ora questo esempio.
La parola inglese *tear* ha due significati differenti in base a come la pronunciamo:

- Se pronunciamo *tear* come [tiar], intendiamo la secrezione acquosa delle ghiandole lacrimali, che serve a inumidire la congiuntiva.
- Se lo pronunciamo [tear], ci riferiamo all'atto del ferire o danneggiare, soprattutto allo strappare, come in "there is a longitudinal *tear* in the posterior horn of the internal meniscus".

Tra i termini medici più frequentemente pronunciati male ce ne sono due che meritano un'attenta analisi poiché i medici li usano (o abusano) quasi ogni giorno della loro vita professionale. Queste due parole sono "*radiology*" e "*image*".

Molti radiologi di tutto il mondo dicono di essere dei [ra-diò-locist], "I am a radiologist," invece di [rei-diò-locist] . Una difficoltà simile si presenta con parole che hanno a che fare con la radiologia, come radiology, radiograph, radiologic...Per favore, d'ora in avanti evitate questo errore incredibilmente frequente.

Image e *images* sono due dei termini medici più comunemente pronunciati male. Riuscite a immaginare quante volte direte *image* e *images* nella vostra vita medica? Per favore non dite [im-èich] o [im-èiches], ma [im-ich] e [im-iches]. Se fate parte del nutrito gruppo di medici che diceva [im-èich] a ogni singola diapositiva di ogni presentazione, allora non dite niente a nessuno e "continuate" a dire [im-ich] "come avete sempre fatto". Non vi preoccupate! Probabilmente non c'è alcuna registrazione delle vostre presentazioni e, se ci fosse, non sarebbe facilmente reperibile.

Il motivo per cui evidenziamo questi due errori più comuni è quello di sottolineare che bisogna evitare gli errori di pronuncia, a partire dalle parole più usuali nella vostra pratica clinica quotidiana. Se non siete un chirurgo toracico e non sapete come si pronuncia, per esempio, "lymphangioleiomyomatosis", non preoccupatevi di questa parola fino a quando non padroneggerete la pronuncia dei vostri usuali termini chirurgici.

Il nostro consiglio è quello di crearvi un elenco delle 100 parole di uso quotidiano più difficili in termini di ortografia. Una volta presa confidenza con esse, allungate l'elenco continuando a leggere ad alta voce quanti più articoli potete. Se siete un chirurgo traumatologico, i depliant e i foglietti illustrativi vi possono tenere aggiornati senza alcuno sforzo e vi aiuteranno a colmare quegli inutili tempi morti tra un paziente e l'altro.

Abbiamo creato una lista composta da alcuni termini chirurgici pronunciati erroneamente. Dal momento che questa lista è arbitraria e potrebbe variare a seconda della lingua madre, vi incoraggiamo a creare la vostra lista.

> *Parenchyma*

Parenchima è, in linea di principio, una parola facile da pronunciare [pa-ren-ki-ma].. L'abbiamo inclusa in questa lista perché abbiamo notato che alcuni relatori, in particolare italiani, tendono a pronunciare [pa-ren-kai-ma].

> La lettera *"h"*

"Non-pronunciata": gli oratori italiani e francesi tendono a ignorare questa lettera, quindi, quando si pronuncia la parola "enhancement", dicono [en-áns-ment] invece di [en-hans-ment]. È' vero che la "h" può essere silente, ma non sempre.

"Troppo-pronunciata": medici spagnoli tendono a pronunciare la lettera "h" quando dovrebbe essere silente.

> *Data*

Anche se alcuni medici americani dicono [data], la pronuncia corretta di questa parola è [dei-ta].

> *Disease/decease*

La pronuncia di *disease* può essere strana, dal momento che, a seconda di come si pronuncia la "s", si può dire *"decease"* che è quello in cui esita un *disease* terminale. La pronuncia corretta di *disease* è [di-ss'ss] con la

"s" liquida; se dite [di-sìs] con una "s" normale, come fanno molti oratori di lingua spagnola e latino-americani, ogni volta che parlerete, per
esempio, dell'*Alzheimer's disease*, parlerete di *Alzheimer's decease* o
morte da Alzheimer.

> *Chamber*

La pronuncia di *chamber* è un po' complicata, in quanto gli oratori francesi tendono a "francesizzarlo", dicendo [cham-bre], mentre alcuni italiani dicono semplicemente [cham-ber] invece di [cheim-ber].

> Parole francesi come *"technique"*

In inglese potete dire [tek-nik], "alla francese", anche se dite *technical*
[tek-ni-cal].

> *Hippocampus*

Il responsabile di questo errore è la mancanza della conoscenza etimolo-
gica di questo termine. Molti medici nel mondo dicono [haippo-campus],
come se stessero parlando dell' hypotalamus [aipo-talamos].
Sfortunatamente, il termine hippocampus non ha nessuna relazione eti-
mologica con i termini hypotalamus o hypotension. Hyppo- significa
cavallo e hippocampus si pronuncia [hippo-campos]

> *Director*

Anche se si può dire sia [di-rect] che [dai-rect], solo [dai-rec-tor] è corretto; non si può dire [di-rec-tor].

> *Anesthesist*

Come chirurghi, userete questo termine quasi ogni giorno della vostra
vita e se non avete familiarità con la sua pronuncia, lo pronuncerete in
maniera errata. Si tratta di una delle parole più difficili da comprendere:
gli oratori di lingua neolatina diranno automaticamente [an_stezist(_)].
La pronuncia corretta è [æ'ni:s_ _ tist/an-aes-thet-ist].

Analizzare tutte le parole potenzialmente difficili in termini di pronuncia
va ben oltre lo scopo di questo manuale; tuttavia, qui di seguito vi offria-
mo un breve elenco di tali parole e vi incoraggiamo ancora una volta a
creare la vostra lista "personale".

> Medulla (Me-dú-la)
> Gynecology (gai-ne-có-lo-gy)
> Edema (i-dima)
> Case report (kéis ri-port, NOT kéis ré-port)

> Multidetector (multi-, NOT mul-tai)
> Oblique (o-blik, NOT o-bláik)
> Femoral (f'-mo-ral)
> Jugular (ju-gu-lar)
> Triquetrum (trai-ki-tram)

Capitolo 9

Terminologia latina e greca

La terminologia latina e greca rappresenta un altro possibile ostacolo da superare per poter diventare padroni dell'inglese medico. I relatori di origine neo-latina (italiani, spagnoli, francesi,...) sono senza dubbio agevolati, sebbene questo vantaggio sia diventato un limite nella pronuncia e, in particolare, nell'uso delle forme plurali delle parole latine e greche.

La maggior parte delle parole latine impiegate nell'inglese medico mantiene la terminazione plurale latina – per esempio, *metastasis,* plurale *metastases*; *viscus,* plurale *viscera* – è, quindi, essenziale conoscere le basi delle regole di utilizzo del plurale in latino.

Tutti i sostantivi e gli aggettivi latini hanno una differente desinenza per ogni genere (maschile, femminile e neutro), numero (singolare/plurale) e caso – il caso è una speciale desinenza della parola che rivela la funzione della parola nella frase. Pertanto, gli aggettivi latini si devono coniugare con il sostantivo in base al caso, numero e genere. Sebbene possiamo appena ricordarcelo dai giorni della scuola superiore, ci sono cinque differenti flessioni di nomi o aggettivi, ciascuna chiamata declinazione.

Il nominativo indica il soggetto della frase, mentre il genitivo denota una specificazione o il possesso. Eliminando la desinenza dal genitivo singolare, si ha la radice a cui si aggiunge la desinenza del nominativo plurale, per formare il plurale dell'inglese medico.
Per esempio:
- *Corpus* (nominativo singolare), *corporis* (genitivo singolare), *corpora* (nominativo plurale). Questo è un sostantivo della terza declinazione neutro, che significa "corpo". Le corrispondenti forme per l'aggettivo

R. Ribes, P. J. Aranda, J. Giba, *Inglese per chirurghi,*
© Springer-Verlag Italia 2012

sono *callosus, callosum* e *callosa,* rispettivamente. Per cui *corpus callosum* (nominativo, singulare, neutro), *corpora callosa* (nominativo, plurale, neutro).

Un altro esempio:
- *Coxa vara* (femminile singolare), *coxae varae* (femminile plurale), ma *genu varum* (neutro, singolare), *genua vara* (neutro, plurale).

In questo capitolo riportiamo un esteso glossario latino/inglese che include il nominativo singolare e plurale, il genitivo singolare e anche la declinazione e il genere di ciascuna parola. In alcuni casi, sono state aggiunte delle parole addizionali, come la desinenza plurale inglese, se largamente accettate (per esempio, *fetus*, latino plurale *feti*; inglese plurale *fetuses*) e terminazioni di origine greca, mantenute in alcune parole latine (per esempio, *thorax,* pl. *thoraces,* gen. *thoracos/thoracis*). Le desinenze di sostantivi latini elencate per caso e declinazione sono riportate nella Tabella 9.1.

Tabella 9.1 Desinenze di sostantivi latini elencate per caso e declinazione

Caso	Declinazione							
	1a	**2a**		**3a**		**4a**		**5a**
	Fem.	**Masc.**	**Neut.**	**Masc./Fem**	**Neut.**	**Masc.**	**Neut**	**Fem.**
Nominativo singolare	*-a*	*-us*	*-um*	//	//	*-us*	*-u*	*-es*
Genitivo singolare	*-ae*	*-i*	*-i*	*-is*	*-is*	*-us*	*-us*	*-ei*
Nominativo plurale	*-ae*	*-i*	*-a*	*-es*	*-a*	*-us*	*-ua*	*-es*

Esempi:
- Prima declinazione:
  Parole femminili plurali:
  - *patella* (nominativo singolare), *patellae* (genitivo), *patellae* (nominativo plurale). Inglese: *patella*

- Seconda declinazione:
  Parole maschili:
  - *humerus* (nom. sing.), *humeri* (gen.), *humeri* (nom. pl.).
  Inglese: *humerus*
  Parole neutre:
  - *interstitium* (nom. sing.), *interstitii* (gen.), *interstitia* (nom. pl.).
  Inglese: *interstice*

- Terza declinazione:
Parole maschili e femminili:
  - *Pars* (nom. sing.), *partis* (gen.), *partes* (nom. pl.). Inglese: *part*

  Parole neutre:
  - *os* (nom. sing.), *oris* (gen.), *ora* (nom. pl.). Inglese: *mouth*

- Quarta declinazione:
Parole maschili:
  - *processus* (nom. sing.), *processus* (gen.), *processus* (nom. pl).
  Inglese: *process*

  Parole neutre:
  - *cornu* (nom. sing.), *cornus* (gen.), *cornua* (nom. pl.).
  Inglese: *horn*

- Quinta declinazione:
Parole femminili:
  - *facies* (nom. sing.), *faciei* (gen.), *facies* (nom. pl.).
  Inglese: *face*

La desinenza degli aggettivi cambia in base a uno di questi due aspetti:
1. Singolare maschile *-us*, fem. *-a*, neut. *-um*
   Plurale maschile *-i*, fem. *-ae*, neut. *–a*
2. Singolare maschile -is, fem. -is, neut. -e
   Plurale maschile -es, fem. -es, neut. -a

Regole del plurale

Non intendiamo sostituire i dizionari medici o i libri di testo di latino e greco. Al contrario, desideriamo solo dare dei suggerimenti sulla terminologia latina e greca che possano essere utili per l'utilizzo.

Il nostro primo suggerimento è: quando dovete scrivere una parola latina o greca, per prima cosa verificatene l'ortografia e, se la parola che dovete utilizzare è un plurale, non inventate. Sebbene "indovina la forma plurale" possa essere un valido esercizio, controllatene sul dizionario medico la correttezza.

Queste regole per ottenere il plurale sono utili perlomeno per aumentare la nostra confidenza nell'uso di parole latine e greche quali, per esempio, *metastasis–metastases*, *pelvis–pelves*, *bronchus–bronchi*, ecc.

Alcuni medici ritengono che i termini *metastasis* e *metastases* siano equivalenti. Questo non è corretto; la differenza tra una singola metastasi epatica e metastasi epatiche multiple non richiede nessun ulteriore commento.

Ci sono molte parole latine e greche la cui forma singolare non è quasi mai impiegata, come anche alcuni termini la cui forma plurale è scritta o detta raramente. Pensiamo ad esempio alla forma singolare di *viscera* (*viscus*). Pochi medici sono a conoscenza del fatto che il fegato è un *viscus*, mentre il fegato e la milza sono delle *viscera*. Da un punto di vista colloquiale, questa discussione può essere considerata futile, ma coloro che scrivono articoli sanno che la terminologia greco/latina è spesso un incubo e richiede particolare attenzione e che i termini che vengono adoperati raramente nel linguaggio di tutti i giorni devono essere scritti in maniera corretta in un articolo scientifico.

Consideriamo ancora la forma plurale di *pelvis* (*pelves*). Parlare di diverse *pelves* è così raro che molti dottori si domandano se esista davvero il termine *pelves*.

Sebbene esistano alcune eccezioni, le seguenti regole generali possono essere utili con i termini plurali:
- Le parole che terminano in -*us* cambiano in -*i* (parole maschili di seconda declinazione):
  - *bronchus – bronchi*

- Le parole che terminano in -*um* cambiano in -*a* (parole neutre di seconda declinazione):
  - *acetabulum – acetabula*

- Le parole che terminano in -*a* cambiano in -*ae* (parole femminili di prima declinazione):
  - *vena - venae*

- Le parole che terminano in -*ma* cambiano in -*mata* or -*mas* (parole neutre di terza declinazione di origine greca):
  - *sarcoma - sarcomata/sarcomas*

- Le parole che terminano in -*is* cambiano in -*es* (parole maschili e femminili di terza declinazione):
  - *metastasis - metastases*

- Le parole che terminano in *-itis* cambiano in *-itides* (parole maschili e femminili di terza declinazione):
  - *arthritis – arthritides*

- Le parole che terminano in *-x* cambiano in *-ces* (parole maschili e femminili di terza declinazione):
  - *pneumothorax – pneumothoraces*

- Le parole che terminano in *-cyx* cambiano in *-cyges* (parole maschili e femminili di terza declinazione):
  - *coccyx – coccyges*

- Le parole che terminano in *-ion* cambiano in *-ia* (parole neutre di seconda declinazione, per la maggior parte di origine greca):
  - *Criterion – criteria*

Elenco di termini latini e greci con i loro plurali e traduzione inglese

Abbreviazioni:

adj.	adjective
Engl.	English
fem.	feminine
gen.	genitive
Gr.	Greek
Lat.	Latin
lit.	literally
m.	muscle
masc.	masculine
neut.	neuter
pl.	plural
sing.	singular

A

- *Abdomen*, pl. *abdomina*, gen. *abdominis*. Abdomen. 3rd declension neut.
- *Abducens*, pl. *abducentes*, gen. *abducentis* (from the verb *abduco*, to detach, to lead away)

- *Abductor*, pl. *abductores*, gen. *abductoris* (from the verb *abduco*, to detach, to lead away). 3rd declension masc.
- *Acetabulum*, pl. *acetabula*, gen. *acetabuli*. Cotyle. 2nd declension neut.
- *Acinus*, pl. *acini*, gen. *acini*. Acinus. 2nd declension masc.
- *Adductor*, pl. *adductores*, gen. *adductoris*. Adductor. 3rd declension masc.
- *Aditus,* pl. *aditus*, gen. *aditus*. Entrance to a cavity. 4th declension masc. *Aditus ad antrum, aditus glottidis inferior*, etc.
- *Agger*, pl. *aggeres*, gen. *aggeris*. Agger (prominence). 3rd declension masc. *Agger valvae venae, agger nasi, agger perpendicularis*, etc.
- *Ala*, pl. *alae*, gen. *alae*. Wing. 1st declension fem.
- *Alveolus*, pl. *alveoli*, gen. *alveoli*. Alveolus (lit. *basin*). 2nd declension masc.
- *Alveus*, pl. *alvei*, gen. *alvei*. Cavity, hollow. 2nd declension masc.
- *Amoeba*, pl. *amoebae*, gen. *amoebae*. Ameba. 1st declension fem.
- *Ampulla*, pl. *ampullae*, gen. *ampullae*. Ampoule, blister. 1st declension fem.
- *Anastomosis*, pl. *anastomoses*, gen. *anastomosis*. Anastomosis. 3rd declension
- *Angulus*, pl. *anguli*, gen. *anguli*. Angle, apex, corner. 2nd declension neut.
- *Annulus*, pl. *annuli*, gen. *annuli*. Ring. 2nd declension masc.
- *Ansa*, pl. *ansae*, gen. *ansae*. Loop, hook, handle. 1st declension fem.
- *Anterior*, pl. *anteriores*, gen. *anterioris*. Foremost, that is before, former. 3rd declension masc.
- *Antrum*, pl. *antra*, gen. *antri*. Antrum, hollow, cave. 2nd declension neut.
- *Anus*, pl. *ani*, gen. *ani*. Anus (lit. *ring*). 2nd declension masc.
- *Aorta*, pl. *Aortae*, gen. *aortae*. Aorta. 1st declension fem.
- *Apex*, pl. *apices*, gen. *apices*. Apex (top, summit, cap). 3rd declension masc.
- *Aphtha*, pl. *aphthae*, gen. *aphthae*. Aphtha (small ulcer). 1st declension fem.
- *Aponeurosis*, pl. *aponeuroses*, gen. *aponeurosis*. Aponeurosis. 3rd declension
- *Apophysis*, pl. *apophyses*, gen. *apophysos/apophysis*. Apophysis. 3rd declension fem.
- *Apparatus*, pl. *apparatus*, gen. *apparatus*. Apparatus, system. 4th declension masc.
- *Appendix*, pl. *appendices*, gen. *appendicis*. Appendage. 3rd declension fem.
- *Area*, pl. *areae*, gen. *areae*. Area. 1st declension fem.

- *Areola*, pl. *areolae*, gen. *areolae*. Areola (lit. *little area*). 1st declension fem.
- *Arrector*, pl. *arrectores*, gen. *arrectoris*. Erector, tilt upwards. 3rd declension masc.
- *Arteria*, pl. *arteriae*, gen. *arteriae*. Artery. 1st declension fem.
- *Arteriola*, pl. *arteriolae*, gen. *arteriolae*. Arteriola (small artery). 1st declension fem.
- *Arthritis*, pl. *arthritides*, gen. *arthritidis*. Arthritis. 3rd declension fem.
- *Articularis*, pl. *articulares*, gen. *articularis*. Articular, affecting the joints. 3rd declension masc. (adj.: masc. *articularis*, fem. *articularis*, neut. *articulare*)
- *Articulatio*, pl. *articulationes*, gen. *articulationis*. Joint. 3rd declension fem.
- *Atlas*, pl. *atlantes*, gen. *atlantis*. First cervical vertebra. 3rd declension masc.
- *Atrium*, pl. *atria*, gen. *atrii*. Atrium. 2nd declension neut.
- *Auricula*, pl. *auriculae*, gen. *auriculae*. Auricula (ear flap). 1st declension fem.
- *Auricularis m.*, pl. *auriculares*, gen. *auricularis*. Pertaining to the ear. 3rd declension masc.
- *Auris*, pl. *aures*, gen. *auris*. Ear. 3rd declension fem.
- *Axilla*, pl. *axillae*, gen. *axillae*. Armpit. 1st declension fem.
- *Axis*, pl. *axes*, gen. *axis*. Second cervical vertebra, axis. 3rd declension masc.

B

- *Bacillus*, pl. *bacilli*, gen. *bacilli*. Stick-shape bacterium (lit. *small stick*). 2nd declension masc.
- *Bacterium*, pl. *bacteria*, gen. *bacterii*. Bacterium. 2nd declension neut.
- *Basis*, pl. *bases*, gen. *basis*. Basis, base. 3rd declension fem.
- *Biceps m.*, pl. *bicipites*, gen. *bicipitis*. A muscle with two heads. 3rd declension masc. Biceps + genitive. Biceps *brachii* (*brachium*. Arm)
- *Borborygmus*, pl. *borborygmi*, gen. *borborygmi*. Borborygmus (gastrointestinal sound). 2nd declension masc.
- *Brachium*, pl. *brachia*, gen. *brachii*. Arm. 2nd declension neut.
- *Brevis*, pl. *breves*, gen. *brevis*. Short, little, small. 3rd declension masc. (adj.: masc. *brevis*, fem. *brevis*, neut. *breve*)
- *Bronchium*, pl. *bronchia*, gen. *bronchii*. Bronchus. 2nd declension neut.
- *Buccinator m.*, pl. *buccinatores*, gen. *buccinatoris*. Buccinator m. (trumpeter's muscle). 3rd declension masc.
- *Bulla*, pl. *bullae*, gen. *bullae*. Bulla. 1st declension fem.
- *Bursa*, pl. *bursae*, gen. *bursae*. Bursa (bag, pouch). 1st declension fem.

C

- *Caecum*, pl. *caeca*, gen. *caeci*. Blind. 2nd declension neut. (adj.: masc. *caecus*, fem. *caeca*, neut. *caecum*)
- *Calcaneus*, pl. *calcanei*, gen. *calcanei*. Calcaneus (from *calx*, heel). 2nd declension masc.
- *Calculus*, pl. *calculi*, gen. *calculi*. Stone (lit. pebble). 2nd declension masc.
- *Calix*, pl. *calices*, gen. *calicis*. Calix (lit. *cup*, *goblet*). 3rd declension masc.
- *Calx*, pl. *calces*, gen. *calcis*. Heel. 3rd declension masc.
- *Canalis*, pl. *canales*, gen. *canalis*. Channel, conduit. 3rd declension masc.
- *Cancellus*, pl. *cancelli*, gen. *cancelli*. Reticulum, lattice, grid. 2nd declension masc.
- *Cancer*, pl. *cancera*, gen. *canceri*. Cancer. 3rd declension neut.
- *Capillus*, pl. *capilli*, gen. *capilli*. Hair. 2nd declension masc.
- *Capitatus*, pl. *capitati*, gen. *capitati*. Capitate, having or forming a head. 2nd declension masc. (adj.: masc. *capitatus*, fem. *capitata*, neut. *capitatum*)
- *Capitulum*, pl. *capitula*, gen. *capituli*. Head of a structure, condyle. 2nd declension neut.
- *Caput*, pl. *capita*, gen. *capitis*. Head. 3rd declension neut.
- *Carcinoma*, pl. Lat. *carcinomata*, pl. Engl. *carcinomas*, gen. *carcinomatis*. Carcinoma (epithelial cancer). 3rd declension neut.
- *Carina*, pl. *carinae*, gen. *carinae*. Carina (lit. *keel*, *bottom of ship*). 1st declension fem.
- *Cartilago*, pl. *cartilagines*, gen. *cartilaginis*. Cartilage. 3rd declension neut.
- *Cauda*, pl. *caudae*, gen. *caudae*. Tail. 1st declension fem. *Cauda equina* (adj.: masc. *equinus*, fem. *equina*, neut. *equinum*. Concerning horses)
- *Caverna*, pl. *cavernae*, gen. *cavernae*. Cavern. 1st declension fem.
- *Cavitas*, pl. *cavitates*, gen. *cavitatis*. Cavity. 3rd declension fem.
- *Cavum*, pl. *cava*, gen. *cavi*. Cavum (hole, pit, depression). 2nd declension neut.
- *Cella*, pl. *cellae*, gen. *cellae*. Cell (lit. *cellar*, *wine storeroom*). 1st declension fem.
- *Centrum*, pl. *centra*, gen. *centri*. Center. 2nd declension neut.
- *Cerebellum*, pl. *cerebella*, gen. *cerebelli*. Cerebellum. 2nd declension neut.
- *Cerebrum*, pl. *cerebra*, gen. *cerebri*. Brain. 2nd declension neut.
- *Cervix*, pl. *cervices*, gen. *cervicis*. Neck. 3rd declension fem.
- *Chiasma*, pl. *chiasmata*, gen. *chiasmatis/chiasmatos*. Chiasm. 3rd declension neut.

- *Choana*, pl. *choanae*, gen. *choanae*. Choana. 1st declension fem. *Choanae narium*. Posterior opening of the nasal fossae (*naris*, gen. *narium*. nose)
- *Chorda*, pl. *chordae*, gen. *chordae*. String. 1st declension fem. *Chorda tympani*. A nerve given off from the facial nerve in the facial canal that crosses over the tympanic membrane (*tympanum*, gen *tympani*. eardrum)
- *Chorion*, pl. *choria*, gen. *chorii*. Chorion (membrane enclosing the fetus). 2nd declension neut.
- *Cicatrix*, pl. *cicatrices*, gen. *cicatricis*. Scar. 3rd declension fem.
- *Cilium*, pl. *cilia*, gen. *cilii*. Cilium (lit. *upper eyelid*). 2nd declension neut.
- *Cingulum*, pl. *cingula*, gen. *cinguli*. Cingulum (belt-shaped structure, lit. *belt*). 2nd declension neut.
- *Cisterna*, pl. *cisternae*, gen. *cisternae*. Cistern. 1st declension fem.
- *Claustrum*, pl. *claustra*, gen. *claustri*. Claustrum. 2nd declension neut.
- *Clitoris*, pl. *clitorides*, gen. *clitoridis*. Clitoris. 3rd declension
- *Clivus*, pl. *clivi*, gen. *clivi*. Clivus (part of the skull, lit. *slope*). 2nd declension masc.
- *Clostridium*, pl. *clostridia*, gen. *clostridii*. Clostridium (genus of bacteria). 2nd declension neut.
- *Coccus*, pl. *cocci*, gen. *cocci*. Coccus (rounded bacterium, lit. *a scarlet dye*). 2nd declension masc.
- *Coccyx*, pl. *coccyges*, gen. *coccygis*. Coccyx. 3rd declension masc.
- *Cochlea*, pl. *cochleae*, gen. *cochleae*. Cochlea (lit. *snail shell*). 1st declension fem.
- *Collum*, pl. *colla*, gen. *colli*. Neck. 2nd declension neut.
- *Comedo*, pl. *comedones*, gen. *comedonis*. Comedo (a dilated hair follicle filled with keratin). 3rd declension masc.
- *Comunis*, pl. *comunes*, gen. *comunis*. Common. 3rd declension masc (adj.: masc./fem. *comunis*, neut. *comune*)
- *Concha*, pl. *conchae*, gen. *conchae*. Concha (shell-shaped structure). 1st declension fem.
- *Condyloma*, pl. *condylomata*, gen. *condylomatis*. Condyloma. 3rd declension neut. *Condyloma acuminatum*
- *Conjunctiva*, pl. *conjunctivae*, gen. *conjunctivae*. Conjunctiva. 1st declension fem.
- *Constrictor*, pl. *constrictores*, gen. *constrictoris*. Sphincter. 3rd declension masc.
- *Conus*, pl. *coni*, gen. *coni*. Cone. 2nd declension masc. *Conus medullaris* (from *medulla*, pl. *medullae*, the tapering end of the spinal cord)
- *Cor*, pl. *corda*, gen. *cordis*. Heart. 3rd declension neut.
- *Corium*, pl. *coria*, gen. *corii*. Dermis (lit. *skin*). 2nd declension neut.

- *Cornu*, pl. *Cornua*, gen. *cornus*. Horn. 4th declension neut.
- *Corona*, pl. *coronae*, gen. *coronae*. Corona (lit. *crown*). 1st declension fem. *Corona radiata*, pl. *coronae radiatae*, gen. *coronae radiatae*
- *Corpus*, pl. *corpora*, gen. *corporis*. Body. 3rd declension neut. *Corpus callosum, corpus cavernosum* (penis)
- *Corpusculum*, pl. *corpuscula*, gen. *corpusculi*. Corpuscle. 2nd declension neut.
- *Cortex*, pl. *cortices*, gen. *corticis*. Cortex, outer covering. 3rd declension masc.
- *Coxa*, pl. *coxae*, gen. *coxae*. Hip. 1st declension fem.
- *Cranium*, pl. *crania*, gen. *cranii*. Skull. 2nd declension neut.
- *Crisis*, pl. *crises*, gen. *crisos/crisis*. Crisis. 3rd declension fem.
- *Crista*, pl. *cristae*, gen. *cristae*. Crest. 1st declension fem. *Crista galli* (from *gallus*, pl. *galli*, rooster. The midline process of the ethmoid bone arising from the cribriform plate)
- *Crus*, pl. *crura*, gen. *cruris*. Leg, leg-like structure. 3rd declension neut. *Crura diaphragmatis*
- *Crusta*, pl. *crustae*, gen. *crustae*. Crust, hard surface. 1st declension fem.
- *Crypta*, pl. *cryptae*, gen. *cryptae*. Crypt. 1st declension fem.
- *Cubitus*, pl. *cubiti*, gen. *cubiti*. Ulna (lit. *forearm*). 2nd declension masc.
- *Cubitus*, pl. *cubitus*, gen. *cubitus*. State of lying down. 4th declension masc. *De cubito supino/prono*
- *Culmen*, pl. *culmina*, gen. *culminis*. Peak, top (*culmen*. Top of cerebellar lobe). 3rd declension neut.
- *Cuneiforme*, pl. *cuneiformia*, gen. *cuneiformis*. Wedge-shaped structure. 3rd declension neut. (adj.: masc. *cuneiformis*, fem. *cuneiformis*, neut. *cuneiforme*)

D

- *Decussatio*, pl. *decussationes*, gen. *decussationis*. Decussation. 3rd declension fem.
- *Deferens*, pl. *deferentes*, gen. *deferentis*. Spermatic duct (from the verb *defero*, to carry). 3rd declension masc.
- *Dens*, pl. *dentes*, gen. *dentis*. Tooth, pl. Teeth. 3rd declension masc.
- *Dermatitis*, pl. *dermatitides*, gen. *dermatitis*. Dermatitis. 3rd declension
- *Dermatosis*, pl. *dermatoses*, gen. *dermatosis*. Dermatosis. 3rd declension
- *Diaphragma*, pl. *diaphragmata*, gen. *diaphragmatis*. Diaphragm. 3rd declension neut.
- *Diaphysis*, pl. *Diaphyses*, gen. *diaphysis*. Shaft. 3rd declension
- *Diarthrosis*, pl. *diarthroses*, gen. *diarthrosis*. Diarthrosis. 3rd declension

- *Diastema*, pl. *diastemata*, gen. *diastematis*. Diastema (congenital fissure). 3rd declension
- *Digastricus m.*, pl. *digastrici*, gen. *digastrici*. Digastric (having two bellies). 2nd declension masc.
- *Digitus*, pl. *digiti*, gen. sing. *digiti*, gen. pl. *digitorum*. Finger. 2nd declension masc. *Extensor digiti minimi, flexor superficialis digitorum*
- *Diverticulum*, pl. *diverticula*, gen. *diverticuli*. Diverticulum. 2nd declension neut.
- *Dorsum*, pl. *dorsa*, gen. *dorsi*. Back. 2nd declension neut.
- *Ductus*, pl. *ductus*, gen. *ductus*. Duct. 4th declension masc. *Ductus arteriosus, ductus deferens*
- *Duodenum*, pl. *duodena*, gen. *duodeni*. Duodenum (lit. *twelve*. The duodenum measures 12 times a finger). 2nd declension neut.

E

- *Ecchymosis*, pl. *ecchymoses*, gen. *ecchymosis*. Ecchymosis. 3rd declension
- *Effluvium*, pl. *effluvia*, gen. *effluvii*. Effluvium (fall). 2nd declension neut.
- *Encephalitis*, pl. *encephalitides*, gen. *encephalitidis*. Encephalitis. 3rd declension fem.
- *Endocardium*, pl. *endocardia*, gen. *endocardii*. Endocardium. 2nd declension neut.
- *Endometrium*, pl. *endometria*, gen. *endometrii*. Endometrium. 2nd declension neut.
- *Endothelium*, pl. *endothelia*, gen. *endothelii*. Endothelium. 2nd declension neut.
- *Epicondylus*, pl. *epicondyli*, gen. *epicondyli*. Epicondylus. 2nd declension masc.
- *Epidermis*, pl. *epidermides*, gen. *epidermidis*. Epidermis. 3rd declension
- *Epididymis*, pl. *epididymes*, gen. *epididymis*. Epididymis. 3rd declension
- *Epiphysis*, pl. *epiphyses*, gen. *epiphysis*. Epiphysis. 3rd declension
- *Epithelium*, pl. *epithelia*, gen. *epithelii*. Epithelium. 2nd declension neut.
- *Esophagus*, pl. *esophagi*, gen. *esophagi*. Esophagus. 2nd declension masc.
- *Exostosis*, pl. *exostoses*, gen. *exostosis*. Exostosis. 3rd declension
- *Extensor*, pl. *extensores*, gen. *extensoris*. A muscle contraction of which stretches out a structure. 3rd declension masc. *Extensor carpi ulnaris m., extensor digitorum communis m., extensor hallucis longus/brevis m.*, etc.
- *Externus*, pl. *externi*, gen. *externi*. External, outward. 2nd declension masc. (adj.: masc. *externus*, fem. *externa*, gen. *externum*)

F

- *Facies*, pl. *facies*, gen. *faciei*. Face. 5th declension fem.
- *Falx*, pl. *falces*, gen. *falcis*. Sickle-shaped structure. 3rd declension fem. *Falx cerebrii*
- *Fascia*, pl. *fasciae*, gen. *fasciae*. Fascia. 1st declension fem.
- *Fasciculus*, pl. *fasciculi*, gen. *fasciculi*. Fasciculus. 2nd declension masc.
- *Femur*, pl. *femora*, gen. *femoris*. Femur. 3rd declension neut.
- *Fenestra*, pl. *fenestrae*, gen. *fenestrae*. Window, hole. 1st declension fem.
- *Fetus*, pl. *feti/fetus*, gen. *feti/fetus*. Fetus. 2nd declension masc./4th declension masc.
- *Fibra*, pl. *fibrae*, gen. *fibrae*. Fiber. 1st declension fem.
- *Fibula*, pl. *fibulae*, gen. *fibulae*. Fibula. 1st declension fem.
- *Filamentum*, pl. *filamenta*, gen. *filamentii*. Filament. 2nd declension neut.
- *Filaria*, pl. *filariae*, gen. *filariae*. Filaria. 1st declension fem.
- *Filum*, pl. *fila*, gen. *fili*. Filamentous structure. 2nd declension neut. *Filum terminale*
- *Fimbria*, pl. *fimbriae*, gen. *fimbriae*. Fimbria (lit. *fringe*). 1st declension fem.
- *Fistula*, pl. *fistulae*, gen. *fistulae*. Fistula (lit. *pipe, tube*). 1st declension fem.
- *Flagellum*, pl. *flagella*, gen. *flagelli*. Flagellum (whip-like locomotory organelle). 2nd declension neut.
- *Flexor*, pl. *flexores*, gen. *flexoris*. A muscle whose action flexes a joint. 3rd declension masc. *Flexor carpi radialis/ulnaris mm., flexor pollicis longus/brevis mm.*, etc.
- *Flexura*, pl. *flexurae*, gen. *flexurae*. Flexure, curve, bow. 1st declension fem.
- *Folium*, pl. *folia*, gen. *folii*. Leaf-shaped structure (lit. *leaf*). 2nd declension neut.
- *Folliculus*, pl. *folliculi*, gen. *folliculi*. Follicle. 2nd declension masc.
- *Foramen*, pl. *foramina*, gen. *foraminis*. Foramen, hole. 3rd declension neut. *Foramen rotundum, foramen ovale. Foramina cribrosa*, pl. (multiple pores in lamina cribrosa)
- *Formula*, pl. *formulae*, gen. *formulae*. Formula. 1st declension fem.
- *Fornix*, pl. *fornices*, gen. *fornicis*. Fornix (arch-shaped structure). 3rd declension masc.
- *Fossa*, pl. *fossae*, gen. *fossae*. Fossa, depression. 1st declension fem.
- *Fovea*, pl. *foveae*, gen. *foveae*. Fovea, depression, pit. 1st declension fem.
- *Frenulum*, pl. *frenula*, gen. *frenuli*. Bridle-like structure. 2nd declension neut.

- *Fungus*, pl. *fungi*, gen. *fungi*. Fungus (lit. *mushroom*). 2nd declension masc.
- *Funiculus*, pl. *funiculi*, gen. *funiculi*. Cord, string. 2nd declension masc.
- *Furfur*, pl. *furfures*, gen. *furfuris*. Dandruff. 3rd declension masc.
- *Furunculus*, pl. *furunculi*, gen. *furunculi*. Furuncle. 2nd declension masc.

G

- *Galea*, pl. *galeae*, gen. *galeae*. Cover, a structure shaped like a helmet (lit. *helmet*). 1st declension fem. *Galea aponeurotica*, pl. *galeae aponeuroticae* (epicranial aponeurosis)
- *Ganglion*, pl. *ganglia*, gen. *ganglii*. Node. 2nd declension masc.
- *Geniculum*, pl. *genicula*, gen. *geniculi*. Geniculum (knee-shaped structure). 2nd declension neut.
- *Geniohyoideus m.*, pl. *geniohyoidei*, gen. *geniohyoidei*. Glenohyoid muscle. 2nd declension masc.
- *Genu*, pl. *genua*, gen. *genus*. Knee. 4th declension neut.
- *Genus*, pl. *genera*, gen. *generis*. Gender. 3rd declension neut.
- *Gestosis*, pl. *gestoses*, gen. *gestosis*. Gestosis (pregnancy impairment). 3rd declension
- *Gingiva*, pl. *gingivae*, gen. *gingivae*. Gum. 1st declension fem.
- *Glabella*, pl. *glabellae*, gen. *glabellae*. Small lump/mass. 1st declension fem.
- *Glandula*, pl. *glandulae*, gen. *glandulae*. Gland. 1st declension fem.
- *Glans*, pl. *glandes*, gen. *glandis*. Glans (lit. *acorn*). 3rd declension fem. *Glans penis*
- *Globus*, pl. *globi*, gen. *globi*. Globus, round body. 2nd declension masc.
- *Glomerulus*, pl. *glomeruli*, gen. *glomeruli*. Glomerule. 2nd declension masc.
- *Glomus*, pl. *glomera*, gen. *glomeris*. Glomus (ball-shaped body). 3rd declension
- *Glottis*, pl. *glottides*, gen. *glottidis*. Glottis. 3rd declension
- *Gluteus m.*, pl. *glutei*, gen. *glutei*. Buttock. 2nd declension masc.
- *Gracilis m.*, pl. *graciles*, gen. *gracilis*. Graceful. 3rd declension masc. (adj.: masc. *gracilis*, fem. *gracilis*, neut. *gracile*)
- *Granulatio*, pl. *granulationes*, gen. *granulationis*. Granulation. 3rd declension
- *Gumma*, pl. *gummata*, gen. *gummatis*. Syphiloma. 3rd declension neut.
- *Gutta*, pl. *guttae*, gen. *guttae*. Gout. 1st declension fem.
- *Gyrus*, pl. *gyri*, gen. *gyri*. Convolution. 2nd declension masc.
- *Gastrocnemius m.*, pl. *gastrocnemii*, gen. *gastrocnemii*. Calf muscle. 2nd declension masc.

H

- *Hallux*, pl. *halluces*, gen. *hallucis*. First toe. 3rd declension masc.
- *Hamatus*, pl. *hamati*, gen. *hamati*. Hamate bone. 2nd declension masc. (adj.: masc. *hamatus*, fem. *hamata*, neut. *hamatum*. Hooked)
- *Hamulus*, pl. *hamuli*, gen. *hamuli*. Hamulus (lit. *small hook*). 2nd declension masc.
- *Haustrum*, pl. *haustra*, gen. *haustri*. Pouch from the lumen of the colon. 2nd declension neut.
- *Hiatus*, pl. *hiatus*, gen. *hiatus*. Gap, cleft. 4th declension masc.
- *Hilum*, pl. *hila*, gen. *hili*. Hilum (the part of an organ where the neurovascular bundle enters). 2nd declension neut.
- *Hircus*, pl. *hirci*, gen. *hirci*. Hircus (armpit hair, lit. *goat*). 2nd declension masc.
- *Humerus*, pl. *humeri*, gen. *humeri*. Humerus. 2nd declension masc.
- *Humor*, pl. *humores*, gen. *humoris*. Humor, fluid. 3rd declension masc.
- *Hypha*, pl. *hyphae*, gen. *hyphae*. Hypha, tubular cell (lit. Gr. *web*). 1st declension fem.
- *Hypophysis*, pl. *hypophyses*, gen. *hypophysis*. Pituitary gland (lit. *undergrowth*). 3rd declension
- *Hypothenar*, pl. *hypothenares*, gen. *hypothenaris*. Hypothenar (from Gr. *thenar*, the palm of the hand). 3rd declension

I

- *Ilium*, pl. *ilia*, gen. *ilii*. Iliac bone. 2nd declension neut.
- *In situ*. In position (from *situs*, pl. *situs*, gen. *situs*, site). 4th declension masc.
- *Incisura*, pl. *incisurae*, gen. *incisurae*. Incisure (from the verb *incido*, cut into). 1st declension fem.
- *Incus*, pl. *incudes*, gen. *incudis*. Incus (lit. *anvil*). 3rd declension fem.
- *Index*, pl. *indices*, gen. *indicis*. Index (second digit, forefinger), guide. 3rd declension masc.
- *Indusium*, pl. *indusia*, gen. *indusii*. Indusium (membrane, amnion). 2nd declension neut.
- *Inferior*, pl. *inferiores*, gen. *inferioris*. Inferior. 3rd declension masc.
- *Infundibulum*, pl. *infundibula*, gen. *infundibuli*. Infundibulum. 2nd declension neut.
- *Insula*, pl. *insulae*, gen. *insulae*. Insula. 1st declension fem.
- *Intermedius*, pl. *intermedii*, gen. *intermedii*. In the middle of. 2nd declension masc. (adj.: masc. *intermedius*, fem. *intermedia*, neut. *intermedium*)
- *Internus*, pl. *interni*, gen. *interni*. Internal. 2nd declension masc. (adj.: masc. *internus*, fem. *interna*, neut. *internum*)

- *Interosseus*, gen. *interossei*, pl. *interossei*. Interosseous. 2nd declension masc. (adj.: masc. *interosseus*, fem. *interossea*, neut. *interosseum*)
- *Intersectio*, pl. *intersectiones*, gen. *intersectionis*. Intersection. 3rd declension fem.
- *Interstitium*, pl. *interstitia*, gen. *interstitii*. Interstice. 2nd declension neut.
- *Intestinum*, pl. *intestina*, gen. *intestini*. Bowel. 2nd declension neut.
- *Iris*, pl. *irides*, gen. *iridis*. Iris. 3rd declension masc.
- *Ischium*, pl. *ischia*, gen. *ischii*. Ischium. 2nd declension neut.
- *Isthmus*, pl. Lat. *isthmi*, pl. Engl. *isthmuses*, gen. *isthmi*. Constriction, narrow passage. 2nd declension masc.

J

- *Jejunum*, pl. *jejuna*, gen. *jejuni*. Jejunum (from Lat. adj. *jejunus*, fasting, empty). 2nd declension neut.
- *Jugular*, pl. *jugulares*, gen. *jugularis*. Jugular vein (lit. relating to the throat, from Lat. *jugulus*, throat). 3rd declension
- *Junctura*, pl. *juncturae*, gen. *juncturae*. Joint, junction. 1st declension fem.

L

- *Labium*, pl. *labia*, gen. *labii*. Lip. 2nd declension neut.
- *Labrum*, pl. *labra*, gen. *labri*. Rim, edge, lip. 2nd declension neut.
- *Lacuna*, pl. *lacunae*, gen. *lacunae*. Pond, pit, hollow. 1st declension fem.
- *Lamellipodium*, pl. *lamellipodia*, gen. *lamellipodii*. Lamellipodium. 2nd declension neut.
- *Lamina*, pl. *laminae*, gen. *laminae*. Layer. 1st declension fem. *Lamina papyracea, lamina perpendicularis*
- *Larva*, pl. *larvae*, gen. *larvae*. Larva. 1st declension fem.
- *Larynx*, pl. Lat. *larynges*, pl. Engl. *larynxes*, gen. *laryngis*. Larynx. 3rd declension
- *Lateralis*, pl. *laterales*, gen. *lateralis*. Lateral. 3rd declension masc. (adj.: masc. *lateralis*, fem. *lateralis*, neut. *laterale*)
- *Latissimus*, pl. *latissimi*, gen. *latissimi*. Very wide, the widest. 2nd declension masc. (adj.: masc. *latissimus*, fem. *latissima*, neut. *latissimum*)
- *Latus*, pl. *latera*, gen. *lateris*. Flank. 3rd declension neut.
- *Latus*, pl. *lati*, gen. *lati*. Wide, broad. 2nd declension masc. (adj.: masc. *latus*, fem. *lata*, neut. *latum*)
- *Lemniscus*, pl. *lemnisci*, gen. *lemnisci*. Lemniscus (lit. *ribbon*). 2nd declension masc.
- *Lentigo*, pl. *lentigines*, gen. *lentiginis*. Lentigo (lit. *lentil-shaped spot*). 3rd declension

- *Levator*, pl. *levatores*, gen. *levatoris*. Lifter (from Lat. verb *levo*, to lift). 3rd declension masc.
- *Lien*, pl. *lienes*, gen. *lienis*. Spleen. 3rd declension masc.
- *Lienculus*, pl. *lienculi*, gen. *lienculi*. Accessory spleen. 2nd declension masc.
- *Ligamentum*, pl. *ligamenta*, gen. *ligamenti*. Ligament. 2nd declension neut.
- *Limbus*, pl. *limbi*, gen. *limbi*. Border, edge. 2nd declension masc.
- *Limen*, pl. *limina*, gen. *liminis*. Threshold. 3rd declension neut.
- *Linea*, pl. *lineae*, gen. *lineae*. Line. 1st declension fem.
- *Lingua*, pl. *linguae*, gen. *linguae*. Tongue. 1st declension fem.
- *Lingualis*, pl. *linguales*, gen. *lingualis*. Relative to the tongue. 3rd declension masc. (adj.: masc. *lingualis*, fem. *lingualis*, neut. *linguale*)
- *Lingula*, pl. *lingulae*, gen. *lingulae*. Lingula (tongue-shaped). 1st declension fem.
- *Liquor*, pl. *liquores*, gen. *liquoris*. Fluid. 3rd declension masc.
- *Lobulus*, pl. *lobuli*, gen. *lobuli*. Lobule. 2nd declension masc.
- *Lobus*, pl. *lobi*, gen. *lobi*. Lobe. 2nd declension masc.
- *Loculus*, pl. *loculi*, gen. *loculi*. Loculus (small chamber). 2nd declension masc.
- *Locus*, pl. *loci*, gen. *loci*. Locus (place, position, point). 2nd declension masc.
- *Longissimus*, pl. *longissimi*, gen. *longissimi*. Very long, the longest. 2nd declension masc. (adj.: masc. longissimus, fem. longissima, neut. longissimum). *Longissimus dorsi/capitis mm.* (long muscle of the back/head)
- *Longus*, pl. *longi*, gen. *longi*. Long. 2nd declension masc. (adj.: masc. *longus*, fem. *longa*, neut. *longum*). *Longus colli m.* (long muscle of the neck)
- *Lumbar*, pl. *lumbares*, gen. *lumbaris*. Lumbar. 3rd declension
- *Lumbus*, pl. *lumbi*, gen. *lumbi*. Loin. 2nd declension masc.
- *Lumen*, pl. *lumina*, gen. *luminis*. Lumen. 3rd declension neut.
- *Lunatum*, pl. *lunata*, gen. *lunati*. Lunate bone, crescent-shaped structure. 2nd declension neut. (adj.: masc. *lunatus*, fem. *lunata*, neut. *lunatum*) Lunula, pl. lunulae, gen. lunulae. Lunula. 1st declension fem.
- *Lymphonodus*, pl. *lymphonodi*, gen. *lymphonodi*. Lymph node. 2nd declension masc.

M

- *Macula*, pl. *maculae*, gen. *maculae*. Macula, spot. 1st declension fem.
- *Magnus*, pl. *magni*, gen. *magni*. Large, great. 2nd declension masc. (adj.: masc. *magnus*, fem. *magna*, neut. *magnum*)

- *Major*, pl. *majores*, gen. *majoris*. Greater. 3rd declension masc./fem.
- *Malleolus*, pl. *malleoli*, gen. *malleoli*. Malleolus (lit. *small hammer*). 2nd declension masc.
- *Malleus*, pl. *mallei*, gen. *mallei*. Malleus (lit. *hammer*). 2nd declension masc.
- *Mamilla*, pl. *mamillae*, gen. *mamillae*. Mamilla. 1st declension fem.
- *Mamma*, pl. *mammae*, gen. *mammae*. Breast. 1st declension fem.
- *Mandibula*, pl. *mandibulae*, gen. *mandibulae*. Jaw. 1st declension fem.
- *Mandibular*, pl. *mandibulares*, gen. *mandibularis*. Relative to the jaw. 3rd declension
- *Manubrium*, pl. *manubria*, gen. *manubrii*. Manubrium (lit. *handle*). 2nd declension neut. *Manubrium sterni*, pl. *manubria sterna* (superior part of the sternum)
- *Manus*, pl. *manus*, gen. *manus*. Hand. 4th declension fem.
- *Margo*, pl. *margines*, gen. *marginis*. Margin. 3rd declension fem.
- *Matrix*, pl. *matrices*, gen. *matricis*. Matrix (formative portion of a structure, surrounding substance). 3rd declension fem.
- *Maxilla*, pl. *maxillae*, gen. *maxillae*. Maxilla. 1st declension fem.
- *Maximus*, pl. *maximi*, gen. *maximi*. The greatest, the biggest, the largest. 2nd declension masc. (adj.: masc. *maximus*, fem. *maxima*, neut. *maximum*)
- *Meatus*, pl. *meatus*, gen. *meatus*. Meatus, canal. 4th declension masc.
- *Medialis*, pl. *mediales*, gen. *medialis*. Medial. 3rd declension masc./fem. (adj.: masc. *medialis*, fem. *medialis*, neut. *mediale*)
- *Medium*, pl. *media*, gen. *medii*. Substance, culture medium, means. 2nd declension neut.
- *Medulla*, pl. *medullae*, gen. *medullae*. Marrow. 1st declension fem. *Medulla oblongata* (caudal portion of the brainstem), *medulla spinalis*
- *Membrana*, pl. *membranae*, gen. *membranae*. Membrane. 1st declension fem.
- *Membrum*, pl. *membra*, gen. *membri*. Limb. 2nd declension neut.
- *Meningitis*, pl. *meningitides*, gen. *meningitidis*. Meningitis. 3rd declension fem.
- *Meningococcus*, pl. *meningococci*, gen. *meningococci*. Meningococcus. 2nd declension masc.
- *Meninx*, pl. *meninges*, gen. *meningis*. Meninx. 3rd declension
- *Meniscus*, pl. *menisci*, gen. *menisci*. Meniscus. 2nd declension masc.
- *Mentum*, pl. *menti*, gen. *menti*. Chin. 2nd declension masc.
- *Mesocardium*, pl. *mesocardia*, gen. *mesocardii*. Mesocardium. 2nd declension neut.

- *Mesothelium*, pl. *mesothelia*, gen. *mesothelii*. Mesothelium. 2nd declension neut.
- *Metacarpus*, pl. *metacarpi*, gen. *metacarpi*. Metacarpus. 2nd declension masc.
- *Metaphysis*, pl. *metaphyses*, gen. *metaphysis*. Metaphysis. 3rd declension
- *Metastasis*, pl. *metastases*, gen. *metastasis*. Metastasis. 3rd declension
- *Metatarsus*, pl. *metatarsi*, gen. *metatarsi*. Metatarsus. 2nd declension masc.
- *Microvillus*, pl. *microvilli*, gen. *microvilli*. Microvillus (from *villus*, hair). 2nd declension masc.
- *Minimus*, pl. *minimi*, gen. *minimi*. The smallest, the least. 2nd declension masc. (adj.: masc. *minimus*, fem. *minima*, neut. *minimum*)
- *Minor*, pl. *minores*, gen. *minoris*. Lesser. 3rd declension masc.
- *Mitochondrion*, pl. *mitochondria*, gen. *mitochondrium*. Mitochondrion. 3rd declension neut.
- *Mitosis*, pl. *mitoses*, gen. *mitosis*. Mitosis. 3rd declension (from Gr. *mitos*, thread)
- *Mons*, pl. *montes*, gen. *montis*. Mons (lit. *mountain*). 3rd declension masc.
- *Mors*, pl. *mortes*, gen. *mortis*, acc. *mortem*. Death. 3rd declension fem.
- *Mucolipidosis*, pl. *mucolipidoses*, gen. *mucolipidosis*. Mucolipidosis. 3rd declension masc./fem.
- *Mucro*, pl. *mucrones*, gen. *mucronis*. Sharp-tipped structure. 3rd declension masc. *Mucro sterni* (sternal xyphoides)
- *Musculus*, pl. *musculi*, gen. *musculi*. Muscle. 2nd declension masc.
- *Mycelium*, pl. *mycelia*, gen. *mycelii*. Mycelium, mass of hyphae. 2nd declension neut.
- *Mycoplasma*, pl. *mycoplasmata*, gen. *mycoplasmatis*. Mycoplasma. 3rd declension neut.
- *Mylohyoideus m.*, pl. *mylohyoidei*, gen. *mylohyoidei*. 2nd declension masc.
- *Myocardium*, pl. *myocardia*, gen. *myocardii*. Myocardium. 2nd declension neut.
- *Myofibrilla*, pl. *myofibrillae*, gen. *myofibrillae*. Myofibrilla. 1st declension fem.
- *Myrinx*, pl. *myringes*, gen. *myringis*. Eardrum. 3rd declension

N

- *Naris*, pl. *nares*, gen. *naris*. Nostril. 3rd declension fem.
- *Nasus*, pl. *nasi*, gen. *nasi*. Nose. 2nd declension masc.
- *Navicularis*, pl. *naviculares*, gen. *navicularis*. Ship shaped. 3rd declension masc.

- *Nebula*, pl. *nebulae*, gen. *nebulae*. Mist, cloud (corneal nebula, corneal opacity). 1st declension fem.
- *Neisseria*, pl. *neisseriae*, gen. *neisseriae*. Neisseria. 1st declension fem.
- *Nephritis*, pl. *nephritides*, gen. *nephritidis*. Nephritis 3rd declension
- *Nervus*, pl. *nervi*, gen. *nervi*. Nerve. 2nd declension masc.
- *Neuritis*, pl. *neuritides*, gen. *neuritidis*. Neuritis. 3rd declension
- *Neurosis*, pl. *neuroses*, gen. *neurosis*. Neurosis. 3rd declension
- *Nevus*, pl. *nevi*, gen. *nevi*. Nevus (*lit. mole on the body, birthmark*). 2nd declension masc.
- *Nidus*, pl. *nidi*, gen. *nidi*. Nidus (lit. *nest*). 2nd declension masc.
- *Nodulus*, pl. *noduli*, gen. *noduli*. Nodule (small node, knot). 2nd declension masc.
- *Nucleolus*, pl. *nucleoli*, gen. *nucleoli*. Nucleolus (small nucleus). 2nd declension masc.
- *Nucleus*, pl. *nuclei*, gen. *nuclei*. Nucleus (central part, core, lit. *inside of a nut*). 2nd declension masc.

O

- *Obliquus*, pl. *obliqui*, gen. *obliqui*. Oblique. 2nd declension masc. (adj.: masc. *obliquus*, fem. *obliqua*, neut. *obliquum*)
- *Occiput*, pl. *occipita*, gen. *occipitis*. Occiput (back of the head). 3rd declension neut.
- *Oculentum*, pl. *oculenta*, gen. *oculenti*. Eye ointment. 2nd declension neut.
- *Oculus*, pl. *oculi*, gen. *oculi*. Eye. 2nd declension masc.
- *Oliva*, pl. *olivae*, gen. *olivae*. Rounded elevation (lit. *olive*). 1st declension fem.
- *Omentum*, pl. *omenta*, gen. *omenti*. Peritoneal fold. 2nd declension neut.
- *Oogonium*, pl. *oogonia*, gen. *oogonii*. Oocyte. 2nd declension neut.
- *Operculum*, pl. *opercula*, gen. *operculi*. Operculum, cover (lit. *lesser lid*). 2nd declension neut.
- *Orbicularis m.*, pl. *orbiculares*, gen. *orbicularis*. Muscle encircling a structure. 3rd declension masc. (adj.: masc. *orbicularis*, fem. *orbicularis*, neut. *orbiculare*)
- *Organum*, pl. *organa*, gen. *organi*. Organ. 2nd declension neut.
- *Orificium*, pl. *orificia*, gen. *orificii*. Opening, orifice. 2nd declension neut.
- *Os*, pl. *ora*, gen. *oris*. Mouth. 3rd declension neut. *Os* + genitive case: *os coccyges* (coccigeal bone), *os ischii* (ischium)
- *Os*, pl. *ossa*, gen. *ossis*. Bone. 3rd declension neut.
- *Ossiculum*, pl. *ossicula*, gen. *ossiculi*. Ossicle, small bone. 2nd declension masc.

- *Ostium*, pl. *ostia*, gen. *ostii*. Opening into a tubular organ, entrance. 2nd declension neut.
- *Ovalis*, pl. *ovales*, gen. *ovalis*. Oval. 3rd declension masc. (adj.: masc. *ovalis*, fem. *ovalis*, neut. *ovale*)
- *Ovarium*, pl. *ovaria*, gen. *ovarii*. Ovary. 2nd declension neut.
- *Ovulum*, pl. *ovula*, gen. *ovuli*. Ovule. 2nd declension neut.

P

- *Palatum*, pl. *palata*, gen. *palati*. Palate. 2nd declension neut.
- *Palma*, pl. *palmae*, gen. *palmae*. Palm. 1st declension fem.
- *Palmaris*, pl. *palmares*, gen. *palmaris*. Relative to the palm of the hand. 3rd declension masc. (adj.: masc. *palmaris*, fem. *palmaris*, neut. *palmare*)
- *Palpebra*, pl. *palpebrae*, gen. *palpebrae*. Eyelid. 1st declension fem.
- *Pancreas*, pl. *pancreates/pancreata*, gen. *pancreatis*. Pancreas. 3rd declension fem./neut.
- *Panniculus*, pl. *panniculi*, gen. *panniculi*. Panniculus (a layer of tissue, from *pannus*, pl. *panni*, cloth). 2nd declension masc.
- *Pannus*, pl. *panni*, gen. *panni*. Pannus (lit. *cloth*). 2nd declension masc.
- *Papilla*, pl. *papillae*, gen. *papillae*. Papilla (lit. *nipple*). 1st declension fem.
- *Paralysis*, pl. *paralyses*, gen. *paralysos/paralysis*. Palsy. 3rd declension fem.
- *Parametrium*, pl. *parametria*, gen. *parametrii*. Parametrium. 2nd declension neut.
- *Paries*, pl. *parietes*, gen. *parietis*. Wall. 3rd declension masc.
- *Pars*, pl. *partes*, gen. *partis*. Part. 3rd declension fem.
- *Patella*, pl. *patellae*, gen. *patellae*. Patella. 1st declension fem.
- *Pectoralis m.*, pl. *pectorales*, gen. *pectoralis*. Pectoralis muscle. 3rd declension masc. (adj.: masc. *pectoralis*, fem. *pectoralis*, neut. *pectorale*)
- *Pectus*, pl. *pectora*, gen. *pectoris*. Chest. 3rd declension neut. *Pectus excavatum, pectus carinatum*
- *Pediculus*, pl. *pediculi*, gen. *pediculi*. 1. Pedicle. 2. Louse. 2nd declension masc.
- *Pedunculus*, pl. *pedunculi*, gen. *pedunculi*. Pedicle. 2nd declension masc.
- *Pelvis*, pl. *pelves*, gen. *pelvis*. Pelvis. 3rd declension fem.
- *Penis*, pl. *penes*, gen. *penis*. Penis. 3rd declension masc.
- *Perforans*, pl. *perforantes*, gen. *perforantis*. Something which pierces a structure. 3rd declension masc.
- *Pericardium*, pl. *pericardia*, gen. *pericardii*. Pericardium. 2nd declension neut.

- *Perimysium*, pl. *perimysia*, gen. *perimysii*. Perimysium (from Gr. *mysia*, muscle). 2nd declension neut.
- *Perineum*, pl. *perinea*, gen. *perinei*. Perineum. 2nd declension neut.
- *Perineurium*, pl. *perineuria*, gen. *perineurii*. Perineurium (from Gr. *neuron*, nerve). 2nd declension neut.
- *Periodontium*, pl. *periodontia*, gen. *periodontii*. Periodontium (from Gr. *odous*, tooth). 2nd declension neut.
- *Perionychium*, pl. *perionychia*, gen. *perionychii*. Perionychium (from Gr. *onyx*, nail). 2nd declension neut.
- *Periosteum*, pl. *periostea*, gen. *periosteii*. Periosteum (from Gr. *osteon*, bone). 2nd declension neut.
- *Periostosis*, pl. *periostoses*, gen. *periostosis*. Periostosis. 3rd declension
- *Peritoneum*, pl. *peritonea*, gen. *peritonei*. Peritoneum. 2nd declension neut.
- *Peroneus m.*, pl. *peronei*, gen. *peronei*. Peroneal bone. 2nd declension masc.
- *Pes*, pl. *pedes*, gen. *pedis*. Foot. 3rd declension masc.
- *Petechia*, pl. *petechiae*, gen. *petechiae*. Petechiae (tiny hemorrhagic spots). 1st declension fem.
- *Phalanx*, pl. *phalanges*, gen. *phalangis*. Phalanx (long bones of the digits). 3rd declension fem. *Os phalangi*, pl. *ossa phalangium*
- *Phallus*, pl. *phalli*, gen. *phalli*. Phallus, penis. 2nd declension masc.
- *Pharynx*, pl. *pharynges*, gen. *pharyngis*. Pharynx. 3rd declension
- *Philtrum*, pl. *philtra*, gen. *philtri*. Philtrum. 2nd declension neut.
- *Phimosis*, pl. *phimoses*, gen. *phimosis*. Phimosis. 3rd declension masc.
- *Phlyctena*, pl. *phlyctenae*, gen. *phlyctenae*. Phlyctena (small blister). 1st declension fem.
- *Pia mater*, pl. *piae matres*, gen. *piae matris*. Pia mater (inner meningeal layer of tissue). 1st declension fem. (adj.: masc. *pius*, fem. *pia*, neut. *pium*, tender)
- *Placenta*, pl. *placentae*, gen. *placentae*. Placenta (lit. *cake*). 1st declension fem.
- *Planta*, pl. *plantae*, gen. *plantae*. Plant, sole. 1st declension fem.
- *Plantar*, pl. *plantaria*, gen. *plantaris*. Relating to the sole of the foot. 3rd declension neut.
- *Planum*, pl. *plana*, gen. *plani*. Plane. 2nd declension neut.
- *Platysma m.*, pl. *platysmata*, gen. *platysmatis*. Platysma. 3rd declension neut.
- *Pleura*, pl. *pleurae*, gen. *pleurae*. Pleura. 1st declension fem.
- *Plica*, pl. *plicae*, gen. *plicae*. Fold. 1st declension fem.
- *Pneumoconiosis*, pl. *pneumoconioses*, gen. *pneumoconiosis*. Pneumoconiosis. 3rd declension

- *Pollex*, pl. *pollices*, gen. *pollicis*. Thumb. 3rd declension masc.
- *Polus*, pl. *poli*, gen. *poli*. Pole. 2nd declension masc.
- *Pons*, pl. *pontes*, gen. *pontis*. Pons (lit. *bridge*). 3rd declension masc.
- *Porta*, pl. *portae*, gen. *portae*. Porta (from Lat. verb *porto*, carry, bring). 1st declension fem.
- *Portio*, pl. *portiones*, gen. *portionis*. Portion. 3rd declension fem.
- *Porus*, pl. *pori*, gen. *pori*. Pore. 2nd declension masc.
- *Posterior*, pl. *posteriores*, gen. *posterioris*. Coming after. 3rd declension
- *Praeputium*, pl. *praeputia*, gen. *praeputii*. Prepuce, foreskin. 2nd declension neut.
- *Princeps*, pl. *principes*, gen. *principis*. Princeps (first, foremost, leading). 3rd declension masc.
- *Processus*, pl. *processus*, gen. *processus*. Process. 4th declension masc.
- *Profunda*, pl. *profundae*, gen. *profundae*. Deep. 1st declension fem. (adj.: masc. *profundus*, fem. *profunda*, neut. *profundum*). *Vena femoralis profunda*, deep femoral vein
- *Prominentia*, pl. *prominentiae*, gen. *prominentiae*. Prominence. 1st declension fem.
- *Promontorium*, pl. *promontoria*, gen. *promontorii*. Promontorium. 2nd declension neut.
- *Pronator*, pl. *pronatores*, gen. *pronatoris*. A muscle that serves to pronate. 3rd declension masc. *Pronator teres m., pronator quadratus m.*
- *Prophylaxis*, pl. *prophylaxes*, gen. *prophylaxis*. Prophylaxis (from Gr. *prophylasso*, take precaution). 3rd declension
- *Proprius*, pl. *proprii*, gen. *proprii*. Own. 2nd declension masc. (adj.: masc. *proprius*, fem. *propria*, neut. *proprium*)
- *Prosthesis*, pl. *prostheses*, gen. *prosthesis*. Prosthesis. 3rd declension fem.
- *Psychosis*, pl. *psychoses*, gen. *psychosis*. Psychosis. 3rd declension fem.
- *Ptosis*, pl. *ptoses*, gen. *ptosis*. Ptosis. 3rd declension
- *Pubes*, pl. *pubes*, gen. *pubis*. Pubis. 3rd declension fem.
- *Pudendum*, pl. *pudenda*, gen. *pudendi*. Relative to the external genitals (lit. *shameful*). 2nd declension neut. (adj.: masc. *pudendus*, fem. *pudenda*, neut. *pudendum*)
- *Puerpera*, pl. *puerperae*, gen. *puerperae*. Puerpera. 1st declension fem.
- *Puerperium*, pl. *puerperia*, gen. *puerperii*. Puerperium. 2nd declension neut.
- *Pulmo*, pl. *pulmones*, gen. *pulmonis*. Lung. 3rd declension masc.
- *Punctata*, pl. *punctatae*, gen. *punctatae*. Pointed. 1st declension fem.
- *Punctum*, pl. *puncta*, gen. *puncti*. Point. 2nd declension neut.
- *Pylorus*, pl. *pylori*, gen. *pylori*. Pylorus. 2nd declension masc.

- *Pyramidalis m.*, pl. *pyramidales*, gen. *pyramidalis*. Pyramidal. 3rd declension masc. (adj.: masc. *pyramidalis*, fem. *pyramidalis*, neut. *pyramidale*)
- *Pyriformis m.*, pl. *pyriformes*, gen. *pyriformis*. Pear-shaped. 3rd declension masc. (adj.: masc. *pyriformis*, fem. *pyriformis*, neut. *pyriforme*)

Q

- *Quadratus*, pl. *quadrati*, gen. *quadrati*. Square. 2nd declension masc. (adj.: masc. *quadratus*, fem. *quadrata*, neut. *quadratum*)
- *Quadrigemina*, pl. *quadrigeminae*, gen. *quadrigeminae*. Fourfold, in four parts. 1st declension fem. (adj.: *quadrigeminus*, fem. *quadrigemina*, neut. *quadrigeminum*)

R

- *Rachis*, pl. Lat. *rachides*, pl. Engl. *rachises*, gen. *rachidis*. Rachis, vertebral column. 3rd declension
- *Radiatio*, pl. *radiationes*, gen. *radiationis*. Radiation. 3rd declension fem.
- *Radius*, pl. *radii*, gen. *radii*. Radius. 2nd declension masc.
- *Radix*, pl. *radices*, gen. *radicis*. Root, base. 3rd declension fem.
- *Ramus*, pl. *rami*, gen. *rami*. Branch. 2nd declension masc.
- *Receptaculum*, pl. *receptacula*, gen. *receptaculi*. Receptacle, reservoir. 2nd declension neut.
- *Recessus*, pl. *recessus*, gen. *recessus*. Recess. 4th declension masc.
- *Rectus*, pl. *recti*, gen. *recti*. Right, straight (adj.: masc. *rectus*, fem. *recta*, neut. *rectum*). Rectus abdominis m.
- *Regio*, pl. *regiones*, gen. *regionis*. Region. 3rd declension fem.
- *Ren*, pl. *renes*, gen. *renis*. Kidney. 3rd declension masc.
- *Rete*, pl. *retia*, gen. *Retis*. Network, net. 3rd declension neut. *Rete mirabilis*
- *Reticulum*, pl. *reticula*, gen. *reticuli*. Reticulum. 2nd declension neut.
- *Retinaculum*, pl. *retinacula*, gen. *retinaculi*. Retinaculum (retaining band or ligament). 2nd declension neut.
- *Rima*, pl. *rimae*, gen. *rima*. Fissure, slit. 1st declension fem.
- *Rostrum*, pl. *rostra*, gen. *rostri*. Rostrum (beak-shaped structure). 2nd declension neut.
- *Rotundum*, pl. *rotunda*, gen. *rotundi*. Round declension (adj.: masc. *rotundus*, fem. *rotunda*, neut. *Ruga*, pl. *rugae*, gen. *rugae*. Wrinkle, fold. 1st declension fem.

S

- *Sacculus*, pl. *sacculi*, gen. *sacculi*. Small pouch. 2nd declension masc.
- *Saccus*, pl. *sacci*, gen. *sacci*. Pouch. 2nd declension masc.

- *Sacrum*, pl. *sacra*, gen. *sacri*. Sacral bone (lit. *sacred vessel*). 2ⁿᵈ declension neut.
- *Salpinx*, pl. *salpinges*, gen. *salpingis*. Fallopian tube. 3ʳᵈ declension
- *Sartorius m.*, pl. *sartorii*, gen. *sartorii*. Sartorius muscle (tailor's muscle). 2ⁿᵈ declension masc.
- *Scalenus m.*, gen. *scaleni*, pl. *scaleni*. Uneven. 2ⁿᵈ declension masc.
- *Scapula*, pl. *scapulae*, gen. *scapulae*. Scapula, shoulder blade. 1ˢᵗ declension fem.
- *Sclerosis*, pl. *scleroses*, gen. *sclerosis*. Sclerosis. 3ʳᵈ declension
- *Scolex*, pl. *scoleces*, gen. *scolecis*. Scolex. 3ʳᵈ declension
- *Scotoma*, pl. *scotomata*, gen. *scotomatis*. Scotoma. 3ʳᵈ declension neut.
- *Scrotum*, pl. *scrota*, gen. *scroti*. Scrotum. 2ⁿᵈ declension neut.
- *Scutulum*, pl. *scutula*, gen. *scutuli*. Scutulum. 2ⁿᵈ declension neut.
- *Scybalum*, pl. *scybala*, gen. *scybali*. Scybalum. 2ⁿᵈ declension neut.
- *Segmentum*, pl. *segmenta*, gen. *segmenti*. Segment. 2ⁿᵈ declension neut.
- *Sella turcica*, pl. *sellae turcicae*, gen. *sellae turcicae*. Turkish chair. 1ˢᵗ declension fem.
- *Semen*, pl. *semina*, gen. *seminis*. Semen. 3ʳᵈ declension neut.
- *Semimembranosus m.*, pl. *semimembranosi*, gen. *semimembranosi*. 2ⁿᵈ declension masc.
- *Semitendinosus m.*, pl. *semitendinosi*, gen. *semitendinosi*. 2ⁿᵈ declension masc.
- *Sensorium*, pl. *sensoria*, gen. *sensorii*. Sensorium. 2ⁿᵈ declension neut.
- *Sepsis*, pl. *sepses*, gen. *sepsis*. Sepsis. 3ʳᵈ declension
- *Septum*, pl. *septa*, gen. *septi*. Septum. 2ⁿᵈ declension neut.
- *Sequela*, pl. *sequelae*, gen. *sequelae*. Sequela. 1ˢᵗ declension fem.
- *Sequestrum*, pl. *sequestra*, gen. *sequestri*. Sequestrum (from sequester, go-between). 2ⁿᵈ declension neut.
- *Serosa*, pl. *serosae*, gen. *serosae*. Serosa. 1ˢᵗ declension fem.
- *Serratus m.*, pl. *serrati*, gen. *serrati*. Serrated, toothed like a saw. 2ⁿᵈ declension masc.
- *Serum*, pl. *sera*, gen. *seri*. Serum (lit. *whey*). 2ⁿᵈ declension neut.
- *Sinciput*, pl. *sincipita*, gen. *sincipitis*. Sinciput. 3ʳᵈ declension neut.
- *Sinus*, pl. *sinus*, gen. *sinus*. Sinus. 4ᵗʰ declension masc.
- *Soleus m.*, pl. *solei*, gen. *solei*. Soleus. 2ⁿᵈ declension masc.
- *Spatium*, pl. *spatia*, gen. *spatii*. Space. 2ⁿᵈ declension neut.
- *Spectrum*, pl. *spectra*, gen. *spectri*. Spectrum. 2ⁿᵈ declension neut.
- *Sphincter*, pl. Lat. *sphincteres*, pl. Engl. *sphincters*, gen. *sphincteris*. Sphincter. 3ʳᵈ declension masc.
- *Spiculum*, pl. *spicula*, gen. *spiculi*. Spike (lit. *sting*). 2ⁿᵈ declension neut.
- *Spina*, pl. *spinae*, gen. *spinae*. Spine. 1ˢᵗ declension fem.

- *Splenium*, pl. *splenia*, gen. *splenii*. Splenium. 2nd declension neut. *Splenius capitis/colli m.*
- *Splenunculus*, pl. *splenunculi*, gen. *splenunculi*. Accessory spleen. 2nd declension masc.
- *Sputum*, pl. *sputa*, gen. *sputi*. Sputum. 2nd declension neut.
- *Squama*, pl. *squamae*, gen. *squamae*. Squama (scale, plate-like structure). 1st declension fem.
- *Stapes*, pl. *stapedes*, gen. *stapedis*. Stapes. 3rd declension masc.
- *Staphylococcus*, pl. *staphylococci*, gen. *staphylococci*. Staphylococcus. 2nd declension masc.
- *Stasis*, pl. *stases*, gen. *stasis*. Stasis. 3rd declension masc.
- *Statoconium*, pl. *statoconia*, gen. *statoconii*. Statoconium. 2nd declension neut.
- *Stenosis*, pl. *stenoses*, gen. *stenosis*. Stenosis. 3rd declension
- *Stereocilium*, pl. *stereocilia*, gen. *stereocilii*. Stereocilium. 2nd declension neut.
- *Sternocleidomastoideus m.*, pl. *sternocleidomastoidei*, gen. *sternocleidomastoidei*. 2nd declension masc.
- *Sternum*, pl. *sterna*, gen. *sterni*. Sternum. 2nd declension neut.
- *Stigma*, pl. *stigmata*, gen. *stigmatis*. Stigma (mark aiding in diagnosis). 3rd declension neut.
- *Stimulus*, pl. *stimuli*, gen. *stimuli*. Stimulus (lit. *spur*). 2nd declension masc.
- *Stoma*, pl. *stomata*, gen. *stomatis*. Stoma, opening, hole. 3rd declension neut.
- *Stratum*, pl. *strata*, gen. *strati*. Stratum. 2nd declension neut.
- *Stria*, pl. *striae*, gen. *striae*. Fluting, channel. 1st declension fem.
- *Stroma*, pl. *stromata*, gen. *stromatis*. Stroma. 3rd declension neut.
- *Struma*, pl. *strumae*, gen. *strumae*. Struma. 1st declension fem.
- *Subiculum*, pl. *subicula*, gen. *subiculi*. Subiculum. 2nd declension neut.
- *Substantia*, pl. *substantiae*, gen. *substantiae*. Substance. 1st declension fem.
- *Sulcus*, pl. *sulci*, gen. *sulci*. Sulcus. 2nd declension masc.
- *Supercilium*, pl. *supercilia*, gen. *supercilii*. Eyebrow. 2nd declension neut.
- *Superficialis*, pl. *superficiales*, gen. *superficialis*. Superficial. 3rd declension masc. (adj.: masc. *superficialis*, fem. *superficialis*, neut. *superficiale*)
- *Superior*, pl. *superiores*, gen. *superioris*. Higher, upper, greater. 3rd declension
- *Sustentaculum*, pl. *sustentacula*, gen. *sustentaculi*. Sustentaculum. 2nd declension neut.
- *Sutura*, pl. *suturae*, gen. *suturae*. Suture. 1st declension fem.

- *Symphysis*, pl. *symphyses*, gen. *symphysis*. Symphysis. 3rd declension
- *Synchondrosis*, pl. *synchondroses*, gen. *synchondrosis*. Synchondrosis. 3rd declension
- *Syncytium*, pl. *syncytia*, gen. *syncytii*. Syncytium. 2nd declension neut.
- *Syndesmosis*, pl. *syndesmoses*, gen. *syndesmosis*. Syndesmosis. 3rd declension
- *Synechia*, pl. *synechiae*, gen. *synechiae*. Synechia. 1st declension fem.
- *Syrinx*, pl. *syringes*, gen. *syringis*. Syrinx. 3rd declension

T

- *Talus*, pl. *tali*, gen. *tali*. Talus. 2nd declension masc.
- *Tarsus*, pl. *tarsi*, gen. *tarsi*. Tarsus. 2nd declension masc.
- *Tectum*, pl. *tecta*, gen. *tecti*. Roof. 2nd declension neut.
- *Tegmen*, pl. *tegmina*, gen. *tegminis*. Roof, covering. 3rd declension neut.
- *Tegmentum*, pl. *tegmenta*, gen. *tegmenti*. Covering. 2nd declension neut.
- *Tela*, pl. *telae*, gen. *telae*. Membrane (lit. *web*). 1st declension fem.
- *Telangiectasis*, pl. *telangiectases*, gen. *telangiectasis*. Telangiectasis. 3rd declension
- *Temporalis m.*, pl. *temporales*, gen. *temporalis*. 3rd declension masc. (adj.: masc. *temporalis*, fem. *temporalis*, neut. *temporale*)
- *Tenaculum*, pl. *tenacula*, gen. *tenaculi*. Surgical clamp. 2nd declension neut.
- *Tendo*, pl. *tendines*, gen. *tendinis*. Tendon, sinew (from verb *tendo*, stretch). 3rd declension masc.
- *Tenia*, pl. *teniae*, gen. *teniae*. Tenia. 1st declension fem.
- *Tensor*, pl. *tensores*, gen. *tensoris*. Something that stretches, that tenses a muscle. 3rd declension masc.
- *Tentorium*, pl. *tentoria*, gen. *tentorii*. Tentorium. 2nd declension neut.
- *Teres*, pl. *teretes*, gen. *teretis*. Round and long. 3rd declension masc.
- *Testis*, pl. *testes*, gen. *testis*. Testicle. 3rd declension masc.
- *Thalamus*, pl. *thalami*, gen. *thalami*. Thalamus (lit. *marriage bed*). 2nd declension masc.
- *Theca*, pl. *thecae*, gen. *thecae*. Theca, envelope (lit. *case*, *box*). 1st declension fem.
- *Thelium*, pl. *thelia*, gen. *thelii*. Nipple. 2nd declension neut.
- *Thenar*, pl. *thenares*, gen. *thenaris*. Relative to the palm of the hand. 3rd declension neut.
- *Thesis*, pl. *theses*, gen. *thesis*. Thesis. 3rd declension fem.
- *Thorax*, pl. *thoraces*, gen. *thoracos/thoracis*. Chest. 3rd declension masc.
- *Thrombosis*, pl. *thromboses*, gen. *thombosis*. Thrombosis. 3rd declension
- *Thrombus*, pl. *thrombi*, gen. *thrombi*. Thrombus, clot (from Gr. *thrombos*). 2nd declension masc.

- *Thymus*, pl. *thymi*, gen. *thymi*. Thymus. 2nd declension masc.
- *Tibia*, pl. *tibiae*, gen. *tibiae*. Tibia. 1st declension fem.
- *Tonsilla*, pl. *tonsillae*, gen. *tonsillae*. Tonsil. 1st declension fem.
- *Tophus*, pl. *tophi*, gen. *tophi*. Tophus. 2nd declension masc.
- *Torulus*, pl. *toruli*, gen. *toruli*. Papilla, small elevation. 2nd declension masc.
- *Trabecula*, pl. *trabeculae*, gen. *trabeculae*. Trabecula (supporting bundle of either osseous or fibrous fibers). 1st declension fem.
- *Trachea*, pl. *tracheae*, gen. *tracheae*. Trachea. 1st declension fem.
- *Tractus*, pl. *tractus*, gen. *tractus*. Tract. 4th declension masc.
- *Tragus*, pl. *tragi*, gen. *tragi*. Tragus, hircus. 2nd declension masc.
- *Transversalis*, pl. *transversales*, gen. *transversalis*. Transverse. 3rd declension (adj.: masc. *transversalis*, fem. *transversalis*, neut. *transversale*)
- *Transversus*, pl. *transversi*, gen. *transversi*. Lying across, from side to side. 2nd declension masc. (adj.: masc. *transversus*, fem. *transversa*, neut. *transversum*)
- *Trapezium*, pl. *trapezia*, gen. *trapezii*. Trapezium bone. 2nd declension neut.
- *Trauma*, pl. *traumata*, gen. *traumatis*. Trauma. 3rd declension neut.
- *Triangularis*, pl. *triangulares*, gen. *triangularis*. Triangular. 3rd declension masc. (adj.: masc. *triangularis*, fem. *triangularis*, neut. *triangulare*)
- *Triceps*, pl. *tricipes*, gen. *tricipis*. Triceps (from *ceps*, pl. *cipes*, gen. *cipis*, headed). 3rd declension masc.
- *Trigonum*, pl. *trigona*, gen. *trigoni*. Trigonum (lit. *triangle*). 2nd declension neut.
- *Triquetrum*, pl. *triquetra*, gen. *triquetri*. Triquetrum, triquetral bone, pyramidal bone. 2nd declension neut. (adj.: masc. *triquetrus*, fem. *triquetra*, neut. *triquetrum*. Three-cornered, triangular)
- *Trochlea*, pl. *trochleae*, gen. *trochleae*. Trochlea (lit. *pulley*). 1st declension fem.
- *Truncus*, pl. *trunci*, gen. *trunci*. Trunk. 2nd declension masc.
- *Tuba*, pl. *tubae*, gen. *tubae*. Tube. 1st declension fem.
- *Tuberculum*, pl. *tubercula*, gen. *tuberculi*. Tuberculum, swelling, protuberance. 2nd declension neut.
- *Tubulus*, pl. *tubuli*, gen. *tubuli*. Tubule. 2nd declension masc.
- *Tunica*, pl. *tunicae*, gen. *tunicae*. Tunic. 1st declension fem.
- *Tylosis*, pl. *tyloses*, gen. *tylosis*. Tylosis (callosity). 3rd declension
- *Tympanum*, pl. *tympana*, gen. *tympani*. Tympanum, eardrum (lit. *Small drum*). 2nd declension neut.

U

- *Ulcus*, pl. *ulcera*, gen. *ulceris*. Ulcer. 3rd declension neut.

- *Ulna*, pl. *ulnae*, gen. *ulnae*. Ulna (lit. *forearm*). 1st declension fem.
- *Umbilicus*, pl. *umbilici*, gen. *umbiculi*. Navel. 2nd declension masc.
- *Uncus*, pl. *unci*, gen. *unci*. Uncus (lit. *hook, clamp*). 2nd declension masc.
- *Unguis*, pl. *ungues*, gen. *unguis*. Nail, claw. 3rd declension masc.
- *Uterus*, pl. *uteri*, gen. *uteri*. Uterus, womb. 2nd declension masc.
- *Utriculus*, pl. *utriculi*, gen. *utriculi*. Utriculus (lit. *wineskin*). 2nd declension masc.
- *Uveitis*, pl. *uveitides*, gen. *uveitidis*. Uve'tis. 3rd declension fem.
- *Uvula*, pl. *uvulae*, gen. *uvulae*. Uvula (lit. *small grape*, from *uva*, pl. *uvae*, grape). 1st declension fem.

V

- *Vagina*, pl. *vaginae*, gen. *vaginae*. Vagina, sheath. 1st declension fem.
- *Vaginitis*, pl. *vaginitides*, gen. *vaginitidis*. Vaginitis. 3rd declension fem.
- *Vagus*, pl. *vagi*, gen. *vagi*. Vagus nerve. 2nd declension masc. (adj.: masc. *vagus*, fem. *vaga*, neut. *vagum*. Roving, wandering)
- *Valva*, pl. *valvae*, gen. *valvae*. Leaflet. 1st declension fem.
- *Valvula*, pl. *valvulae*, gen. *valvulae*. Valve. 1st declension fem.
- *Varix*, pl. *varices*, gen. *varicis*. Varix, varicose vein. 3rd declension masc.
- *Vas*, pl. *vasa*, gen. *vasis*. Vessel. 3rd declension neut. *Vas deferens, vasa recta, vasa vasorum*
- *Vasculum*, pl. *vascula*, gen. *vasculi*. Small vessel. 2nd declension neut.
- *Vastus*, pl. *vasti*, gen. *vasti*. Vast, huge. 2nd declension neut. (adj.: masc. *vastus*, fem. *vasta*, neut. *vasti*) *Vastus medialis/intermedius/lateralis m.*
- *Vasum*, pl. *vasa*, gen. *vasi*. Vessel. 2nd declension neut.
- *Velum*, pl. *veli*, gen. *veli*. Covering, curtain (lit. *sail*). 2nd declension neut.
- *Vena*, pl. *venae*, gen. *venae*. Vein. 1st declension fem. *Vena cava*, pl. *venae cavae*, gen. *venae cavae* (from adj. *cavus/a/um*, hollow)
- *Ventriculus*, pl. *ventriculi*, gen. *ventriculi*. Ventricle (lit. *small belly*). 2nd declension masc.
- *Venula*, pl. *venulae*, gen. *venulae*. Venule. 1st declension fem.
- *Vermis*, pl. *vermes*, gen. *vermis*. Worm. 3rd declension masc.
- *Verruca*, pl. *verrucae*, gen. *verrucae*. Wart. 1st declension fem.
- *Vertebra*, pl. *vertebrae*, gen. *vertebrae*. Vertebra. 1st declension fem.
- *Vertex*, pl. *vertices*, gen. *verticis*. Vertex (lit. *peak, top*). 3rd declension masc.
- *Vesica*, pl. *vesicae*, gen. *vesicae*. Bladder. 1st declension fem.
- *Vesicula*, pl. *vesiculae*, gen. *vesiculae*. Vesicle (lit. *lesser bladder*). 1st declension fem.
- *Vestibulum*, pl. *vestibula*, gen. *vestibuli*. Entrance to a cavity. 2nd declension neut.

- *Villus*, pl. *villi*, gen. *villi*. Villus (shaggy hair). 2nd declension masc.
- *Vinculum*, pl. *vincula*, gen. *vinculi*. Band, band-like structure (lit. *chain, bond*). 2nd declension neut.
- *Virus*, pl. Lat. *viri*, pl. Engl. *viruses*, gen. *viri*. Virus. 2nd declension masc.
- *Viscus*, pl. *viscera*, gen. *visceris*. Viscus, internal organ. 3rd declension neut.
- *Vitiligo*, pl. *vitiligines*, gen. *vitiligis*. Vitiligo. 3rd declension masc.
- *Vomer*, pl. *vomeres*, gen. *vomeris*. Vomer bone. 3rd declension masc.
- *Vulva*, pl. *vulvae*, gen. *vulvae*. Vulva. 1st declension fem.

Z

- *Zona*, pl. *zonae*, gen. *zonae*. Zone. 1st declension fem.
- *Zonula*, pl. *zonulae*, gen. *zonulae*. Small zone. 1st declension fem.
- *Zygapophysis*, pl. *zygapophyses*, gen. *zygapophysis*. Vertebral articular apophysis. 3rd declension fem.

Desinenze

- **ectomy** significa la rimozione chirurgica di qualcosa, per esempio l'appendice in **appendectomy** o **appendicectomy**.
- **otomy** fa riferimento all'atto del tagliare o affettare una parte del corpo, per esempio **laparotomy**, operazione che consiste nell'aprire l'addome.
- **stomy** consiste nella creazione di un'apertura artificiale, come in **colostomy**, un'apertura del colon attraverso la parete addominale per deviare le feci all'esterno.
- **pathy** si riferisce a una malattia, come in **neurophaty**, patologia che colpisce i nervi.
- **itis** significa infiammazione, come in **gastritis**, infiammazione dello stomaco.
- **emesis** sta per vomito, come in **Hematemesis**, che significa vomitare sangue.

Capitolo 10

Acronimi e abbreviazioni in chirurgia e in medicina

Introduzione

"The patient went from the ER to the OR and then to the ICU". Indubbiamente il lessico dei medici è ricco di abbreviazioni, tanto che gli operatori della sanità in generale e i chirurghi in particolare adoperano perlomeno dieci abbreviazioni per minuto (questa è una statistica fatta in casa, non citatela).

Vi sono diversi "tipi" di abbreviazioni:
- abbreviazioni dirette
- abbreviazioni immediate
- abbreviazioni che espandono il termine
- abbreviazioni che risparmiano energia
- abbreviazioni a doppio senso
- abbreviazioni che espandono la mente

Iniziamo dalle più simpatiche; le chiamiamo abbreviazioni dirette perché sono quelle in cui esiste un'equivalenza di termini tra l'italiano e l'inglese; in questi casi, non ci sono difficoltà. È necessario solo invertire l'ordine delle parole, identificare le abbreviazioni e impararle.
Vediamo alcuni esempi, così che possiate godere delle cose semplici della vita...fino a che potete!

HRT	Hormone-replacement therapy
LVOT	Left ventricle outflow tract
ASD	Atrial septal defect
VSD	Ventricular septal defect
TEE	Transesophageal echocardiography
LAD	Left anterior descending artery
ACE	Angiotensin-converting enzyme

R. Ribes, P. J. Aranda, J. Giba, *Inglese per chirurghi*,
© Springer-Verlag Italia 2012

Le abbreviazioni immediate sono impiegate più frequentemente per farmaci e sostanze chimiche il cui nome possiede tre o quattro sillabe di troppo. Le chiamiamo immediate perché in genere sono le stesse in diverse lingue. Vediamo un esempio:

CPK   Creatin phosphokinase

Di seguito riportiamo alcuni esempi di abbreviazioni largamente impiegate nella lingua inglese, ma in genere utilizzate nella loro forma esplicita in altre lingue. Siccome la lingua è in continuo cambiamento, siamo sicuri che questi termini possano avere un'abbreviazione nelle diverse lingue; tuttavia, vengono perlopiù impiegati nella loro forma esplicita.

NSCLC Non-small-cell lung cancer
PBSC   Peripheral blood stem cells

Esiste un altro gruppo di abbreviazioni, quelle "che risparmiano energia". Queste sono abbreviazioni che in molte lingue vengono mantenute nella forma inglese, per cui, quando vengono espanse, la prima lettera di ciascuna parola non combacia con l'abbreviazione. Le possiamo chiamare "abbreviazioni che risparmiano energia" in quanto non è così difficile arrivare all'abbreviazione "nazionale" di questi termini. In questi esempi, possiamo notare che la maggior parte dei nomi degli ormoni vengono abbreviati con sigle che risparmiano energia:

FSH   Follicle-stimulating hormone
TNF   Tumor necrosis factor
PAWP   Pulmonary arterial wedge pressure

Esiste un altro tipo di abbreviazioni, che chiamiamo "a doppio senso". In questi casi, un'abbreviazione si riferisce a due diversi termini. Il contesto aiuta, ovviamente, nell'individuare il significato reale; tuttavia, è importante fare particolare attenzione, in quanto un errore interpretativo può portare a situazioni anche imbarazzanti:

- PCR
  - Polymerase chain reaction
  - Plasma clearance rate
  - Pathological complete response
  - Protein catabolic rate

- HEV
    - Human enteric virus
    - Hepatitis E virus

- PID
    - Pelvic inflammatory disease
    - Prolapsed intervertebral disc

- CSF
    - Colony-stimulating factor
    - Cerebrospinal fluid

Le abbreviazioni più strane sono quelle in cui la pronuncia dell'acronimo ricorda una parola che non ha nessuna relazione con il significato dell'abbreviazione. Noi chiamiamo questo gruppo "le abbreviazioni che espandono la mente".

Il *cabbage* in inglese è il cavolo, un ortaggio dotato di proprietà gasogenica; tuttavia, quando un chirurgo dice "This patient is a clear candidate for cabbage" non indica che cosa il paziente debba mangiare, ma piuttosto sta suggerendo il tipo di chirurgia a cui il paziente debba essere sottoposto, che è quella del CABG (*coronary artery bypass grafting*; bypass aorto-coronarico).
Se vi capita di ascoltare per caso un oncologo che dice: "I think your patient needs a CHOP," vi chiederete camminando lungo il corridoio se la nuova terapia alternativa consiste in una braciola di maiale o di agnello. Ma subito dopo capirete che lo specialista si riferiva al CHOP (uno schema chemioterapico contenente ciclofosfamide, idrossidaunomicina, oncovin e prednisone).
Ci sono ancora molte altre abbreviazioni e tante altre ancora ce ne saranno nel futuro. Di sicuro la professione medica ci terrà impegnati nell'inseguire tutte le sue incursioni nella creatività linguistica.

Indipendentemente dal tipo di abbreviazione che avete di fronte, diamo tre suggerimenti:

1. identificate le abbreviazioni;
2. leggete le abbreviazioni nei vostri elenchi;
3. iniziate con gli elenchi delle abbreviazioni della vostra sottospecialità chirurgica.

Leggete le abbreviazioni nei vostri elenchi.
Leggete le abbreviazioni nei vostri elenchi in maniera naturale; tenete presente che essere capaci di riconoscere delle abbreviazioni scritte potrebbe non essere sufficiente.
Da questo punto di vista ci sono tre tipi di abbreviazioni:

1. abbreviazioni di cui fare lo spelling.
2. abbreviazioni da leggere (acronimi).
3. abbreviazioni in parte da leggere e in parte di cui fare lo spelling.

Per abbreviazioni di cui fare lo spelling, intendiamo dire che ogni lettera va letta singolarmente. La maggior parte delle abbreviazioni va letta in questo modo. Pensate per esempio a PCR- se non c'è nessun vocale non si può costruire una parola in Inglese. Pensate per esempio a COPD (*chronic obstructive pulmonary disease*; BPCO) e tentate di leggerne l'abbreviazione; non adoperate la "forma esplicita" (*chronic obstructive pulmonary disease*) di una classica abbreviazione come questa perché suonerebbe terribilmente innaturale.
Alcune abbreviazioni sono diventate acronimi e per questo devono essere lette. L'ordine stesso delle loro lettere ci permette di leggerle. LAM appartiene a questo gruppo.
Nessuno capirebbe un'abbreviazione della quale va fatto lo spelling se la leggeste come una parola, così come nessuno capirebbe una parola che va letta come tale se voi ne faceste lo spelling.
 Lasciateci chiarire questo concetto con un esempio:
LAM sta per lymphangiomyomatosis e va letto "lam", pronunciato allo stesso modo di "lamb". Al contrario, nessuno vi capirebbe se pronunciaste L–A–M.
Il terzo gruppo è costituito da abbreviazioni come CPAP (*continuous positive air way pressure*; ventilazione meccanica a pressione positiva delle vie aeree) che deve essere pronunciato *C-pap*. Se voi ne fate lo spelling C-P-A-P nessuno vi capirà.

Rivedete l'elenco delle abbreviazioni della vostra sottospecialità.
Rivedete quanti più elenchi di abbreviazioni possibile della vostra specialità e ripetetele finché non acquisirete familiarità con il significato e con la pronuncia.
Sebbene ognuno debba approntare i propri elenchi di abbreviazioni, ve ne proponiamo alcune classificate per specializzazione.
Per iniziare, controllate che l'elenco della vostra specialità sia incluso, altrimenti iniziate a scriverlo da soli. Siate pazienti…questo compito può durare per il resto della vostra carriera.

Elenchi di abbreviazioni

Elenco generale

5FU	5-Fluorouracil
ABPA	Allergic bronchopulmonary aspergillosis
ACE	Angiotensin-converting enzyme
aCL	Antibodies to cardiolipin
ACTH	Adrenocorticotropic hormone
ADH	Antidiuretic hormone
ADPKD	Autosomal dominant polycystic kidney disease
AF	Atrial fibrillation
AFP	Alpha fetoprotein
AJCC	American Joint Cancer Commission
ALT	Alanine aminotransferase
α1AT	α1-Antitrypsin
AML	Acute myeloid leukemia
ANA	Antinuclear antibodies
APCs	Atrial premature complexes
API	Arterial pressure index
APUD	Amine precursor uptake and decarboxylation system
ARDS	Acute respiratory distress syndrome
ARF	Acute renal failure
AS	Ankylosing spondylitis
AST	Aspartate aminotransferase
ATN	Acute tubular necrosis
AVP	Arginine vasopressin
BAL	Bronchoalveolar lavage
BCC	Basal cell carcinoma
BCG	Bacillus Calmette-Guérin
BMT	Bone marrow transplant
BP	Bullous pemphigoid
BPF	Brazilian purpuric fever
CBD	Common bile duct
CCK	Cholecystokinin
CD	Crohn disease
CEA	Carcinoembryonic antigen
CF	Cystic fibrosis
CML	Chronic myeloid leukemia
CMML	Chronic myelomonocytic leukemia

COPD	Chronic obstructive pulmonary disease
CP	Cicatricial pemphigoid
CRF	Chronic renal failure
CRH	Corticotropin-releasing hormone
CSF	Colony stimulating factor
CT	Computed tomography
CTX	Cholera toxin
CUPS	Cancer of unknown primary site
CWP	Coal workers' pneumoconiosis
CXR	Chest X-ray
DCIS	Ductal carcinoma in situ
DLE	Discoid lupus erythematosus
DGI	Disseminated gonococcal infection
DH	Dermatitis herpetiformis
DISH	Diffuse idiopathic skeletal hyperostosis
DPB	Diastolic blood pressure
DRA	Dialysis-related amyloidosis
DRE	Digital rectal examination
DU	Duodenal ulcer
DVT	Deep venous thrombosis
EBA	Epidermolysis bullosa acquisita
EBV	Epstein Barr virus
ECG	Electrocardiogram
EGD	Esophagogastroduodenoscopy
ERCP	Endoscopic retrograde cholangiopancreatography
ESRD	End-stage renal disease
FAP	Familial amyloid polyneuropathies
FEV1	Forced expiratory volume in one second
FMF	Familial Mediterranean fever
FSGS	Focal and segmental glomerulosclerosis
FSH	Follicle-stimulating hormone
GBM	Glomerular basement membrane
GCT	Germ cell tumor
GFR	Glomerular filtration rate
GGT	γ-Glutamyltranspeptidase, γ-glutamyltransferase
GH	Growth hormone
GHRH	Growth hormone-releasing hormone
GI	Gastrointestinal
GIP	Gastrin inhibitory peptide
GU	Gastric ulcer
HBV	Hepatitis B virus
hCG	Human chorionic gonadotropin

HCV	Hepatitis C virus
HIVAN	Human immunodeficiency virus-associated nephropathy
HOA	Hypertrophic osteoarthropathy
HP	Hypersensitivity pneumonitis
HPV	Human papilloma virus
HRT	Hormone replacement therapy
HSC	Hematopoietic stem cell
HUS	Hemolytic uremic syndrome
IBD	Inflammatory bowel disease
IBS	Irritable bowel syndrome
IL	Interleukin
ILD	Interstitial lung disease
IPSID	Immunoproliferative small intestinal disease (Mediterranean lymphoma)
ITP	Idiopathic thrombocytopenic purpura
JN	Juvenile nephronophthisis
LA	Lupus anticoagulant
LBBB	Left bundle branch block
LCDD	Light chain deposition disease
LDH	Lactate dehydrogenase
LES	Lower esophageal sphincter
LH	Luteinizing hormone
LIP	Lymphoid interstitial pneumonitis
MAC	*Mycobacterium avium* complex
MALT	Mucosa-associated lymphoid tissue
MCD	Medullary cystic disease
MCD	Minimal change disease
MCHC	Mean corpuscular hemoglobin concentration
MCTD	Mixed connective tissue disease
MCV	Mean corpuscular volume
MEN1	Type 1 multiple endocrine neoplasia
MPGN	Membranoproliferative glomerulopathies
MR	Magnetic resonance
MRI	Magnetic resonance imaging
NSAIDs	Nonsteroidal anti-inflammatory drugs
NUD	Non-ulcer dyspepsia
OA	Osteoarthritis
OCG	Oral cholecystography
ODTS	Organic dust toxic syndrome
OSA	Obstructive sleep apnea
PAH	Primary alveolar hypoventilation

PAN	Polyarteritis nodosa
PAP	Pulmonary alveolar proteinosis
PBC	Primary biliary cirrhosis
PCI	Prophylactic cranial irradiation
PCP	*Pneumocystis carinii* pneumonia
PDR	Physicians' desk reference (vademecum)
PEG	Percutaneous endoscopic gastrostomy
PF	Pemphigus foliaceus
PG	Pemphigoid gestations
PIF	Prolactin inhibitory factor
PML	Progressive multifocal leukoencephalopathy
PNET	Peripheral primitive neuroectodermal tumor
PRA	Plasma renin activity
PRL	Prolactin
PSA	Prostate-specific antigen
PsA	Psoriatic arthritis
PTC	Percutaneous transhepatic cholangiography
PTE	Pulmonary thromboembolism
PTH	Parathyroid hormone
PV	Pemphigus vulgaris
RA	Rheumatoid arthritis
RBBB	Right bundle branch block
RBC	Red blood cell
RF	Rheumatoid factor
RMSF	Rocky mountain spotted fever
RPGN	Rapidly progressive glomerulonephritis
RPRF	Rapidly progressive renal failure
RTA	Renal tubular acidosis
RV	Residual volume
RVT	Renal vein thrombosis
SBC	Secondary biliary cirrhosis
SBP	Systolic blood pressure
SCC	Squamous cell carcinoma
SCID	Severe combined immunodeficiency
SCLE	Subacute cutaneous lupus erythematosus
SI	Serum iron
SIADH	Syndrome of inappropriate secretion of antidiuretic hormone
SLE	Systemic lupus erythematosus
SPB	Spontaneous bacterial peritonitis
SSc	Systemic sclerosis
SVCS	Superior vena cava syndrome

TB	Tuberculosis
TBB	Transbronchial biopsy
TGFβ	Transforming growth factor β
TIBC	Transferrin iron-binding capacity
TIPS	Transjugular intrahepatic portosystemic shunt
TLC	Total lung capacity
TNF	Tumor necrosis factor
TRH	Thyrotropin-releasing hormone
TSH	Thyroid-stimulating hormone
TTA	Transtracheal aspiration
TTP	Thrombotic thrombocytopenic purpura
UC	Ulcerative colitis
US	Ultrasonography
VATS	Video-assisted thoracic surgery
VC	Vital capacity
VF	Ventricular fibrillation
VIP	Vasoactive intestinal peptide
VPCs	Ventricular premature complexes
WBC	White blood cell
WDHA	syndrome Watery diarrhea, hypokalemia, and achlorhydria syndrome (Verner-Morrison)
ZES	Zollinger–Ellison syndrome
Wt	Weight

Liste per specialità

Anatomia

AC	Acromioclavicular joint
ACL	Anterior cruciate ligament
ACS	Anterior cervical space
ARA	Anorectal angle
ATA	Anterior tibial artery
BNA	Basle Nomina Anatomica
CBD	Common bile duct
CFA	Common femoral artery
CHA	Common hepatic artery
CHD	Common hepatic duct
CN	Cranial nerve
CNS	Central nervous system

CS	Carotid space
DCF	Deep cervical fascia
DLDCF	Deep layer of the deep cervical fascia
DRUJ	Distal radioulnar joint
ECU	Extensor carpi ulnaris
EEL	External elastic lamina
GB	Gallbladder
GDA	Gastroduodenal artery
GE	Gastroesophageal junction
GI	Gastrointestinal
IANC	International anatomical nomenclature
ICA	Internal carotid artery
ICRP	International Commission on Radiological Protection
IEL	Internal elastic lamina
IHBD	Intrahepatic biliary ducts
IMA	Inferior mesenteric artery
ITB	Iliotibial band
IVC	Inferior vena cava
JV	Jugular vein
LA	Left atrium
LAA	Left atrial appendage
LAD	Left anterior descending coronary artery
LCL	Lateral collateral ligament
LCX	Left circumflex coronary artery
LES	Lower esophageal sphincter
LGA	Left gastric artery
LHA	Left hepatic artery
LHD	Left hepatic duct
LHV	Left hepatic vein
LIMA	Left internal mammary artery
LLL	Left lower lobe (of lung)
LLQ	Left lower quadrant (of abdomen)
LPV	Left portal vein
LUCL	Lateral ulnar collateral ligament
LUL	Left upper lobe (of lung)
LUQ	Left upper quadrant (of abdomen)
LV	Left ventricle
LVOT	Left ventricular outflow tract
MCL	Medial collateral ligament
MCP	Metacarpophalangeal
MHV	Middle hepatic artery
MLDCF	Middle layer of the deep cervical fascia

MS	Masticator space
MTP	Metatarsophalangeal
NA	Nomina anatomica
OM	Obtuse marginal branch
PCL	Posterior cruciate ligament
PCS	Posterior cervical space
PDA	Posterior descending anterior coronary artery, patent ductus arteriosus
PDV	Pancreaticoduodenal vein
PHA	Proper hepatic artery
PICA	Posteroinferior cerebellar artery
PMS	Pharyngeal mucosal space
PS	Parotid space
PTA	Posterior tibial artery
PV	Portal vein
RA	Right atrium
RAS	Reticular activating system
RCL	Radial collateral ligament
RDPA	Right descending pulmonary artery
RHA	Right hepatic artery
RHD	Right hepatic duct
RHV	Right hepatic vein
RIMA	Right internal mammary artery
RL	Right lower lobe (of lung)
RLQ	Right lower quadrant (of abdomen)
RPS	Retropharyngeal space
RPV	Right portal vein
RUL	Right upper lobe (of lung)
RUQ	Right upper quadrant (of abdomen)
RV	Right ventricle
RVOT	Right ventricular outflow tract
SCF	Superficial cervical fascia
SCM	Sternocleidomastoid muscle
SCV	Subclavian vein
SFA	Superficial femoral artery
SLS	Sublingual space
SMA	Superior mesenteric artery
SMC	Smooth muscle cell
SMS	Submandibular space
SMV	Superior mesenteric vein
ST	Scapulothoracic
STT	Scaphoid–trapezium–trapezoideum

SVC	Superior vena cava
TE	Tracheoesophageal
TFCC	Triangular fibrocartilage complex
TMJ	Temporomandibular joint
TMT	Tarsometatarsal
UCL	Ulnar collateral ligament
UES	Upper esophageal sphincter
UPJ	Ureteropelvic junction
UVJ	Ureterovesical junction
VS	Visceral space

Anamnesi

AU	Auris auterque (each ear)
ABCD	Airway, breathing, circulation, defibrillate in cardiopulmonary resuscitation
ABSYS	Above symptoms
AC	a.c. Antecibum (before a meal)
ad lib.	Ad libitum (as desired; for example, a patient may be permitted to move out of bed freely and orders would, therefore, be for activities to be ad lib)
ADR	Adverse drug reaction
ANV	Nausea and vomiting symptoms
AVPU	Alert, responsive to verbal stimuli, responsive to painful stimuli, and unresponsive (assessment of mental status)
AWS	Alcohol withdrawal symptoms a/g ratio Albumin to globulin ratio
ACL	Anterior cruciate ligament (one of the most common ligament injuries to the knee; the ACL can be sprained or completely torn from trauma and/or degeneration)
AKA	Above the knee amputation
BC, BLCO, cbc	(Complete) blood count
BID, b.i.d.	Bis in die (twice a day)
BIO	Biochemistry
BIPRO	Biochemistry profile
BP	Blood pressure
BUCR	BUN and creatinine
BUN/Cr, BUCR	Blood urea nitrogen/creatinine Bandemia Slang for elevated level of band forms of white blood cells

BKA	Below the knee amputation
BMP	Basic metabolic panel: electrolytes (potassium, sodium, carbon dioxide, and chloride) and creatinine and glucose
BP	Blood pressure (blood pressure is recorded as part of the physical examination)
BSO	Bilateral salpingo-oophorectomy (a BSO is the removal of both of the ovaries and adjacent fallopian tubes and is often performed as part of a total abdominal hysterectomy)
CC	Chief complaint
CCCR	Calculated creatinine clearance
Ch D	Chirugiae doctor, surgery doctor
Cib.	Cibus (food)
COEPS	Cortically originating extrapyramidal symptoms
CPE, CPX	Complete physical examination
CR	Creatinine
CrCl	Creatinine clearance
CVS	Current vital signs
C&S	Culture and sensitivity, performed to detect infection
C/O	Complaint of (the patient's expressed concern)
Cap	Capsule
CBC	Complete blood count
CC	Chief complaint (the patient's main concern)
Cc	Cubic centimeters (e.g., the amount of fluid removed from the body is recorded in ccs)
Chem panel	Chemistry panel (a comprehensive screening blood test that indicates the status of the liver, kidneys, and electrolytes)
COPD	Chronic obstructive pulmonary disease
CVA	Cerebrovascular accident (stroke)
d.	Dexter (right)
D/D, DDX	Differential diagnosis
DIFFRLS	Differentials
DM	Diastolic murmur
DNR	Do not resuscitate
DOA	Dead on arrival
DRE	Digital rectal examination
DTR	Deep tendon reflex
D/C or DC	Discontinue or discharge (e.g., a doctor will D/C a drug; alternatively, the doctor might DC a patient from the hospital)

DM	Diabetes mellitus
DNC, D&C, or D and C	Dilation and curettage. Widening the cervix and scraping with a curette for the purpose of removing tissue lining the inner surface of the womb (uterus)
DOE	Dyspnea on exertion (shortness of breath with activity)
DTR	Deep tendon reflexes (these are reflexes that the doctor tests by tapping the tendons with a rubber hammer)
DVT	Deep venous thrombosis (blood clot in large vein)
E/A	Emergency admission
EAU	Emergency admission unit
EPMS	Extrapyramidal motor symptoms
ESR	Erythrocyte sedimentation rate
ETOH	Alcohol (ETOH intake history is often recorded as part of a patient history)
FCUS	First-catch urine sediment
FEN	Fluid, electrolytes, and nutrition
FH, FAHX	Family history
FH+/FH-	Family history positive/negative
FHA/FHHD	Family history of alcoholism/heavy drinking
FHCa	Family history of cancer
FHEH	Family history of essential hypertension
FHMI	Family history of mental illness
FHSF	Family history symptom free
FHVD	Family history of vascular disease
FX	Fracture
GERS	Gastroesophageal reflux symptoms
GISYS	Gastrointestinal symptoms
GP	General practitioner
GOMER	Slang for "get out of my emergency room"
gtt	Drops
H&P	History and physical examination
HARPPS	Heat, absence of use, redness, pain, pus, swelling (symptoms of infections)
H&H	Hemoglobin and hematocrit (when the H&H is low, the patient has anemia; the H&H can be elevated in persons who have lung disease from long-term smoking or from disease, such as polycythemia rubra vera)
h.s.	At bedtime (as in taking a medicine at bedtime)
H/O or h/o	History of (a past event that occurred…)
HA	Headache
HTN	Hypertension
IBSY	Irritable bowel symptoms

IRSS	Illness-related symptoms
IV, i.v.	Intravenous
I&D	Incision and drainage
IM	Intramuscular (this is a typical notation when noting or ordering an injection (shot) given into muscle, such as with B12 for pernicious anemia)
IMP	Impression (this is the summary conclusion of the patient's condition by the healthcare practitioner at that particular date and time)
in vitro	In the laboratory
in vivo	In the body
IU	International units
JT	Joint
K	Potassium (an essential electrolyte frequently monitored regularly in intensive care)
KCL	Potassium chloride
LUQ	Left upper quadrant (of the abdomen)
LUTS	Lower urinary tract symptoms
LBP	Low back pain (LBP is one of most common medical complaints)
LLQ	Left lower quadrant (diverticulitis pain is often located in the LLQ of the abdomen)
LUQ	Left upper quadrant (the spleen is located in the LUQ of abdomen)
Lytes Electrolytes	(potassium, sodium, carbon dioxide, and chloride)
M.D.	Medicinae doctor
MOUS	Multiple occurrence of unexplained symptoms
MCL	Medial collateral ligament
mg	Milligrams
ml	Milliliters
MVP	Mitral valve prolapse
NFH	Negative family history
NIS	No inflammatory signs
NNS	Non-specific symptoms
NOHF	No heart failure symptoms
NOSYS	No symptoms
NPO	Nil per os (nothing by mouth)
NPx	Neurologist's physical examination
NSAD	No signs of acute disease
NSI	No signs of infection/inflammation
NVS	Neurological vital signs
NVS	No visual symptoms

N/V	Nausea or vomiting
Na	Sodium
OD	Oculus dexter (right eye), overdose
OI	Oculus sinister (left eye)
OPEX	On physical examination
O&P	Ova and parasites (stool O&P is tested in the laboratory to detect parasitic infection in persons with chronic diarrhea)
O.U.	Both eyes
ORIF	Open reduction and internal fixation (such as with the orthopedic repair of a hip fracture)
p.c.	Post cibum (after meals)
p.r.n.	Pro re nata (according to circumstances, may require)
p.v.	Per vaginam
PC	Present complaint
PCA	Patient-controlled analgesia
PCLS	Persistent cold-like symptoms
PE, Pex, Px, PHEX	Physical examination
PESS	Problem, etiology, signs, and symptoms
PFH	Positive family history
PH, PHx	Past history
PHI	Past history of illness
PMS	Premenstrual symptoms
PO	Per os (by mouth, oral)
POMR	Problem-oriented medical record
PPES	Peer physical examinations
ppm	Parts per million
PRE	Progressive-resistance exercise
PRSCJ, PS	Prescription
PT	Physical therapy/therapist
P	Pulse
p.r.n.	As needed (so that something is done only when the situation calls for it; for example, administering a pain killer only when the patient is in pain)
PCL	Posterior cruciate ligament
PERRLA	Pupils equal, round, and reactive to light and accommodation
Plt	Platelets (one of the elements making up blood along with the white and red blood cells)
PMI	Point of maximum impulse of the heart when felt during examination (as in beats against the chest)
q.2h.	Quaque secunda hora (every 2 h)

q.3h.	Quaque tertia hora (every 3 h)
q.d.	Quaque die (every day)
q.h.	Quaque hora (every hour)
q.i.d.	Quater in die (four times daily)
q.v.	Quantum vis (as much as desired)
qAM	Each morning (as in taking a medicine each morning)
qhs	At each bedtime (as in taking a medicine each bedtime)
qod	Every other day (as in taking a medicine every other day)
qPM	Each evening (as in taking a medicine each evening)
RBC	Red blood count
RDA	Recommended daily allowance
RESP	Respiratory symptoms
RLL	Right lower lobe (of lung)
RLQ	Right lower quadrant (of abdomen)
RML	Right middle lobe (of lung)
RMSD	Rheumatic-musculoskeletal symptoms/diseases
RS	Review of symptoms
RUL	Right upper lobe (of lung)
RUQ	Right upper quadrant (of abdomen; the liver is located in the RUQ of the abdomen)
Rx	Prescribe, prescription drug
R/O	Rule out (doctors frequently will rule out various possible diagnoses when figuring out the correct diagnosis)
REB	Rebound (as in rebound tenderness of the abdomen when pushed in and then released)
ROS	Review of systems (an overall review relating to the organ systems, such as the respiratory, cardiovascular, and nervous systems)
S&S, S/S, SS	Signs and symptoms
SASR	Symptoms of acute stress reaction
si op. sit, si opus sit	If necessary
SM	Systolic murmur
SOAP	Subjective, objective, assessment, and plan (used in problem-oriented records)
SQ	Subcutaneous
SSHF	Signs and symptoms of heart failure
SUS	Stained urinary sediment
Sx	Signs
s/p	Status post (e.g., a person who had a knee operation would be s/p a knee operation)

SOB	Shortness of breath = dyspnea
SQ	Subcutaneous (this is a typical notation when noting or ordering an injection (shot) given into the fatty tissue under the skin, such as with insulin for diabetes mellitus)
t.i.d.	Ter in die (three times daily)
TFTS	Thyroid function tests
TINFHO/NFHO	(There is) no family history of …
TPN	Total parenteral nutrition
TRINS	Totally reversible ischemic neurological symptoms
TWBC	(Total) white blood count
T	Temperature (recorded as part of the physical examination; it is one of the "vital signs")
T&A	Tonsillectomy and adenoidectomy
tab	Tablet
TAH	Total abdominal hysterectomy
THR	Total hip replacement
TKR	Total knee replacement
U&E	Urea and electrolytes
UEE	Urinary excretion of electrolytes
UGIS	Upper gastrointestinal symptoms
UGS	Urogenital symptoms
URELS	Urine electrolytes
UA or u/a	Urinalysis (a typical part of a comprehensive physical examination)
URI	Upper respiratory infection (such as sinusitis or the common cold)
ut dict	As directed (as in taking a medicine according to the instructions that the healthcare practitioner gave in the office or in the past)
UTI	Urinary tract infection
VR	Vocal resonance
VS, vs	Vital signs
VSA	Vital signs absent
VSOK	Vital signs normal
WRS	Work-related symptoms

Ospedale

CCU	Coronary care unit
CCU	Critical care unit

ICF	Intermediate care facility
ICU	Intensive care unit
ECU	Emergency care unit
EMS	Emergency medical service
ER	Emergency room
OT	Operating theatre (UK) = OR operating room (US)

Radiologia

Computed Tomography (CT), Image Reconstruction and Reformation

CAT	Computed axial tomography
CECT	Contrast-enhanced CT
CPR	Curved planar reformation
CT	Computed tomography
CTA	CT angiography, CT arteriography
CTAP	CT during arterial portography
CTC	CT cholangiography
CTDI	CT dose index
CTHA	CT hepatic arteriography
CTM	CT myelography
CTP	CT perfusion imaging
CVS	Continuous volume scanning
DCTM	Delay CT myelography
DEQCT	Dual-energy CT
EBCT	Electron beam CT
EBT	Electron beam tomography
FOV	Field of view
FWAHM	Full width at half maximum
FWATA	Full width at tenth area
HRCT	High-resolution CT
HU	Hounsfield units
LI	Linear interpolation
MCTM	Metrizamide CT myelography
MIP	Maximum intensity projection
mIP, minIP	Minimum intensity projection
MLI	Multislice linear interpolation
MPR	Multiplanar reformation or multiplanar reconstruction
MTT	Mean transit time

Nr-MIP	Noise-reduced maximum intensity projection
QCT	Quantitative CT
ROI	Region of interest
SC	Slice collimation
SEQCT	Single-energy CT
SFOV	Scan field of view
SNR	Signal-to-noise ratio
SSD	Shaded surface display
SSP	Section sensitivity profile
SVS	Step volume scanning (EBCT)
TF	Table feed
UFCT	Ultrafast CT
VOI	Volume of interest
VRT	Volume rendering technique

Conventional Radiology

ABER	Abduction and external rotation
ACR	American College of Radiology
ALARA	As low as reasonably achievable (radiation dosages)
AP	Anteroposterior
ASNR	American Society of Neuroradiology
ASSR	American Society of Spine Radiology
At Wt, AW	Atomic weight
BE	Barium enema
Bol	Bolus
Bq	Becquerel
BS	Cervical/esophageal barium swallows
C/C	Cholecystectomy and operative cholangiogram
CAG, CHGM	Cholangiogram
CAG, CHGRY	Cholangiography
CDG	Conventional dacryocystography
CPR	Curved planar reformation
CRT	Cathode ray tube
CSG, CG, CCG	Cholecystography or cholecystogram
CXR	Chest X-ray
DC	Double contrast
DCG	Dacryocystography
DCSA	Double-contrast shoulder arthrography
DFCG	Digital fluorocholangiogram
DICOM	Digital imaging and communications in medicine

DLP	Dose–length product
DSAR	Digital subtraction arthrography
FOV	Field of view
FWAHM	Full width at half maximum
FWATA	Full width at tenth area
H/S	Hysterosalpingography
HOCA	High osmolar contrast agent
ICRP	International Commission on Radiological Protection
IOCG	Intraoperative cholangiogram
IVCH	Intravenous cholangiogram
IVP	Intravenous pyelogram
IVU	Intravenous urogram
KeV	Kiloelectron-volt
KUB	Kidney ureters bladder (plain abdominal radiography)
kV	Kilovolt
LAO	Left anterior oblique position
LAP	Late arterial phase
LMM	Lumbar metrizamide myelography
LOCM	Low osmolar contrast medium
LPO	Left posterior oblique position
LUT	Look-up table
MCU	Micturating cystography
MCUG	Micturating cystourethrogram
MLG	Myelography
Nr-MIP	Noise-reduced maximum intensity projection
OCC	Oral cholecystography
OCG	Oral cholangiogram
PA	Posteroanterior
PACS	Picture archive and communication system
PFMM	Plain film metrizamide myelography
PMG	Pneumomyelography
PS	Parotid sialography
PVP	Portal venous phase
RAO	Right anterior oblique
RC	Retrograde cystogram
REP	Retrograde pyelogram
RGP	Retrograde pyelography
ROI	Region of interest
RPO	Right posterior oblique
RU	Retrograde urogram
RUG	Retrograde urethrogram, retrograde urethrography
RUP	Retrograde ureteropyelography, retrograde pyelogram

S/N, SNR	Signal to noise ratio
SBFT	Small-bowel follow-through examination
SC	Single contrast
SCGC	Single-contrast graded-compression technique (GI radiology)
SCVIR	Society of cardiovascular and interventional radiology
SFOV	Scan field of view
SOL	Space-occupying lesion
SSD	Shaded surface display
TTC	T tube cholangiogram
TTP	Time to peak
UCG, UCR	Urethrocystography
UGI	Upper gastrointestinal series
UGI, IGIS	Upper gastrointestinal series/upper gastrointestinal DC/SC examination
VCG	Voiding cystography, voiding cystourethrography
VCU, VCUG	Voiding cystourethrogram, voiding cystourethrography
VOI	Volume of interest
VR	Volume rendering
VRT	Volume rendering technique
WSM	Water-soluble myelography
XR	X-ray

Interventional Radiology

BN	Bird's nest filter
CVA	Central venous access
DSA	Digital subtraction angiography
EAP	Early arterial phase
ERC	Endoscopic retrograde cholangiography
F	French (unit of a scale for denoting size of catheters etc.)
FNAC	Fine-needle aspiration cytology
FWHM	Full width at half maximum
HDAF	Hemodynamic access fistula
IACB	Intraaortic counterpulsation balloon pump
LAP	Late arterial phase
LP	Lumbar puncture
PC	Percutaneous cholecystostomy
PCD	Percutaneous drainage
PCN	Percutaneous nephrostomy

PCWP	Pulmonary capillary wedge pressure
PEG	Percutaneous endoscopic gastrostomy
PEI	Percutaneous ethanol injection
PFG	Percutaneous fluoroscopic gastrostomy
PICC	Peripherally inserted central catheter
PTA	Percutaneous transluminal angioplasty
PTBD	Percutaneous transhepatic biliary drainage
PTC	Percutaneous transhepatic cholangiography
PTFE	Polytetrafluoroethylene
PTHC	Percutaneous transhepatic cholangiography
PVP	Portal venous phase, percutaneous vertebroplasty
Rt-PA	Recombinant tissue plasminogen activator
SCVIR	Standards of Practice Guidelines on Angioplasty
SK	Streptokinase
TACE	Transcatheter arterial chemoembolization
TIPS	Transjugular intrahepatic portosystemic shunt
TNB	Transthoracic needle biopsy
tPA	Tissue plasminogen activator
TTP	Time to peak
UK	Urokinase
VT	Vena-Tech filter

Magnetic Resonance Imaging (MRI)

CHESS	Chemical shift selective pulses
CME-MRI	Contrast medium-enhanced MRI
CNR	Contrast to noise ratio
COPE	Centrally ordered phase encoding
CSI	Chemical shift imaging (magnetic resonance spectroscopy Method)
CVMR	Cardiovascular magnetic resonance
DNMR	Dynamic nuclear magnetic resonance
DTPA	Diethylene triamine pentaacetic acid (a binding substance for Both Gd and 99m-Tc)
DWI	Diffusion-weighted image
EMRI	Electron MRI
EPI	Echoplanar imaging
EPMR	Echoplanar magnetic resonance
EP-MRSI	Echoplanar magnetic resonance spectroscopic imaging
ERSC-MRI	Endorectal surface coil MRI
ESR	Electron spin resonance

ETL	Echo train length
FAST	Fourier-acquired steady-state technique
FC	Flow compensation
FID	Free induction decay
FISP	Fast imaging with steady-state precession
FLASH	Fast low-angle shot
fMRI	Functional MRI
FMRIB	Functional MRI of the brain
FS	Fast saturation
FSE	Fast spin-echo
FT	Fourier transform
FTNMR	Fourier transform nuclear magnetic resonance
Gd-DTPA	Gadolinium-diethylenetriamine pentaacetic acid
Gd-MRA	Gadolinium-enhanced magnetic resonance arteriography
GE	Gradient echo
GEMRA	Gadolinium-enhanced magnetic resonance angiography
GRASS	Gradient-recalled acquisition in steady-state
GRE	Gradient-recalled echo, gradient echo
GRM	Gradient rephasing motion
HASTE	Half Fourier acquisition single-shot turbo spin-echo
I-MR	Interventional MRI
IR	Inversion recovery
ISMRM	International Society for Magnetic Resonance in Medicine
MAS NMR	Magic angle spinning nuclear magnetic resonance
MOTSA	Multiple overlapping thin-slab acquisition
MPGR	Multiplanar two-dimensional gradient echo
MRA	Magnetic resonance angiography
MRA	Magnetic resonance arthrography
MRCP	Magnetic resonance cholangiopancreatography
MRE	Magnetic resonance elastography, magnetic resonance enteroclysis
MRI	Magnetic resonance imaging
MRM	Magnetic resonance myelography
MRS	Magnetic resonance spectroscopy
MRU	Magnetic resonance urography
MRV	Magnetic resonance venography/venogram
MT	Magnetization transfer pulse
MTF	Modulation transfer function
NAA	N-Acetyl aspartate (MR spectroscopy)

NAQ	Number of acquisitions
NEX	Number of excitations
NMRI	Nuclear MRI
PC	Phase contrast
PMR	Proton magnetic resonance
PWI	Perfusion-weighted imaging
RF	Radiofrequency
ROPE	Respiratory-ordered phase encoding
SAR	Specific absorption rate
SE	Spin-echo
SENSE	Sensitivity encoding for MRI
SLS	Interslice spacing
SLTHK	Slice thickness
SMASH	Simultaneous acquisition of spatial harmonics
SMRI	Society of Magnetic Resonance Imaging
SPGR	Spoiled gradient recalled acquisition in steady state, spoiled gradient-recalled echo
SPIO	Superparamagnetic iron oxide (particles)
SPIR	Spectral presaturation by inversion recovery
SSFP	Steady-state free precession
SSNMR	Solid-state nuclear magnetic resonance
STEAM	Stimulated-echo acquisition mode
STIR	Short-tau inversion recovery, short T1 inversion recovery
T1-W	T1-weighted image
T2-W	T2-weighted image
TE	Time to echo (echo time)
TI	Inversion time
TOF	Time of flight
TR	Time of repetition (repetition time)
TSE	Turbo spin echo
USPIO	Ultrasmall superparamagnetic particles
VENC-MR	Velocity-encoded cine MRI

Nuclear Medicine

AXL	Axillary lymphoscintigraphy
CPDS	Computer processed dynamic scintigraphy
CS	Cerebral scintigraphy
DIC	Direct isotope cystography
DMSA	99m-Tc-dimercaptosuccinic acid scintigraphy

DPLS	Dynamic perfusion lung scintigraphy
DRC, DRCG,DRNC	Direct radionuclide cystography
DRVC	Direct radionuclide voiding cystography
DTMS	Dipyridamole-thallium myocardial scintigraphy
EMPS	Exercise myocardial perfusion scintigraphy
HBFS	Hepatobiliary functional scintigraphy
HIDA	Hepatobiliary scintigraphy with dimethyliminodi-acetic acid
IMP	I-123-isopropyliodoamphetamine (radiolabeled agent for brain perfusion SPECT)
IRC	Indirect radionuclide cystography
IVCU	Isotope-voiding cystourethrogram
MPS	Myocardial perfusion scintigraphy
PET	Positron emission tomography
Rcbf	Regional cerebral blood flow
RIA	Radioimmunoassay
RNVC, RNC	Radionuclide voiding cystography
SCINT	Scintigraphy
SESC	Sestamibi scan
SPECT	Single photon emission computed tomography
SRS	Somatostatin receptor scintigraphy
SSMM	Sestamibi scintimammography
Tc-99m-ECD-bicisate	Technetium-99m bicisate ethyl cysteinate dimer (radio-labeled agent for brain perfusion SPECT)
Tc-99m-HMPAO	Technetium-99m-hexamethyl propylamine oxime (radiolabeled agent for Brain Perfusion SPECT)
Tc-99mI-123-QNB	Technetium-99m-iodine-123-quinuclidinyl-iodoben-zylate
Tc-99m-labeled RBCs	Red blood cell scan (Meckel's scan)
TMS	Thallium myocardial scintigraphy
TPBS	Three-phase dynamic bone scintigraphy
V/Q scanning	Ventilation-perfusion scintigraphy
WBC scans	White blood cell scans
WBS	Whole body scintigraphy
WCS	White cell scintigraphy

Ultrasonography

3D US	Three-dimensional ultrasound
AD	Acoustic densitometry (ultrasound)
B-mode	Brightness-mode

BPD	Bi-parietal diameter (ultrasound measurement of the head of a fetus)
CCUS	Complete compression ultrasound
CDI	Color Doppler imaging
CEUS	Contrast-enhanced ultrasound
CRL	Crown rump length (ultrasound fetal measurement)
CW	Doppler Continuous wave Doppler
DPVTI	Doppler power velocity time integral
DR	Dynamic range
EDV	End diastolic velocity
EFOV	Extended field of view
EJU	European Journal of Ultrasound
ELB	Echolucent band
ERUS, EUS	Endorectal ultrasonography, endorectal ultrasound
ESB	Echostrong band
EUS	Endovascular ultrasonography, endoscopic ultrasound
EVS	Endovaginal sonography
EVUS	Endovaginal ultrasound
ISUOG	International Society of Ultrasound in Obstetrics and Gynecology
IVUS	Intravascular ultrasound
PDI	Power Doppler imaging
PI	Pulsatility index
PIM	Pulse inversion mode
PNU	Prenatal ultrasonography
PRF	Pulse repetition frequency
PSV	Peak systolic velocity
PWD	Pulsed-wave Doppler
QUI	Quantitative ultrasound index (bone density)
QUS	Quantitative ultrasound
RI	Resistivity index
RTU	Real-time ultrasound
SVU	Society for Vascular Ultrasound
TAUS	Transabdominal ultrasonography
TEE	Transesophageal echocardiography
TGC	Time-gain compensation
THI	Time harmonic imaging
TRUS	Transrectal ultrasound
TULIP	Transurethral ultrasound-guided laser-induced prostatectomy
TUS	Transabdominal ultrasound
ULTIMA	Ultrasound imaging with an intelligent 2D array

US	Ultrasound, ultrasonography
USB	Ultrasound-guided aspiration biopsy
USG	Ultrasonography
USMF	Ultrasound multi-frame (images)
VUS	Voiding urosonography

Esercizi: frasi comuni contenenti abbreviazioni

In questa parte, riportiamo alcune frasi d'uso comune in lingua inglese contenenti alcune delle abbreviazioni sopra descritte.

Frasi:
> A 40-year-old man was diagnosed with Felty's syndrome because he had splenomegaly and pancytopenia as well as definite RA.
> MCV, MCHC, LDH, ANA, and RF values are normal.
> The platelet and WBC counts exceeded their normal ranges. He was diagnosed with ... (ITP, CMML, AML, CML). Two months later, he received a BMT.
> Foreign bodies display variable signal intensity on both T1- and T2-weighted images. MR shows an inflammatory response while CT can show the retained foreign body. US evaluation could be useful in selected patients.
> COPD is a risk factor for TB.
> Cholera can be diagnosed by the presence of CTX in the stool.
> A 16-year-old girl with fever, chills, rash, and multiple nodular opacities on CXR was diagnosed with ... (RMSF, BPF, DGI).
> An ECG showed ... (RBBB, LBBB, APCs, VPCs, AF, VF).
> He is currently under treatment with ACEI. Ten years ago he underwent PTCA after three AMIs.
> RA and SSc are more common in females.
> PCP and PML are two of the complications that can affect AIDS patients.
> Cutaneous manifestations of SLE can be divided into SCLE (acute) and DLE (chronic).
> The key to the diagnosis of septic arthritis is joint aspiration. Septic joint fluid is opaque and has a WBC count greater than 100,000.
> Clinical signs of skeletal metastases include hypercalcemia and the syndrome known as HPO.

❯ Prolonged morning stiffness helps to distinguish a truly inflammatory arthritis such as RA from non-inflammatory arthritides such as OA.

❯ The typical attack of acute gouty arthritis is a painful monoarthritis, most often in the first MTP joint (podagra).

❯ Scaphoid fractures exhibit a high rate of non-union and AVN.

❯ Water is arbitrarily assigned a value of 0 HU.

❯ MRI is the imaging modality of choice for the CNS.

❯ The aorta is normally visible on PA and lateral chest radiographs.

❯ Generally, a PT of below 15 s, a PTT within 1.2 times control, and a platelet count greater than 75,000/ml will be acceptable.

❯ TIPS is a relatively new technique for the treatment of patients with portal hypertension.

❯ To rule out the presence of DVT, a lower extremity ultrasound examination should be performed.

❯ Approximately 1% of cardiac muscle cells, including those in the SA and AV nodes, are autorhythmic.

❯ In the chronic form of mitral regurgitation, clinical monitoring focuses on the evaluation of left ventricular function, with treatment of CHF.

❯ The RCA supplies the right ventricle and the AV node.

❯ The LCA divides into the anterior descending and circumflex arteries.

❯ In the ARDS, an increase in capillary permeability occurs.

❯ SOB can usually be attributed to one of two fundamental categories of disease, cardiac or pulmonary.

❯ In patients with documented DVT or PE in whom anticoagulation is contraindicated, percutaneous placement of an IVC filter in the angiography suite may be warranted.

❯ The azygos vein provides venous drainage into the SVC.

❯ NHL carries a less-favorable prognosis than Hodgkin's disease.

❯ There is a strong association between thymoma and MG.

❯ Neurofibromas and schwannomas are more common in patients with NF-1.

❯ KS remains the most common malignancy in HIV disease and constitutes an AIDS-defining illness.

❯ LIP is an AIDS-defining illness in children.

❯ One of the classic differential diagnoses in radiology is that of the SPN.

❯ The SMA supplies the bowel between the duodenojejunal junction and the splenic flexure of the colon.

❯ CT scanning has replaced DPL for detecting and evaluating free fluid within the abdominal cavity.

❯ The pelvis joins the ureter at the UPJ, a common site of obstruction.

> The higher incidence of UTIs in young women is attributed to the relatively short female urethra.
> When an ACE inhibitor is administered, glomerular filtration is reduced.
> Intrinsic renal causes of acute renal failure include ATN and acute glomerulonephritis.
> A clue to the prerenal nature of the failure is contained in the ratio of serum BUN to creatinine.
> The standard screening mammogram includes two views of each breast: the CC view and the MLO view.
> Hydrocephalus is called obstructive when there is a blockage of normal flow of CSF.
> Fetal growth is assessed by measurement of abdominal circumference, which is important in detecting IUGR.
> The transitional zone represents the site of BPH.
> Strokes are sometimes preceded clinically by so-called TIAs.
> The most common location of stroke is in the MCA distribution.
> ACA occlusion may cause contralateral foot and leg weakness.
> A small infarction in some portions of the PCA territory may have catastrophic consequences.
> HMD is the most common cause of neonatal respiratory distress.
> An important complication of long-term ventilatory support is BPD.
> TTN occurs when there is inadequate or delayed clearance of the fluid at birth, resulting in a "wet lung."
> EA and TEF both result from anomalies in the development of the primitive foregut.
> NEC occurs primarily in premature neonates exposed to hypoxic stress.
> DDH is suspected clinically in newborns with a breech presentation.
> PVL is the result of prenatal or neonatal hypoxic-ischemic insult.
> An AVM is a congenital lesion resulting from persistent fetal capillaries.

Definizioni:

ACA	Anterior cerebral artery
ACE	Angiotensin-converting enzyme
ACEI	Angiotensin-converting enzyme inhibitor
AF	Atrial fibrillation
AIDS	Acquired immunodeficiency syndrome
AMI	Acute myocardial infarction
AML	Acute myeloid leukemia
ANA	Antinuclear antibodies

APCs	Atrial premature complexes
ARDS	Acute respiratory distress syndrome
ATN	Acute tubular necrosis
AV	Atrioventricular
AVM	Arteriovenous malformation
AVN	Avascular necrosis
BMT	Bone marrow transplantation
BPD	Bronchopulmonary dysplasia
BPF	Brazilian purpuric fever
BPH	Benign prostatic hyperplasia
BUN	Blood-urea nitrogen
CC	Craniocaudal
CHF	Congestive heart failure
CML	Chronic myeloid leukemia
CMML	Chronic myelomonocytic leukemia
CNS	Central nervous system
COPD	Chronic obstructive pulmonary disease
CSF	Cerebrospinal fluid
CT	Computed tomography
CTX	Cholera toxin
CXR	Chest X-ray
DDH	Developmental dysplasia of the hip
DGI	Disseminated gonococcal infection
DLE	Discoid lupus erythematosus
DPL	Diagnostic peritoneal lavage
DVT	Deep venous thrombosis
EA	Esophageal atresia
ECG	Electrocardiogram
HIV	Human immunodeficiency virus
HMD	Hyaline membrane disease
HPO	Hypertrophic pulmonary osteoarthropathy
HU	Hounsfield units
ITP	Idiopathic thrombocytopenic purpura
IUGR	Intrauterine growth retardation
IVC	Inferior vena cava
KS	Kaposi's sarcoma
LBBB	Left bundle branch block
LCA	Left coronary artery
LDH	Lactate dehydrogenase
LIP	Lymphocytic interstitial pneumonitis
MCA	Middle cerebral artery

MCHC	Mean corpuscular hemoglobin concentration
MCV	Mean corpuscular volume
MG	Myasthenia gravis
MLO	Mediolateral oblique
MR	Magnetic resonance
MRI	Magnetic resonance imaging
MTP	Metatarsophalangeal
NEC	Necrotizing enterocolitis
NF-1	Neurofibromatosis type 1
NHL	Non-Hodgkin's lymphoma
OA	Osteoarthritis
PA	Posteroanterior
PCA	Posterior cerebral artery
PCP	Pneumocystis carinii pneumonia
PE	Pulmonary embolism
PML	Progressive multifocal leukoencephalopathy
PT	Prothrombin time
PTCA	Percutaneous transluminal coronary angioplasty
PTT	Partial thromboplastin time
PVL	Periventricular leukomalacia
RA	Rheumatoid arthritis
RBBB	Right bundle branch block
RCA	Right coronary artery
RF	Rheumatoid factor
RMSF	Rocky mountain spotted fever
SA	Sinoatrial
SCLE	Subacute cutaneous lupus erythematosus
SLE	Systemic lupus erythematosus
SMA	Superior mesenteric artery
SOB	Shortness of breath
SPN	Solitary pulmonary nodule
SSc	Systemic sclerosis
SVC	Superior vena cava
TB	Tuberculosis
TEF	Tracheoesophageal fistula
TIA	Transient ischemic attack
TIPS	Transjugular intrahepatic portosystemic shunting
TTN	Transient tachypnea of the newborn
UPJ	Ureteropelvic junction
US	Ultrasonography
UTI	Urinary tract infection

VF	Ventricular fibrillation
VPCs	Ventricular premature complexes
WBC	White blood cell

Capitolo 11

Glossario dei termini chirurgici

Poiché siamo certi che abbiate confidenza con la maggior parte della terminologia inglese relativa alla vostra specializzazione, vi proponiamo questo capitolo allo scopo di offrirvi non una traduzione dei termini chirurgici elencati ma una loro definizione in inglese, che vi tornerà utile sia nella pratica clinica quotidiana, ad esempio nella comunicazione con il paziente o con i parenti, sia nella vostra attività scientifica. A causa dello spazio limitato, avrete bisogno di un buon dizionario medico di inglese o di un traduttore computerizzato per controllare alcune parole.

Nonostante alcuni termini siano comuni alla maggior parte delle specialità, essi sono raggruppati in gruppi specifici.

Glossario dei termini comuni a tutte le specialità chirurgiche

Abscess: A localized collection of pus.

Aneurysm: Dilatation of an artery.

Antegrade/anterograde: Going in the direction of flow.

Diverticulum: Plural, diverticula (hence, use of the term "diverticulae" is erroneous).

Embolus: A blood clot, normally coming from the heart, that becomes lodged in a blood vessel and blocks circulation.

Fistula: A pipe or tube (Latin), plural fistulae. An abnormal communication between two hollow viscera, or one hollow viscera and the skin. Also a communication between an artery and a vein.

R. Ribes, P. J. Aranda, J. Giba, *Inglese per chirurghi*,
© Springer-Verlag Italia 2012

Gangrene: Death of tissue with putrefaction, sometimes referred to as "wet" gangrene (infected) or "dry" (mummified).

Hernia: The abnormal protrusion of the contents of a cavity beyond the normal confines of that cavity.

Ischemia: An inadequate supply of blood to a part of the body caused by blockage of an artery.

Keloid: An area of raised pink or red fibrous scar tissue at the edges of a wound or incision.

Necrosis: Death of tissue with structural evidence of such death.

Retrograde: Going in a direction against flow, e.g., endoscopic retrograde cholangiopancreatogram (ERCP).

Sinus: A blind tract lined with granulation tissue, hollow or solid.

Slough: A piece of dead soft tissue or water (Old English sloh, a hole or low area in the ground filled with mud).

Stent: An artificial tube inserted into a tubular organ to keep it open.

Stoma: Surgical opening: an artificial opening made in an organ, especially an opening in the colon (colostomy) or ileum (ileostomy) made via the abdomen. (Greek, "mouth"). Plural: stomata.

Subacute: Used to describe a medical condition that develops less rapidly and with less severity than an acute condition.

Thrombus: A blood clot that forms in a blood vessel and remains at the site of formation.

Ulcer: A discontinuity of an epithelial surface.

Next, you will find a list of common terms grouped by surgical specialty. This is intended to be a guide to spelling more than a guide to meaning (you will very likely know all of them). In any case, we recommend you acquire a good medical dictionary to complement this book.

Glossario dei termini relativi alla chirurgia addominale

Abdominal hysterectomy: The uterus is removed through the abdomen via a surgical incision.

Abdominoscopy: A type of surgery using a laparoscope, which is inserted into one or more small incisions, to examine the abdominal cavity.

Acute appendicitis: Acute inflammation of the appendix due to infection.

Advance directives: Legal documents stating a patient's medical preferences in the event the patient should become incapable of voicing his/her opinion.

Appendectomy: Surgical removal of the appendix to treat acute appendicitis.

Cholecystectomy: Surgery to remove the gallbladder.

Colectomy: Partial or complete removal of the large bowel or colon.

Colonoscopy: Test to look into the rectum and colon. The doctor uses a long, flexible, narrow tube with a light and a lens on the end (instrument: colonoscope).

Colposcopy: Visual examination of the cervix and vagina using a lighted magnifying instrument (colposcope).

Debridement: The surgical removal of foreign material and/or dead, damaged or infected tissue from a wound or burn (most common: Friedrich).

Deep vein thrombosis: Blood clotting that occurs within the deep venous system.

Diathermy machine or electrocautery: A piece of equipment used in the operating room to control bleeding.

Dilation and curettage (D&C): A common gynecological surgery consisting in widening the cervical canal with a dilator and scraping the uterine cavity with a curette.

Elective surgery: An operation the patient chooses to have done, which may not be essential to continuation of quality of life (see also "Optional surgery").

Electrocoagulation: Electrosurgery which helps harden tissue.

Emergency surgery: An operation performed immediately as a result of an urgent medical condition (see also "Urgent surgery").

Endoscopy: Visual examination of the interior of a hollow body organ by use of an endoscope.

Epidural anesthetic: An anesthetic which is injected into the "epidural space" in the middle and lower back, just outside the spinal space, to numb the lower extremities.

Free skin graft: The detaching of healthy skin from one part of the body to repair areas of lost or damaged skin in another part of the body. If it has its own blood supply, it is a pedicled skin graft.

Gastrectomy: Complete or partial removal of the stomach.

Gastroscopy: Examining the lining of the esophagus, stomach, and the first part of the small intestine with a long viewing tube.

General anesthetic: An anesthetic that causes the patient to become unconscious during surgery.

Hemorrhoidectomy: The removal of hemorrhoids.

Hemorrhoids: Distended veins in the lining of the anus.

Hysterectomy: Surgical removal of the uterus.

Inguinal hernias: Protrusions of part of the intestine into the muscles of the groin.

Infection: Invasion of the body by microorganisms that cause disease.

Informed consent form: A form signed by the patient prior to surgery that explains everything involved in the surgery, including its risks.

Inpatient surgery: Surgery which requires the patient to be admitted and to stay in the hospital.

Laparoscope: A type of endoscope consisting of an illuminated tube with an optical system.

Laparoscopic cholecystectomy: An operation to remove the gallbladder via a minimally invasive technique.

Laparoscopic lymphadenectomy: Removal of pelvic lymph nodes with a laparoscope done through four small incisions in the lower abdominal region.

Laparoscopy: A type of surgery using a laparoscope, which is inserted into one or more small incisions, to examine the abdominal cavity.

Laser surgery: Using a device that emits a beam of light radiation, surgeons can cauterize a wound, repair damaged tissue, or cut through tissue.

Living will: A legal document which states your medical preferences for treatment and resuscitation in the event you can no longer speak for yourself.

Local anesthesia: Anesthetic medicine injected into the site of the operation to temporarily numb that area.

Lumpectomy: A surgical procedure to remove a tumor and surrounding tissue.

Mastectomy: The removal of all or part of the breast.

Minimally invasive surgery: Any surgical technique that does not require a large incision.

Modified radical mastectomy: Surgical removal of the entire breast and the ancillary lymph nodes.

Nephrectomy: Surgical removal of the kidney.

Needle aspiration (of the breast): Uses a thin needle and syringe to collect tissue or drain a lump after using a local anesthetic.

Needle biopsy (of the breast): A procedure to remove a small piece of breast tissue using a needle with a special cutting edge, after using a local anesthetic.

Optional surgery: An operation the patient chooses to have done, which may not be essential to continuation or quality of life (see also "Elective surgery").

Outpatient surgery: Surgery that allows the patient to go home the same day.

Partial colectomy: The removal of part of the large intestine.

Peritoneal adhesions: The peritoneum is a two-layered membrane that lines the wall of the abdominal cavity and covers abdominal organs.

Plasma: Cell-free portion of the blood with coagulation factors.

Post-anesthesia care unit: The area a patient is brought to after surgery to recover. Also called recovery room.

Radical mastectomy: Surgical removal of the entire breast, the pectoral muscles, and the ancillary lymph nodes.

Regional anesthetic: An anesthetic used to numb a portion of the body.

Required surgery: An operation which is necessary to continue quality of life. Unlike emergency surgery, required surgery may not have to be done immediately.

Salpingectomy: Surgical removal of a fallopian tube.

Sigmoidoscopy: Examining the rectum and sigmoid colon.

Simple mastectomy: Surgical removal of the breast and possibly a few of the axillary lymph nodes close to the breast.

Spinal anesthetic: An anesthetic that is injected into the spinal canal fluid for surgery in the lower abdomen, pelvis, rectum, or other lower extremities.

Splenectomy: Surgical removal of the spleen.

Subtotal or partial gastrectomy: Surgical removal of a portion of the stomach.

Total gastrectomy: Complete removal of the stomach.

Total hysterectomy with bilateral salpingo-oophorectomy: The entire uterus, fallopian tubes, and the ovaries are surgically removed.

Total hysterectomy: The entire uterus is surgically removed, including the cervix; the fallopian tubes and the ovaries remain.

Urgent surgery: An operation performed immediately as a result of an urgent medical condition (see also "Emergency surgery").

Urinary retention: Inability to empty the bladder.

Uterus: The hollow, muscular organ of the female reproductive system.

Wedge resection: A small, localized section of the viscera is removed – often for a biopsy.

Glossario dei termini cardiovascolari (cardiologia e cardiochirurgia)

Abdominal aorta: The portion of the aorta in the abdomen.

Ablation: Elimination or removal.

ACE (angiotensin-converting enzyme) inhibitor: A medicine that lowers blood pressure by interfering with the breakdown of a protein-like substance involved in blood pressure regulation.

Aneurysm: A sac-like protrusion from a blood vessel or the heart, resulting from a weakening of the vessel wall or heart muscle.

Angina or angina pectoris: Chest pain that occurs when diseased blood vessels restrict blood flow to the heart.

Angiography: An X-ray technique where dye is injected into the chambers of the heart or the arteries that lead to the heart (the coronary arteries).

Angioplasty: A nonsurgical technique for treating diseased arteries by temporarily inflating a balloon inside an artery.

Angiotensin II receptor blocker: A medicine that lowers blood pressure by blocking the action of angiotensin II, a chemical in the body that causes the blood vessels to tighten (constrict).

Annulus: The ring around a heart valve where the valve leaflet merges with the heart muscle.

Antiarrhythmics: Medicines used to treat patients who have irregular heart rhythms.

Anticoagulant: Any medicine that keeps blood from clotting. Also "blood thinner."

Antihypertensive: Any medicine or other therapy that lowers blood pressure.

Aorta: The largest artery in the body and the initial vessel to supply blood from the heart.

Arrhythmia (or dysrhythmia): An abnormal heartbeat.

Arrhythmogenic right ventricular dysplasia (ARVD): ARVD is a type of cardiomyopathy with no known cause. It appears to be a genetic condition (passed down through a family's genes). ARVD causes ventricular arrhythmias.

Arteriography: A test that is combined with cardiac catheterization to visualize an artery or the arterial system after injection of a contrast dye.

Arteriosclerosis: A disease process, commonly called "hardening of the arteries."

Ascending aorta: The first portion of the aorta, emerging from the heart's left ventricle.

Aspirin: Acetylsalicylic acid; a medicine used to relieve pain, reduce inflammation, and impair platelet aggregation.

Atherosclerosis: A disease process that leads to the buildup of a waxy substance, called plaque, inside blood vessels.

Atrium (right and left): The two upper or holding chambers of the heart (together referred to as atria).

Atrial tachycardia: A type of arrhythmia that begins in the atria and causes a very fast heart rate of 160–200 beats per min.

Atrioventricular block: An interruption or disturbance of the electrical signal between the atria and lower two chambers the ventricles.

Atrium: Either one of the heart's two upper chambers.

Bacterial endocarditis: A bacterial infection of the lining of the heart's chambers (called the endocardium) or the heart's valves.

Balloon catheter: A device with a small balloon on the end that can be threaded through an artery. Used in angioplasty or valvuloplasty.

Balloon valvuloplasty: A procedure to open a closed heart valve through a catheter.

Beta-blocker: An antihypertensive medicine that limits the activity of epinephrine, a hormone that increases blood pressure.

Biopsy: The process by which a small sample of tissue is taken for examination.

Blalock-Taussig procedure: A shunt between the subclavian and pulmonary arteries used to increase the supply of oxygen-rich blood in "blue babies."

Blue babies: Babies who have a blue tinge to their skin (cyanosis) resulting from insufficient oxygen in the arterial blood.

Body mass index (BMI): A number that doctors use to determine the risk of cardiovascular disease created by a person being overweight. BMI is calculated using a formula of weight in kilograms divided by height in meters squared (BMI =W [kg]/H [m2]).

Bradycardia: Abnormally slow heartbeat.

Bruit: A sound made in the blood vessels resulting from turbulence, perhaps because of a buildup of plaque or damage to the vessels.

Bundle branch block: A condition in which parts of the intraventricular conduction system are defective and unable to conduct the electrical signal normally, causing an irregular heart rhythm (arrhythmia).

Bypass: Surgery that can improve blood flow to the heart (or other organs and tissues) by providing a new route, or "bypass," around a section of clogged or diseased artery.

Cardiac arrest: The stopping of the heartbeat, usually because of interference with the electrical signal.

Cardiac output: The amount of blood the heart pumps through the circulatory system in 1 min.

Cardiopulmonary bypass: The process by which a machine is used to do the work of the heart and lungs so the heart can be stopped during surgery.

Cardiopulmonary resuscitation (CPR): An emergency measure that can maintain a person's breathing and heartbeat.

Cardioversion: A technique of applying an electrical shock to the chest to convert an abnormal heartbeat to a normal rhythm.

Cerebrovascular: Pertaining to the blood vessels of the brain.

Cerebrovascular accident: Also called cerebral vascular accident, apoplexy, or stroke. Blood supply to some part of the brain is slowed or stopped, resulting in injury to brain tissue.

Claudication: A tiredness or pain in the arms and legs caused by an inadequate supply of oxygen to the muscles, usually due to narrowed arteries.

Collateral circulation: Blood flow through small, nearby vessels in response to blockage of a main blood vessel.

Commissurotomy: A procedure used to widen the opening of a heart valve that has been narrowed by scar tissue. First developed to correct rheumatic heart disease.

Congenital heart defects: Malformation of the heart or of its major blood vessels present at birth.

Coronary artery bypass (CAB): Surgical rerouting of blood around a diseased vessel that supplies blood to the heart.

Coronary artery disease (CAD): A narrowing of the arteries that supply blood to the heart. The condition results from a buildup of plaque and greatly increases the risk of a heart attack.

Coronary thrombosis: Formation of a clot in one of the arteries carrying blood to the heart muscle. Also called coronary occlusion.

Cryoablation: The removal of tissue using an instrument called a cold probe. Also a method to ablate the pulmonary veins as a surgical treatment to atrial fibrillation.

Cyanosis: Blueness of the skin caused by a lack of oxygen in the blood.

Cyanotic heart disease: A birth defect of the heart that causes oxygen-poor (blue) blood to circulate to the body without first passing through the lungs.

Death rate (age-adjusted): A death rate that has been standardized for age so different populations can be compared or the same population can be compared over time.

Deep vein thrombosis: A blood clot in a deep vein in the calf.

Defibrillator: A machine that helps restore a normal heart rhythm by delivering an electric shock.

Dissecting aneurysm: A condition in which the layers of an artery separate or are torn, causing blood to flow between the layers.

Doppler ultrasound: A technology that uses sound waves to assess blood flow within the heart and blood vessels and to identify leaking valves.

Dyspnea: Shortness of breath.

Ejection fraction: A measurement of blood that is pumped out of a filled ventricle. The normal rate is 50% or more.

Electrocardiogram (ECG or EKG): A test in which several electronic sensors are placed on the body to monitor electrical activity associated with the heartbeat.

Electroencephalogram (EEG): A test that can detect and record the brain's electrical activity. The test is done by attaching metal discs, called electrodes, to the scalp.

Electrophysiological study (EPS): A test that uses cardiac catheterization to study patients who have arrhythmias.

Embolus: Also called embolism; a blood clot that forms in a blood vessel in one part of the body and travels to another part.

Endarterectomy: Surgical removal of plaque deposits or blood clots in an artery.

Endocardium: The smooth membrane covering the inside of the heart. The innermost lining of the heart.

Endothelium: The smooth inner lining of many body structures, including the heart (endocardium) and blood vessels.

Exercise stress test: A common test for diagnosing coronary artery disease, especially in patients who have symptoms of heart disease.

Familial hypercholesterolemia: A genetic predisposition to dangerously high cholesterol levels.

Fibrillation: Rapid, uncoordinated contractions of individual heart muscle fibers.

First-degree heart block: When an electrical impulse from the heart's upper chambers (the atria) is slowed as it moves through the atria and atrioventricular (AV) node.

Flutter: The rapid, ineffective contractions of any heart chamber. A flutter is considered to be more coordinated than fibrillation.

Fusiform aneurysm: A tube-shaped aneurysm that causes the artery to bulge outward. Involves the entire circumference (outside wall) of the artery.

Heart assist device: A mechanical device that is surgically implanted to ease the workload of the heart.

Heart block: General term for conditions in which the electrical impulse that activates the heart muscle cells is delayed or interrupted somewhere along its path.

Heart failure: See "congestive heart failure."

Heart–lung machine: Apparatus that oxygenates and pumps blood to the body during open heart surgery.

Heart murmur: An abnormal heart sound caused by turbulent blood flow.

Heredity: The genetic transmission of a particular quality or trait from parent to child.

High blood pressure: A chronic increase in blood pressure above its normal range.

Holter monitor: A portable device for recording heartbeats over a period of 24 h or more.

Hypertension: High blood pressure.

Hypertrophic obstructive cardiomyopathy (HOCM): An overgrown heart muscle that creates a bulge into the ventricle and impedes blood flow.

Hypertrophy: Enlargement of tissues or organs because of increased workload.

Hypoglycemia: Low levels of glucose (sugar) in the blood.

Hypotension: Abnormally low blood pressure.

Hypoxia: Less than normal content of oxygen in the organs and tissues of the body.

Idiopathic: No known cause.

Immunosuppressants: Any medicine that suppresses the body's immune system

Impedance plethysmography: A noninvasive diagnostic test used to evaluate blood flow through the leg.

Incompetent valve: Also called insufficiency or regurgitation; a valve that is not working properly, causing it to leak blood back in the wrong direction.

Infarct: The area of heart tissue permanently damaged by an inadequate supply of oxygen.

Introducer sheath: A catheter-like tube that is placed inside a patient's vessel during an interventional procedure to help the doctor with insertion and proper placement of the actual catheter. Also called a sheath.

Ischemia: Decreased blood flow to an organ, usually due to constriction or obstruction of an artery.

Left ventricular assist device (LVAD): A mechanical device that can be placed outside the body or implanted inside the body. A LVAD does not replace the heart—it "assists" or "helps" it pump oxygen-rich blood from the left ventricle to the rest of the body.

Lumen: The hollow area within a tube, such as a blood vessel.

Maze surgery: A type of heart surgery that is used to treat chronic atrial fibrillation by creating a surgical "maze" of new electrical pathways to let electrical impulses travel easily through the heart.

Mitral stenosis: A narrowing of the mitral valve, which controls blood flow from the heart's upper left chamber (the left atrium) to its lower left chamber (the left ventricle).

Mitral valve regurgitation: Failure of the mitral valve to close properly, causing blood to flow back into the left atrium.

Necrosis: Refers to the death of tissue within a certain area.

Pacemaker: A surgically implanted electronic device that helps regulate the heartbeat.

Patent ductus arteriosus: A congenital defect in which the opening between the aorta and the pulmonary artery does not close after birth.

Percutaneous coronary intervention (PCI): Any of the noninvasive procedures usually performed in the cardiac catheterization laboratory. Angioplasty is an example of a percutaneous coronary intervention. Also called a transcatheter intervention.

Percutaneous transluminal coronary angioplasty (PTCA): See "angioplasty."

Pericarditis: Inflammation of the outer membrane surrounding the heart.

Pericardiocentesis: A diagnostic or therapeutic procedure that uses a needle to withdraw fluid from the pericardium.

Pericardium: The outer fibrous sac that surrounds the heart.

Positron emission tomography (PET): A test that uses information about the energy of certain elements in your body to show whether parts of the heart muscle are alive and working.

Prevalence: The total number of cases of a given disease that exist in a population at a specific time.

Radionuclide imaging: A test in which a harmless radioactive substance is injected into the bloodstream to show information about blood flow through the arteries.

Regurgitation: Backward flow of blood through a defective heart valve.

Renal: Pertaining to the kidneys.

Restenosis: The reclosing or renarrowing of an artery after an interventional procedure such as angioplasty or stent placement.

Revascularization: A procedure to restore blood flow to the tissues.

Right ventricular assist device (RVAD): A mechanical device that can be placed outside the body or implanted inside the body. An RVAD does not replace the heart—it "assists" or "helps" it pump oxygen-poor blood from the right ventricle to the lungs.

Saccular aneurysm: A round aneurysm that bulges out from an artery. Involves only part of the circumference (outside wall) of the artery.

Septal defect: A hole in the wall of the heart separating the atria or in the wall of the heart separating the ventricles.

Septum: The muscular wall dividing a chamber on the left side of the heart from the chamber on the right.

Sheath: A catheter-like tube that is placed inside a patient's vessel during an interventional procedure to help with the proper placement of the actual catheter. Also called an introducer sheath.

Shock: A condition in which body function is impaired because the volume of fluid circulating through the body is insufficient to maintain normal metabolism.

Shunt: A connector that allows blood to flow between two locations.

Sick sinus syndrome: The failure of the sinus node to regulate the heart's rhythm.

Silent ischemia: Episodes of cardiac ischemia that are not accompanied by chest pain.

Sphygmomanometer: An instrument used to measure blood pressure.

Stenosis: The narrowing or constriction of an opening, such as a blood vessel or heart valve.

Stethoscope: An instrument for listening to sounds within the body.

Streptococcal infection ("strep" infection): An infection, usually in the throat, resulting from the presence of streptococcus bacteria.

Sternum: The breastbone.

Sudden death: Death that occurs unexpectedly and instantaneously or shortly after the onset of symptoms.

Transcatheter intervention: Any of the noninvasive procedures usually performed in the cardiac catheterization laboratory.

Transplantation: Replacing a failing organ with a healthy one from a donor.

Tricuspid valve: The structure that controls blood flow from the heart's upper right chamber (the right atrium) into the lower right chamber (the right ventricle).

Valvuloplasty: Reshaping of a heart valve with surgical or catheter techniques.

Varicose vein: Any vein that is abnormally dilated.

Ventricular fibrillation: A condition in which the ventricles contract in a rapid, unsynchronized fashion.

Glossario dei termini oculistici

Ablation zone: The area of tissue that is removed during laser surgery.

Accommodation: The ability of the eye to change its focus from distant objects to near objects.

Acuity: Sharpness of vision.

Astigmatism: A distortion of the image on the retina caused by irregularities in the cornea or lens.

Cornea: The clear, front part of the eye.

Diopter: The measurement of refractive error. A negative diopter value signifies an eye with myopia and a positive diopter value signifies an eye with hyperopia.

Dry eye syndrome: A common condition that occurs when the eyes do not produce enough tears to keep the eye moist and comfortable.

Endothelium: The inner layer of cells on the inside surface of the cornea.

Epithelium: The outermost layer of cells of the cornea and the eye's first defense against infection.

Excimer laser: An ultraviolet laser used in refractive surgery to remove corneal tissue.

Farsightedness: The common term for hyperopia.

FDA: Abbreviation for the Food and Drug Administration, the U.S. governmental agency responsible for the evaluation and approval of medical devices.

Flap & Zap: A slang term for LASIK.

Ghost image: A fainter second image of the object that is being viewed.

Glare: Scatter from bright light that decreases vision.

Halos: Rings around lights due to optical imperfections in or in front of the eye.

Haze: Corneal clouding that causes the sensation of looking through smoke or fog.

Higher order aberrations: Refractive errors, other than nearsightedness, farsightedness, and astigmatism, that cannot be corrected with glasses or contact lenses.

Hyperopia: The inability to see near objects as clearly as distant objects, and the need for accommodation to see distant objects clearly.

Inflammation: The body's reaction to trauma, infection, or a foreign substance, often associated with pain, heat, redness, swelling, and/or loss of function.

Iris: The colored ring of tissue suspended behind the cornea and immediately in front of the lens.

Keratectomy: Surgical removal of corneal tissue.

Keratotomy: Surgical incision (cut) of the cornea.

Keratitis: Inflammation of the cornea.

Kerato-: Prefix indicating relationship to the cornea.

Keratoconus: A disorder characterized by an irregular corneal surface (coneshaped) resulting in blurred and distorted images.

Keratomileusis: Carving of the cornea to reshape it.

Laser: The acronym for "light amplification by stimulated emission of radiation." A laser is an instrument that produces a powerful beam of light that can vaporize tissue.

LASIK: The acronym for "laser-assisted in situ keratomileusis," which refers to creating a flap in the cornea with a microkeratome and using a laser to reshape the underlying cornea.

Lens: A part of the eye that provides some focusing power. The lens is able to change shape allowing the eye to focus at different distances.

Microkeratome: A surgical device that is affixed to the eye by use of a vacuum ring. When secured, a very sharp blade cuts a layer of the cornea at a predetermined depth.

Monovision: The purposeful adjustment of one eye for near vision and the other eye for distance vision.

Myopia: The inability to see distant objects as clearly as near objects.

Nearsightedness: The common term for myopia.

Ophthalmologist: A medical doctor specializing in the diagnosis and medical or surgical treatment of visual disorders and eye disease.

Optician: An expert in the art and science of making and fitting glasses who may also dispense contact lenses.

Optometrist: A primary eye care provider who diagnoses, manages, and treats disorders of the visual system and eye diseases.

Overcorrection: A complication of refractive surgery where the achieved amount of correction is more than desired.

PRK: Abbreviation for photorefractive keratectomy.

Presbyopia: The inability to maintain a clear image (focus) as objects are moved closer. Presbyopia is due to reduced elasticity of the lens with increasing age.

Pupil: A hole in the center of the iris that changes size in response to changes in lighting. It gets larger in dim lighting conditions and gets smaller in brighter lighting conditions.

Radial keratotomy: Commonly referred to as RK; a surgical procedure designed to correct myopia (nearsightedness) by flattening the cornea using radial cuts.

Refraction: A test to determine the refractive power of the eye; also, the bending of light as it passes from one medium into another.

Refractive errors: Imperfections in the focusing power of the eye, for example, hyperopia, myopia, and astigmatism.

Refractive power: The ability of an object, such as the eye, to bend light as light passes through it.

Retina: A layer of fi ne sensory tissue that lines the inside wall of the eye.

Sclera: The tough, white, outer layer (coat) of the eyeball that, along with the cornea, protects the eyeball.

Snellen Visual Acuity Chart: One of many charts used to measure vision.

Stroma: The middle, thickest layer of tissue in the cornea.

Undercorrection: A complication of refractive surgery where the achieved amount of correction is less than desired.

Visual acuity: The clearness of vision; the ability to distinguish details and shapes.

Vitreous humor: The transparent, colorless mass of gel that lies behind the lens and in front of the retina and fills the center of the eyeball.

Wavefront: A measure of the total refractive errors of the eye, including nearsightedness, farsightedness, astigmatism, and other refractive errors that cannot be corrected with glasses or contact lenses.

Glossario dei termini ginecologici

Amniocentesis: Laboratory analysis of amniotic fluid. The test, typically performed during the second trimester, is extremely reliable and can also be used to determine the baby's sex.

Antepartum: Before labor or delivery.

Anti-D Gamma Globulin: Immunoglobulin for prevention of Rh-sensitization.

Apgar Score: Physical assessment of a newborn baby; usually conducted at 1 min and 5 min after birth.

Basal body temperature (BBT): A woman's body temperature at rest; used for detection of ovulation.

Breakthrough bleeding: Nonorganic endometrial bleeding during the use of oral contraceptives.

Cervical ectropion or eversion: Migration of cells from the lining of the endocervical canal (endocervix) to the outer portion of the cervix (ecto-cervix).

Cesarean section: A surgical procedure during which the fetus is delivered through an incision in the lower abdomen and the uterine wall.

Colposcopy: Examination of the vagina and cervix by using an instrument that provides low magnification.

Embryo: A developing baby during the first trimester.

Epidural: Type of anesthesia administered through the back during labor. Not the same as a "spinal."

Estimated date of confinement (EDC): Also known as the due date. Calculated as 40 weeks—about 9 months—from the first day of the last menstrual period (LMP).

Fecal occult blood test: Test in which a stool sample is checked for blood that could indicate colon or rectal cancer.

Fetus: A developing baby after the first trimester.

Gestation: Pregnancy.

Gynecology: The branch of medicine that involves care of woman's health, including the reproductive system and breasts.

Laparoscopy: Direct visualization of the peritoneal cavity, ovaries, and the outer surfaces of the fallopian tubes and uterus by using a laparoscope.

LMP: First day of a woman's last menstrual period before pregnancy; important to know when calculating the estimated date of confinement (the "due date").

Mammography (mammogram): An X-ray of the breast, used to detect breast cancer.

Menopause: Permanent cessation of the menses, either naturally caused by ovarian failure or resulting from surgical removal of the ovaries.

Obstetrics: Branch of medicine that involves care of a woman during pregnancy, labor, childbirth, and after the baby is born.

Osteoporosis: Atrophy of bone caused by demineralization.

Pap test: A test in which cells are taken from the cervix and examined in a laboratory for abnormalities that could signal cancer.

Preeclampsia: A dangerous condition unique to pregnancy, characterized by elevated blood pressure, protein in the urine, and severe swelling (edema).

Post partum: After delivery or childbirth.

RhoGAM: Rh immunoglobulin (RhIg), also known as RhoGAM, is a special blood product that can prevent an Rh-negative mother's antibodies from reacting to Rh-positive cells.

Salpingectomy: Surgical removal of a fallopian tube.

Salpingo-oophorectomy: Surgical removal of a fallopian tube and ovary.

Sexually transmissible disease: A disease that spreads by sexual contact, including chlamydia infection, gonorrhea, genital warts, herpes, syphilis, and infection with human immunodeficiency virus.

Schiller test: Application of a solution of iodine to the cervix.

Sigmoidoscopy: Test in which a slender device is placed into the rectum and lower colon to look for cancer.

Trimester: A time period of 3 calendar months. *Gestation* is divided into three trimesters.

Tubal ligation: Permanent sterilization by surgically cutting and tying the fallopian tubes.

Urinalysis: A test for signs of chemical changes in the urine that can signal a health problem.

Urine dip-stick: A chemically sensitive strip that can be immersed in a urine sample to provide immediate test results; used to screen for such conditions as diabetes, infection, or preeclampsia.

Varicella: Virus that causes chicken pox.

Vulva: The lips of the external female genital area.

Glossario dei termini neurochirurgici

Abscess: A circumscribed collection of pus.

Acoustic Neurinomas: Benign tumor of the hearing nerve (eighth nerve).

Acromegaly: Disorder marked by progressive enlargement of the head, face, hands, feet, and thorax, due to the excessive secretion of growth hormone.

Adenoma: A benign growth formed of glandular tissue.

Agnosia: Absence of the ability to recognize the form and nature of persons and things.

Agraphia: Loss of the power of writing due either to muscular incoordination or to an inability to phrase thought.

Amaurosis: Loss of vision without discoverable lesion in the eye structures or optic nerve.

Amaurosis fugax: Temporary blindness occurring in short periods.

Amenorrhea: Absence of the menses due to causes other than pregnancy or advancing age.

Amnesia: Loss of memory caused by brain damage or by severe emotional trauma.

Analgesia: Loss of sensibility to pain, loss of response to a painful stimulus.

Anaplasia: In the case of a body cell, a reversion to a more primitive condition. A term used to denote the alteration in cell character that constitutes malignancy.

Anastomosis: A communication, direct or indirect: a joining together. In the nervous system a joining of nerves or blood vessels.

Anencephaly: Absence of the greater part of the brain, often with skull deformity.

Anorexia: Loss of appetite; a condition marked by loss of appetite leading to weight loss.

Anosmic: Without the sense of smell.

Anoxia: Total lack of oxygen supply.

Aphasia: Difficulty with, or loss of use of, language, in any of several ways including reading, writing, or speaking. Failure of understanding of the written, printed, or spoken word not related to intelligence but to specific lesions in the brain.

Apnea: Cessation of respiration; inability to get one's breath.

Apoplexy: A sudden event. Often used as equivalent to stroke.

Arachnoid: Middle layer of membranes covering the brain and spinal cord.

Arachnoiditis: Inflammation of the arachnoid membrane, most commonly seen within the spinal cord around the spinal cord and cauda equina.

Arteriovenous malformation: Collection of blood vessels with one or several abnormal communications between arteries and veins which may cause hemorrhage or seizures.

Astrocyte: Cell that supports the nerve cells (neurons) of the brain and spinal cord.

Astrocytoma: Tumor within the substance of the brain or spinal cord made up of astrocytes; often classified from Grade I (slow-growing) to Grade III (rapid-growing).

Ataxia: A loss of muscular coordination, abnormal clumsiness.

Athetosis: A condition in which there is a succession of slow, writhing, involuntary movements of the fingers and hands, and sometimes of the toes and feet.

Atrophy: A wasting of the tissues of a body part.

Autonomic nervous system: Involuntary nervous system, also termed the vegetative nervous system. A system of nerve cells whose activities are beyond voluntary control.

Avascular: Nonvascular, not provided with blood vessels.

Axon: The part of a nerve cell that usually sends signals to other nerves or structures.

Bactericidal: Causing the death of bacteria.

Bacteriostatic: Inhibiting or retarding the growth of bacteria.

Bell's palsy: Paralysis of facial muscles (usually one side) due to facial nerve dysfunction of unknown cause.

Biopsy: Removal of a small portion of tissue, usually for the purpose of making a diagnosis.

Blood–brain barrier: The barrier that exists between the blood and the cerebrospinal fluid which prevents the passage of various substances from the bloodstream to the brain.

Bradycardia: Slowness of the heart rate.

Bradykinesia: Slowness in movement.

Brown-Sequard's syndrome: Loss of sensation of touch, position sense, and movement on the side of a spinal cord lesion, with loss of pain sensation on the other side. Caused by a lesion limited to one side of the spinal cord.

Carcinoma: Cancer, a malignant growth of epithelial or gland cells.

Carotid artery: Large artery on either side of the neck which supplies most of the cerebral hemisphere.

Carotid sinus: Slight dilatation on the common carotid artery at its bifurcation containing nerve cells sensitive to blood pressure. Stimulation can cause slowing of the heart, vasodilatation, and a fall in blood pressure.

Carpal tunnel: Space under a ligament in the wrist through which the median nerve enters the palm of the hand.

Cauda equina: The bundle of spinal nerve roots arising from the end of the spinal cord and filling the lower part of the spinal canal (from approximately the thoracolumbar junction down).

Caudate nucleus: part of the basal ganglia, which are brain cells that lie deep in the brain.

Cerebellum: The lower part of the brain which is beneath the posterior portion of the cerebrum and regulates unconscious coordination of movement.

Cerebrospinal fluid: Water-like fluid produced in the brain that circulates around and protects the brain and spinal cord.

Cerebrum: The principal portion of the brain, which occupies the major portion of the interior of the skull and controls conscious movement, sensation, and thought.

Cervical: Of or relating to the neck.

Chiasm (optic): Crossing of visual fibers as they head toward the opposite side of the brain. For each optic nerve most of the visual fibers cross to the opposite side, some run directly backward on each side without crossing.

Chorea: A disorder, usually of childhood, characterized by irregular, spasmodic involuntary movements of the limbs or facial muscles.

Choroid plexus: A vascular structure in the ventricles of the brain which produces cerebrospinal fluid.

Coccyx: The small bone at the end of the spinal column in man, formed by the fusion of four rudimentary vertebrae. The "tail bone."

Coma: A state of profound unconsciousness from which one cannot be roused.

Computed tomography (CT) scan: A diagnostic imaging technique in which a computer reads X-rays to create a three-dimensional map of soft tissue or bone.

Concussion: A disruption, usually temporary, of neurological function resulting from a blow or violent shaking.

Contrast medium: Any material (usually opaque to X-rays) employed to delineate or defi ne a structure during a radiologic procedure.

Contusion: A bruise; an area in which blood that has leaked out of blood vessels is mixed with brain tissue.

Coronal suture: The line of junction of the frontal bones and the parietal bones of the skull.

Cortex: The external layer of gray matter covering the hemispheres of the cerebrum and cerebellum.

Cranium: The part of the skull that holds the brain.

Craniectomy: Excision of a portion of the skull.

Craniopharyngioma: Congenital tumor arising from the embryonic duct between the brain and pharynx.

Cranioplasty: The operative repair of a defect of the skull.

Craniosynostosis: Premature closure of cranial sutures, limiting or distorting the growth of the skull.

Craniotomy: Opening of the skull, usually by creating a flap of bone.

CSF: Cerebrospinal fluid.

Depressed skull fracture: A break in the bones of the head in which some bone is pushed inward, possibly pushing on or cutting into the brain.

Diabetes insipidus: Excretion of large amounts of urine of low specific gravity. The inability to concentrate urine.

Diffuse axonal injury: Damage to the axons of many nerve cells that lie in different parts of the brain.

Diffuse brain injury: Damage to the brain that can affect many parts of the brain, often in a subtle fashion; examples include diffuse axonal injury and inadequate blood flow.

Diphenylhydantoin: Dilantin; a medication used to control seizures.

Diplopia: Double vision, usually due to weakness or paralysis of one or more of the extra-ocular muscles.

Disc: The intervertebral disc—cartilaginous cushion found between the vertebrae of the spinal column. It may bulge beyond the vertebral body and compress the nearby nerve root, causing pain. The terms "slipped disc," "ruptured disc," and "herniated disc" are often used interchangeably even though there are subtle differences.

Dome: The round balloon-like portion of an aneurysm which usually arises from the artery from a smaller portion called the neck of the aneurysm.

Dura: Dura mater.

Dura mater: A tough fibrous membrane which covers the brain and spinal cord, but is separated from them by a small space.

Dysesthesia: A condition in which a disagreeable sensation is produced by ordinary touch, temperature, or movement.

Dysphasia: Difficulty in the use of language due to a brain lesion without mental impairment.

Dystonia musculorum deformans: An affliction occurring especially in children, marked by muscular contractions producing distortions of the spine and hips.

Electroencephalography (EEG): The study of the electrical currents set up by brain actions; the record made is called an electroencephalogram.

Electromyography (EMG): A method of recording the electrical currents generated in a muscle during its contraction.

Endarterectomy: Removal of fatty or cholesterol plaques and calcified deposits from the internal wall of an artery.

Endocrine gland: A gland that furnishes an internal secretion, usually having an effect on another organ.

Endocrinopathy: Any disease due to abnormality of quantity or quality in one or more of the internal glandular secretions.

Ependyma: The membrane lining the cerebral ventricles of the brain and central canal of the spinal cord.

Ependymoma: A growth in the brain or spinal cord arising from ependymal tissue.

Epidural: Immediately outside the dura mater. Same as extradural.

Epidural hematoma: A blood clot between the dura mater and the inside of the skull.

Epilepsy: Disorder characterized by abnormal electrical discharges in the brain, causing abnormal sensation, movement, or level of consciousness.

Falx (cerebri): An extension of the dura between the right and left hemispheres of the brain.

Fontanelle: Normal openings in the skull of infants; the largest of these is the anterior fontanel or "soft spot" in the middle of the head.

Foraminotomy: Surgical opening or enlargement of the bony opening traversed by a nerve root as it leaves the spinal canal.

Fusiform aneurysm: A sausage-like enlargement of the vessel.

Galactorrhea: The discharge of milk from the breasts.

Gamma knife: Equipment that precisely delivers a concentrated dose of radiation to a predetermined target using gamma rays.

GCS: Glasgow Coma Scale.

Glasgow Coma Scale: The most widely used system of classifying the severity of head injuries or other neurologic diseases.

Glasgow Outcome Scale: A widely used system of classifying outcome after head injury or other neurologic diseases.

Glia (also termed neuroglia): The major support cells of the brain. These cells are involved in the nutrition and maintenance of the nerve cells.

Glioma: A tumor formed by glial cells.

Glioblastoma: A rapidly growing tumor composed of primitive glial cells, mainly arising from astrocytes.

Globus pallidus: Part of the basal ganglia, which are brain cells that lie deep in the brain.

Hemangioma: An aggregation of multiple, dilated, blood vessels.

Hematoma: A blood clot.

Hemianopia: Loss of vision of one-half of the visual field.

Hemiatrophy: Atrophy of half of an organ or half of the body.

Hemiplegia: Paralysis of one side of the body.

Hemorrhage: Bleeding due to the escape of blood from a blood vessel.

Herniated nucleus pulposus (HNP): Extrusion of the central portion of an intervertebral disc through the outer cartilaginous ring. The material can compress the spinal cord or nerves in or exiting the spinal canal.

Hydrocephalus: A condition, often congenital, marked by abnormal and excessive accumulation of cerebrospinal fluid in the cerebral ventricles. This dilates the ventricles and in infants and young children causes the head to enlarge.

Hydromyelia: Expansion of the spinal cord due to increased size of the central canal of the cord which is filled with CSF.

Hyperacusis: Abnormal acuteness of hearing or auditory sensation.

Hyperesthesia: Excessive sensibility to touch, pain, or other stimuli.

Hypertension: High blood pressure.

Hypothalamus: A collection of specialized nerve cells at the base of the brain which controls the anterior and posterior pituitary secretions, and is involved in other basic regulatory functions such as temperature control and attention.

Infundibulum: A stalk extending from the base of the brain to the pituitary gland.

Intracerebral hematoma: A blood clot within the brain.

Intracranial pressure (ICP): The overall pressure inside the skull.

Intraoperative cisternography: administration of a contrast dye into the ventricles, which are chambers in the brain that contain brain fluid.

Ischemia: Inadequate circulation of blood generally due to a blockage of an artery.

Labyrinth: The internal ear, comprising the semicircular canals, vestibule, and cochlea.

Lamina: The flattened or arched part of the vertebral arch, forming the roof of the spinal canal.

Laminectomy: Excision of one or more laminae of the vertebrae.

Laminotomy: An opening made in a lamina.

Leptomeninges: Two thin layers of fi ne tissue covering the brain and spinal cord (the pia mater and arachnoid).

Leptomeningitis: Inflammation of the membranes covering the brain and spinal cord.

Leukodystrophy: Disturbance of the white matter of the brain.

Leukoencephalitis: An inflammation of the white matter of the brain.

Linear accelerator: Equipment that precisely delivers a concentrated dose of radiation to a predetermined target using X-rays.

Lipoma: A benign fatty tumor, usually composed of mature fat cells.

Lordosis: Curvature of the spine with the convexity forward.

Lumbar drain: A device (usually a long, thin, flexible tube) inserted through the skin into the cerebrospinal fluid space of the lower back; provides a method of draining cerebrospinal fluid.

Median nerve: The nerve formed from the brachial plexus that supplies muscles in the anterior forearm and thumb, as well as sensation of the hand. It may be compressed or trapped at the wrist in carpal tunnel syndrome.

Medulloblastoma: Tumor composed of medulloblasts, which are cells that develop in the roof of the fourth ventricle (medullary velum).

Meninges: The three membranes covering the spinal cord and brain termed dura mater, arachnoid mater, and pia mater.

Meningioma: A firm, often vascular, tumor arising from the coverings of the brain.

Meningitis: An infection or inflammation of the membranes covering the brain and spinal cord.

Meningocele: A protrusion of the coverings of the spinal cord or brain through a defect in the skull or vertebral column.

Meningoencephalitis: An inflammation or infection of the brain and meninges.

Meningoencephalocele: A protrusion of both the meninges and brain tissue through a skull defect.

Myelin: The fat-like substance that surrounds the axon of nerve fibers and forms an insulating material.

Myelogram: An X-ray of the spinal canal following injection of a contrast material into the surrounding cerebrospinal fluid spaces.

Myelopathy: Any functional or pathologic disturbance in the spinal cord.

Myelomeningocele: A protrusion of the spinal cord and its coverings through a defect in the vertebral column.

Myopathy: Any disease of muscle.

Neuralgia: A paroxysmal pain extending along the course of one or more nerves.

Neurectomy: Excision of part of a nerve.

Neuritis: Inflammation of a nerve; may also be used to denote non-inflammatory nerve lesions of the peripheral nervous system.

Neuroblastoma: Tumor of sympathetic nervous system origin, found mostly in infants and children.

Neurofibroma: A tumor of the peripheral nerves due to an abnormal collection of fibrous and insulating cells.

Neurofibromatosis: A familial condition characterized by developmental changes in the nervous system, muscles, and skin, marked by numerous tumors affecting these organ systems.

Neurohypophysis: The posterior lobe of the pituitary gland.

Neurolysis: Removal of scar or reactive tissue from a nerve or nerve root.

Neuroma: A tumor or new growth largely made up of nerve fibers and connective tissue.

Neuropathy: Any functional or pathologic disturbance in the peripheral nervous system.

Nystagmus: Involuntary rapid movement of the eyes in the horizontal, vertical, or rotary planes of the eyeball.

Occiput: The back part of the head.

Oligodendroglia: Non-nerve cells (see glia), forming part of the supporting structure of the central nervous system.

Oligodendroglioma: A growth of new cells derived from the oligodendroglia.

Ophthalmoplegia: Paralysis of one or more of the eye muscles.

Osteoma: A benign tumor of bone.

Osteomyelitis: Inflammation of bone due to infection, which may be localized or generalized.

Papilledema: Swelling of the optic nerve head, which can be seen in the back of the retina during eye examination.

Paraplegia: Paralysis of the lower part of the body including the legs.

Pituitary: Gland at the base of the brain which secretes hormones into the blood stream (those hormones that regulate other glands including the thyroid, adrenals, and gonads). The "master gland."

Polyneuritis: Inflammation of two or more nerves simultaneously.

Porencephaly: Abnormal cavity within brain tissue, usually resulting from outpouching of a lateral ventricle.

Post-ictal: State following a seizure, often characterized by altered function of the limbs and/or mentation.

Proprioception: Sensation concerning movements of joints and position of the body in space.

Pseudotumor cerebri: Raised intracranial pressure, usually causing only headache and papilledema. No clear underlying structural abnormality.

Pupil: The black part of the eye through which light enters; enlarges in dim light and decreases in size in bright light.

Quadrantanopia: Defect in vision or blindness in one fourth of the visual field.

Quadriplegia: Paralysis of all four limbs.

Rachischisis: Abnormal congenital opening of the vertebral column.

Radiation oncologist: A medical doctor who has received advanced training in the treatment of persons undergoing radiotherapy for an illness.

Radiologist: A medical doctor who has received specialized training in interpreting X-rays, CTs, MRIs, and in performing angiography.

Radiotherapy: Treatment of a lesion with radiation.

Saccular aneurysm: A balloon-like outpouching of a vessel (the most common type of aneurysm).

Scotoma: An area of decreased vision surrounded by an area of less depressed or normal vision.

Shunt: A tube or device implanted in the body (usually made of Silastic) to redivert excess cerebrospinal fluid away from the brain to another place in the body. Also an abnormal communication between vessels.

Spina bifida: A congenital defect of the spine marked by the absence of a portion of the spine.

Spinal fusion: Operative method of strengthening and limiting motion of the spinal column. Can be performed with a variety of metal instruments and bone grafts, or bone grafts alone.

Spondylolisthesis: Forward displacement of one vertebra on another.

Spondylosis: Degenerative bone changes in the spine usually most marked at the vertebral joints.

Stereotactic: Originated from the Greek words *stereo* meaning three-dimensional and *tactos* meaning touched.

Stereotactic radiosurgery: The precise delivery of radiation to a prese-lected stereotactically localized target.

Strabismus: Deviation of eye movement which prevents the two eyes from moving in a parallel fashion.

Subarachnoid hemorrhage: Blood in, or bleeding into, the space under the arachnoid membrane, most commonly from trauma or from rupture of an aneurysm.

Subdural hematoma: A collection of blood (clot) trapped under the dura mater, the outermost membrane surrounding the brain and spinal cord.

Syringomyelia: A fluid-filled cavity in the spinal cord.

Teratoma: Tumor or growth made up of several different types of tissue (fat, bone, muscle, skin).

Thrombus: A blood clot attached to the wall of an artery.

Thalamus: Brain cells which lie in the upper part of the brainstem.

Tic douloureux: See "Trigeminal neuralgia."

Transsphenoidal approach: Operative method of reaching the pituitary gland or skull base traversing the nose and sinuses.

Trigeminal neuralgia: Paroxysmal pain in the face. Pain may be so severe that it causes an involuntary grimace or "tic" (tic douloureux).

Ventricle: The cavities or chambers within the brain which contain the cerebrospinal fluid.

Ventriculitis: Inflammation and/or infection of the ventricles.

Ventriculogram: An X-ray study of the ventricles.

Ventriculostomy: An opening into the ventricles of the brain, such as by inserting a small, thin, hollow catheter.

Ventricular drainage: Insertion of a small tube into the ventricles to drain cerebrospinal fluid, usually when pressure is increased.

Vermis: Middle part of the cerebellum between the two hemispheres.

Vertigo: An abnormal sensation of rotation or movement of one's self or the environment.

Glossario dei termini relativi alla chirurgia plastica

Abdominoplasty: A surgical procedure, also known as tummy tuck, to correct the apron of excess skin hanging over the abdomen.

Augmentation mammaplasty: Breast enlargement by surgery.

Bilateral gynecomastia: A condition of over-developed or enlarged breasts affecting both breasts in men.

Blepharoplasty: Eyelid surgery to improve the appearance of the upper eyelids, lower eyelids, or both.

"Botox," Botulinum toxin: Injected to temporarily relax facial muscles to eliminate wrinkles for 3–6 months.

Brachioplasty: A surgical procedure, also known as arm lift, to correct sagging of the upper arms.

Brow lift: A surgical procedure to correct a low-positioned or sagging brow.

Cheek/chin augmentation: Surgery where implants are placed in the cheeks or chin to improve bone structure and support sagging, soft tissues.

Chemical peels: Resurfacing of the skin with an acid solution that peels the top layers and allows smoother, regenerated skin to emerge; an effective treatment for wrinkles caused by sun damage, mild scarring, and certain types of acne.

Circumferential thigh lift: A surgical procedure to correct sagging of the outer and mid-thigh.

Collagen implant: An injection of natural protein that raises skin tissue to smooth skin and make wrinkles and scars appear less visible.

Dermabrasion: A facial sanding technique used to treat deep scars and wrinkles, raised scar tissue, and some severe cases of cystic acne; top layers of skin are "sanded" off with a high-speed rotating brush or a diamond-coated wheel.

Facial reconstruction: Surgery to repair or reconstruct facial features in victims of cancer, facial trauma, and birth defects.

Filler injections: Most commonly collagen—a gel-like substance derived from purified animal tissue, and fat—which is harvested from the patient's thigh or abdomen and then injected to plump up facial areas or "fill" wrinkled areas (see also Botox).

Forehead lift: Surgery to minimize forehead lines and wrinkles, and to elevate brows to reduce lid drooping.

General anesthesia: Drugs and/or gases used during an operation to relieve pain and alter consciousness.

Hair replacement: Surgery to redistribute hair to hide the appearance of hair loss.

Human fat: Harvested from the patient's own body and used as an injectable filler for soft-tissue augmentation.

Injectable fillers: Substances used to restore volume and youthful appearance.

Intravenous sedation: Sedatives that are administered by injection into a vein to help the patient relax.

Laser resurfacing/laserbrasion surgery: Light beams vaporize top layers of the skin to lessen the appearance of wrinkles, scars, or birthmarks or to generally resurface facial skin.

Lipoplasty: Another term for liposuction.

Liposuction: Also called lipoplasty or suction lipectomy, this procedure vacuums out fat from beneath the skin's surface to reduce fullness.

Local anesthesia: A drug that is injected directly to the site of an incision during an operation to relieve pain.

Lower body lift: Surgical procedure to correct sagging of the abdomen, buttocks, groin, and outer thighs.

Mastectomy: The removal of a breast, typically to rid the body of cancer.

Medial thigh lift: A surgical procedure to correct sagging of the inner thigh.

Mentoplasty: Surgery to balance a profile by enlarging, reducing, or reshaping the chin.

Microdermabrasion: A mini-peeling with minimal risk of dyspigmentation or scarring that is achieved by projecting aluminum micro-crystals onto the skin (also referred as the "Power Peel," "Euro Peel," "Parisian Peel," and "Derma Peel"); safe for all skin types.

Mini- or micro-grafting: A hair replacement technique where transplanted pieces of hair-bearing skin are placed between the original "plugs" to refine the overall appearance.

MRI: Magnetic resonance imaging; a painless test to view tissue, similar to an X-ray.

Nasolabial fold: Deep creases between the nose and mouth.

Orthognathic surgery: To alleviate problems with a patient's "bite" or jaw alignment (performed in cooperation with a patient's dentist, orthodontist, or oral maxillofacial surgeon).

Otoplasty: Surgery of the ear where protruding or deformed ears can be "pinned back" by reshaping the cartilage.

PMMA: A widely used implant material formed into tiny microspheres and suspended in a collagen gel for use as a wrinkle filler.

Reduction mammaplasty: The surgical removal of breast tissue to reduce the size of breasts.

Rhinoplasty: Aesthetic surgery of the nose where cartilage and bone are reshaped and reconstructed; excess bone or cartilage may be removed.

Rhytidectomy: A surgical procedure, also known as facelift, to reduce sagging of the mid-face, jowls, and neck.

Saline implants: Breast implants filled with a salt-water solution.

Scalp flap surgery: A hair replacement method that involves rotating strips of hair-bearing scalp from the side and back of the head to the front and top; restores the hairline while maintaining normal hair density.

Scalp reduction surgery: Surgery to reduce the size of the bald area.

Scar revision surgery: Procedures to help minimize visible facial scars.

Septorhinoplasty: A form of rhinoplasty that is performed to reconstruct the nasal passage or to relieve obstructions inside the nose to correct breathing problems; the obstruction is removed through internal incisions and the interior of the nose is restructured.

Silicone implants: Breast implants filled with an elastic gel solution.

Skin resurfacing: Removal of the outer layer of the skin using abrasion, chemicals, or a laser, resulting in smoother and less wrinkled skin.

Soft-tissue augmentation: The use of injectable fillers to restore volume and youthful appearance.

Suction lipectomy: Another term for liposuction.

Sutures: Stitches used by surgeons to hold skin and tissue together.

Tumescent or super-wet liposuction: Requires an infusion of saline solution with adrenaline and possibly anesthetic prior to removal of excess fat.

Tummy tuck: A surgical procedure to correct the apron of excess skin hanging over the abdomen.

Unilateral gynecomastia: A condition of over-developed or enlarged breasts affecting just one breast in men.

Ultrasound: A diagnostic procedure that projects high-frequency sound waves into the body and changes the echoes into pictures.

Ultrasound-assisted lipoplasty: Uses ultrasonic energy to liquefy excess fat prior to surgical suctioning.

Glossario dei termini relativi alla chirurgia toracica

Achalasia: A condition characterized by loss of synchronized muscle contraction in the esophagus and failure of the lower esophageal muscle to relax with swallowing.

Ablation: The removal or destruction of tissue.

Acute: Abrupt onset that usually is severe; happens for a limited period of time.

Adjuvant therapy: Treatment provided in addition to the primary treatment to prevent cancer recurrence.

Advance directives: Legal documents including the Living Will and Durable Power of Attorney for Health Care. A Living Will states what type of treatment you wish to receive in the event that you become physically or mentally unable to communicate your wishes. A Durable Power of Attorney for Health Care authorizes another person to make medical decisions for you when you are unable to do so for yourself.

Allograft (allogenic graft or homograft): An organ or tissue transplanted from one individual to another of the same species, i.e., human to human.

Alveoli: Thin-walled, small sacs located at the ends of the smallest airways in the lungs where the exchange of oxygen and carbon dioxide takes place.

Aortic dissection: The aorta is made up of many layers. In certain circumstances, a tear develops in the middle layer, which allows blood to travel down the layer, setting up two channels.

Aspiration pneumonia: A condition that occurs when the contents of the stomach or esophagus are breathed into the airways.

Asthma, chronic: A disease of the air passages that carry air in and out of the lungs. Asthma causes the airways to narrow, the lining of the airways to swell, and the cells that line the airways to produce more mucus. These changes make breathing difficult and cause a feeling of not getting enough air into the lungs. Common symptoms include shortness of breath, wheezing, and excess mucus production.

Atelectasis: Partial or complete collapse of the lung, usually due to a blockage of the air passages with fluid, mucus, or infection. Symptoms include dry cough, chest pain, and mild shortness of breath.

Attending or primary physician: The doctor who has the main responsibility for your care while you are in the hospital. There may be other doctors caring for you such as consulting doctors, resident doctors, and medical students.

Balloon (pneumatic) dilation: A nonsurgical treatment for achalasia.

Barium swallow test: A test in which the patient swallows a barium sulfate preparation (liquid or other form), and its movement through the esophagus is evaluated using X-ray technology.

Barrett's esophagus: A condition that develops in some people who have chronic gastroesophageal reflux disease (GERD) or inflammation of the esophagus.

Biopsy: The removal of a sample of tissue via a small needle. The tissue is removed for examination to determine a diagnosis.

BIPAP (bi-level positive airway pressure) machine: A breathing machine that uses two pressure levels (inspiratory and expiratory) to provide breathing assistance. This machine is often used for patients with sleep apnea or respiratory failure.

Botox (botulinum toxin) injections: A treatment for some patients with achalasia.

Botox is a protein made by the bacteria that cause botulism.

Breathing rate: the number of breaths per minute.

Breathing tube (endotracheal tube): A temporary tube put into the nose or mouth. Anesthesia or air and oxygen pass through the tube allowing artificial breathing.

Bronchi: A pair of breathing tubes that connect the trachea to the lungs. Oxygen and carbon dioxide travel in opposite directions through the bronchi.

Bronchial tubes: Branches of the airways (air passages) in the lungs.

Bronchioles: The smallest branches of the airways in the lungs. They connect to the alveoli (air sacs).

Bronchitis, chronic: Irritation and inflammation of the lining of the bronchial tubes. Bronchodilator: Medication used to relax the muscle bands that tighten around the airways to increase air flow. Bronchodilators also help clear mucus from the lungs.

Bronchoscope: A long, thin tube with a small camera at the end that is used to evaluate the airways. The bronchoscope is passed through the nose or mouth, past the vocal chords and down the airway as far as necessary. The camera transmits the images on a television monitor. Bronchoscopy can be used to remove objects or mucus blocking the airway, or to remove growths in the airway.

Bronchoscopy: A diagnostic test used to view the inside of the airway. The test can be performed to diagnose lung diseases or locate the source of a problem by visualizing the throat, larynx, trachea, and lungs and to collect tissue samples for biopsy.

Bronchospasm: The sudden tightening of the bands of muscle that surround the airways, causing the airways to become narrower. Bronchospasm may result in wheezing.

Bronchus: Singular of bronchi.

Cannula: A small plastic tube used to supply extra oxygen through the nose.

Carbon dioxide: A colorless, odorless gas that is formed in tissues of the body and is delivered to the lungs for removal.

Carcinogen: Cancer-causing substance.

Chest X-ray: Procedure used to view the lungs and lower respiratory tract. A chest X-ray may be used for diagnosis and therapy.

Chronic: Continuing over a certain period of time; long-term.

Cilia: Hair-like structures that line the airways in the lungs and help to clean out the airways.

Clinical trials: Research programs conducted with patients to evaluate a new medical treatment, drug, or device.

Computed tomography (CT) scan: An X-ray procedure that combines many X-ray images with the aid of a computer to generate cross-sectional views of the body.

Contraindication: Any condition which indicates that a particular course of treatment (or exercise) would be inadvisable or cause harm.

COPD (chronic obstructive pulmonary disease): A general term used to describe several lung diseases. The most common diseases in this group include chronic bronchitis and emphysema. Chronic asthma may also be included. COPD worsens gradually, causing limited airflow in and out of the lungs.

Cor pulmonale: Enlargement of the right side of the heart. Cor pulmonale weakens the heart and causes increased shortness of breath and swelling in the feet and legs. Patients who have chronic COPD with low oxygen levels may develop this condition.

CPAP (continuous positive airway pressure) machine: A breathing machine that provides pressure to keep the upper airways open during breathing. This machine is often used for patients with obstructive sleep apnea.

Diaphragm: The thin muscle below the lungs and heart that separates the chest cavity from the abdomen. The diaphragm is the most efficient breathing muscle.

Diaphragmatic surgery: Surgery performed on the diaphragm. Diaphragmatic surgery may be performed to treat a hernia or any other conditions that affect the diaphragm.

Diffusion capacity: A measurement of how much oxygen is carried from your lungs into your bloodstream.

Dysphagia: Difficulty swallowing.

Dysplasia: Abnormal or precancerous cells or tissue.

Dyspnea: Shortness of breath, difficulty breathing.

Edema: Swelling that may occur in the ankles, feet, or legs.

Emphysema: A degenerative disease characterized by the destruction, or breakdown, of the walls of the alveoli (air sacs) located at the end of the bronchial tubes.

Empyema: A collection of pus in the pleural space (the cavity between the lung and the membrane that surrounds it).

Endoscopic screenings: A diagnostic procedure used to view the lining of the esophagus, stomach, small bowel, or colon.

Esophageal cancer: The uncontrolled growth of abnormal cells in the esophagus. The uncontrolled reproduction of cells results in the formation of tumors that can block or compress the esophagus.

Esophageal diverticulum: A sac or pouch protruding from the esophagus.

Esophageal manometry: A test that measures the timing and strength of the contractions of the esophagus and the relaxations of the lower esophageal sphincter valve.

Esophageal perforation: A tear in the esophagus that requires emergency surgical treatment.

Esophageal pH test: A test that measures the pH in the esophagus to determine if you have GERD.

Esophagectomy: Also called esophageal resection surgery. Surgical removal of the esophagus. An esophagectomy may be performed as a treatment for highgrade dysplasia or cancer.

Esophagitis: An inflammation of the lining of the esophagus.

Esophagoscopy: A diagnostic test in which a flexible, narrow tube called an endoscope is passed through the mouth or nose into the esophagus to produce images of the inside of the esophagus. This video examination projects images onto a screen.

Esophagogastrectomy: The removal of a portion of the lower esophagus and part of the stomach for treatment of tumors or strictures of those organs.

Esophagus: The muscular tube that extends from the neck to the abdomen and connects the throat to the stomach.

Exacerbation: Worsening.

Gastroesophageal reflux disease (GERD): A condition that occurs when the contents of the stomach travel back up into the esophagus. When stomach acid enters the lower part of the esophagus, it can produce a burning sensation, commonly referred to as heartburn.

Gastrostomy: An artificial opening from the stomach to a hole (stoma) in the abdomen where a feeding tube is inserted. The feeding tube allows the delivery of nutrients directly into the small intestine, bypassing the stomach. A feeding may be needed temporarily after certain surgeries to allow recovery. See also enteral nutrition.

H2-receptor antagonists: Also called H2 receptor blockers or histamine receptor blockers. Medications that control or eliminate acid, but may not be as effective as proton pump inhibitors. H2-receptor antagonists may be used to treat gastroesophageal reflux disease (GERD) and include cimetidine (Tagamet HB), famotidine (Pepcid AC), nizatidine (Axid AR), and ranitidine (Zantac 75). Some of these medications are available over-the-counter, but should not be used for more than a few weeks at a time.

Heartburn: A burning sensation in the chest that may occur after eating, bending, stretching, or exercise and sometimes at night when lying down. Heartburn symptoms are usually relieved by antacids and may be more frequent or worse at night.

Heller myotomy: A surgical treatment for achalasia in which the muscles of the valve between the esophagus and the stomach are cut.

Hiatus: An opening in the diaphragm—the muscular wall separating the chest cavity from the abdomen.

Hiatal hernia: Also called hiatus hernia. An area of the stomach that bulges up into the chest through the hiatus. Normally, the esophagus (food pipe) goes through the hiatus to drain into the stomach. In a hiatal hernia, the stomach bulges up into the chest through that opening.

Hyperhidrosis: A medical condition in which a person sweats excessively and unpredictably. People with hyperhidrosis can sweat even when the temperature is cool, and when they are at rest.

Hyperventilation: Excessive rate and depth of breathing.

Hypoxia: Insufficient oxygen in the tissues, even though blood flow is adequate.

I/E ratio: Inhalation/exhalation ratio, or the relative length of inhalation (breathing in) compared to exhalation (breathing out).

Incentive spirometer: A device that is used to encourage deep inspiration to expand the lungs and improve cough effectiveness.

Inflammation: One of the body's defense mechanisms, inflammation results in increased blood flow in response to infection and certain chronic conditions.

Intensive care unit: A special nursing area that provides continuous and immediate care to patients recovering right after surgery or to seriously ill patients.

Intubation: Placing a tube in the trachea (wind pipe) to enable artificial breathing.

Jejunostomy tube (J-tube): A feeding tube that is inserted through the skin on the abdomen into the small intestine.

Laparoscopic surgery: A minimally invasive surgical technique.

Laparoscopic antireflux surgery: See Nissen fundoplication.

Laparoscopic Heller myotomy: A minimally invasive surgical procedure used to treat achalasia. This surgical treatment opens up the lower valve (lower esophageal sphincter) so that food passes from the mouth to the stomach by gravity.

Laparoscopic hiatal hernia repair: A minimally invasive procedure to correct a defect in the diaphragm.

Laparoscopy: An evaluation that involves looking into the abdominal cavity with a special camera (called a laparoscope).

Lobectomy: Removal of a lobe of the lung. Lobectomy is the most common surgery performed to treat lung cancer. Also see video-assisted lobectomy surgery.

Lower esophageal sphincter (LES): A valve located at the end of the esophagus that controls the passage of food from the esophagus to the stomach during swallowing.

Lung biopsy: A procedure in which several small samples of lung tissue are removed through a small incision between the ribs.

Lung transplant: A surgical procedure in which a healthy lung from a donor replaces the recipient's unhealthy lung. Lung transplant is a treatment option reserved for selected patients with chronic lung diseases.

Lung volume reduction surgery: A surgical procedure performed to remove diseased, emphysematous lung tissue.

Lymphoma: Cancer that occurs in cells of the lymphatic system. Lymphoma includes Hodgkin's disease and non-Hodgkin's lymphoma.

Mediastinal tumor: A benign or cancerous growth that forms in the area of the chest that separates the lungs (mediastinum).

Mediastinoscopy: A minimally invasive surgical technique used to diagnose and sometimes treat some mediastinal tumors. This test is performed under general anesthesia in the operating room of a hospital and takes 1–2 h (same-day procedure).

Mediastinum: The area of the chest that separates the lungs. It is surrounded by the breastbone in the front, the spine in the back, and the lungs on each side. It contains the heart, aorta, esophagus, thymus, and trachea.

Minimally invasive thoracic surgery (MIS): See video-assisted thoracic surgery.

Motility disorder: Also called esophageal motor disorder. A disorder affecting the movement of food from the esophagus to the stomach.

Mucus clearing device: Also called a PEP device. A device used to loosen mucus in the airways so it can be coughed up more easily.

Myasthenia gravis: A chronic disease characterized by weakness and rapid fatigue of the voluntary muscles.

Nissen fundoplication: A minimally invasive procedure that corrects gastroesophageal reflux by creating an effective valve mechanism at the bottom of the esophagus.

Odysphagia: Pain when swallowing.

Parenteral nutrition: A method of providing food through a tube placed in the nose, the stomach, or the small intestine. A tube in the nose is called a nasogastric or nasoenteral tube. A tube that goes through the skin into the stomach is called a gastrostomy or percutaneous endoscopic gastrostomy (PEG). A tube into the small intestine is called a jejunostomy or percutaneous endoscopic jejunostomy (PEJ) tube. Also called tube feeding. See also gastrostomy and jejunostomy.

Pectus excavatum: A congenital chest wall deformity in which several ribs and the sternum grow abnormally, producing a concave, or caved-in, appearance to the front of the chest wall (also known as sunken or funnel chest).

Pericardial effusion: Presence of an abnormal amount and/or type of fluid in the pericardial space.

Pericardial space: The space between the layers of the pericardium. It contains fluid that lubricates the membrane surfaces and allows easy heart movement.

Pericardium: The sac that surrounds the heart.

Peritoneum: The inner lining of the abdomen.

Pleura: The thin membrane that lines the outside of the lungs and the inside of the chest cavity. The pleura acts as a lubricant to help you breathe easily. Normally, very little fluid is present in the pleura.

Pleural effusion: An excessive build-up of fluid between the layers of the pleura.

Pleural mesothelioma: A rare form of cancer in which tumors form in the sac lining the chest (the pleura) or the abdomen (the peritoneum).

Pleural space: The cavity between the lung and the membrane that surrounds it.

Pleuroscopy: Another term for minimally invasive thoracic surgery. See videoassisted thoracic surgery (VATS).

Pneumonectomy: Surgical removal of a lung, usually as a treatment for cancer.

Pneumonia: A group of diseases that cause infection or inflammation (swelling) in the lungs.

Pneumothorax: A collection of air or gas in the space surrounding the lungs.

Pulmonary function test: A test used to reveal lung capacity and function, and to determine the blood's capacity to transport oxygen.

Pulmonary hypertension: A rare lung disorder in which the arteries in the lungs have become narrowed, making it difficult for blood to flow through the vessels.

Pulmonary rehabilitation: A program that can help a patient learn how to breathe easier and improve quality of life. It includes treatment, exercise training, education, and counseling.

Pulmonologist: A doctor who specializes in caring for people with lung diseases and breathing problems.

Regurgitation: The uncontrolled flow of stomach contents back into the esophagus and mouth.

Rejection: Transplant rejection may occur when immune cells recognize the transplanted organ as different from the rest of the body and attempt to destroy it. This is the body's way of not accepting the new organ. Fortunately, rejection can be treated, especially if the signs of rejection are recognized early.

Sleep apnea: A sleep disorder in which a person's breathing stops in intervals that may last from 10 s to 1 min or longer. When an apneic event occurs, air exchange may be impaired.

Spirometry test: A breathing test that provides information about lung function and the extent of a patient's lung disease.

Sternotomy: A type of surgical procedure in which an incision is made along the sternum, after which the sternum itself is divided, or "cracked." This procedure provides access to the heart and lungs for surgical procedures.

Thoracentesis: Procedure used to drain fluid from the chest, such as a pleural effusion.

Thoracic outlet syndrome: A group of distinct disorders that affect the nerves in the brachial plexus and blood vessels between the base of the neck and axilla, mediastinum (space behind the sternum, the spine, and in between the lungs), and diaphragm (thin muscle below the lungs and heart that separates the chest from the abdomen).

Thoracoscopy: Another term for minimally invasive thoracic surgery. Also called thorascopy. See "Video-assisted thoracic surgery" (VATS).

Thorascope: Small video-scope used during video-assisted thoracic surgery to project images on a video screen for the surgeon to view during the procedure.

Thoracotomy surgery: A type of surgery in which an incision is made on the side of the chest between the ribs.

Thoracosotomy, chest tube: A procedure performed to drain fluid, blood, or air from the space around the lungs (pleural space).

Thorax: Area of the body located between the neck and abdomen. The thorax contains the heart, lungs, esophagus, and great vessels surrounded by the breastbone or sternum in front, the ribs on each side, and the spine in the back.

Thymoma: Disease in which cancerous (malignant) cells are found in the tissues of the thymus.

Thymus: Small organ located in the upper/front portion of the chest, extending from the base of the throat to the front of the heart.

Total lung capacity test: a test that measures the amount of air in the lungs after a person has breathed in as much as possible.

Trachea: Also called the "windpipe." The main airway (windpipe) supplying air to both lungs.

Tracheal stricture: A narrowing in the trachea that restricts airflow to the lungs.

Tracheostomy: Small opening or incision made in the throat. Through the tracheostomy, a tube is placed to aid breathing for patients who may need to be supported longer than expected with mechanical ventilation. Instead of breathing through the nose and mouth, the patient then breathes through the tracheostomy or "trach" (pronounced "trake").

Upper GI (gastrointestinal) series: A series of X-rays used to evaluate the upper gastrointestinal system (the esophagus, stomach, and part of the small intestine) to detect abnormalities.

Video-assisted thoracic surgery (VATS): Surgery of the chest that is performed with a thoracoscope (small video-scope) using small incisions and special instruments to minimize trauma.

Video-assisted lobectomy surgery (VATS lobectomy): A minimally invasive surgical technique that is less invasive than traditional thoracotomy surgery.

Wedge resection: Surgical removal of a wedge-shaped portion of tissue from one, or both, lungs. A wedge resection is typically performed for the diagnosis or treatment of small lung nodules.

Glossario dei termini ortopedici

Achilles tendonitis: Inflammation of the heel cord that is the extension from the triceps surae group of muscles.

ACL: Anterior cruciate ligament.

ALPSA lesion: Anterior labrum periosteal sleeve avulsion.

Arthritis: Inflammation of a joint, usually accompanied by pain, swelling, and sometimes change in structure.

Arthroscopy: A surgical procedure used to visualize, diagnose, and treat problems inside a joint.

Ankylosing spondylitis: A rheumatoid arthritis-type disease causing spontaneous fusion of the spine.

Arthritis: Inflammation of a joint.

Arthroplasty: Reconstructive surgery of a joint or joints to restore motion because of ankylosis or trauma or to prevent excessive motion.

Atrophy: Reduction in size of an anatomic structure, frequently related to disuse or decreased blood supply.

Bennet lesion: Posterior glenoid defect associated with overhead throwing injuries.

Bone metastases: The spread of malignant cancer cells to bone.

Brachial plexus palsy: Excessive lateral flexion of the head on the trunk during delivery of the shoulders or delivery of the head in a traction injury to one or more components of the brachial plexus.

Brachytherapy: Radiotherapy treatment with ionizing radiation whose source is applied to the surface of the skin.

Bunion: An inflammation and thickening of the bursa in the joint of the big toe.

Bursa: A sac filled with fluid located between a bone and a tendon or muscle.

Bursitis: Repeated small stresses and overuse that cause the bursa to swell and become irritated.

Carpal tunnel syndrome: Loss of sensation and sometimes motor control if the median nerve is cut off at the wrist because of compression of the nerve at the carpal ligament.

Cartilage: A smooth material that covers bone ends of a joint to cushion the bone and allow the joint to move easily without pain.

Cerebral palsy: A general term applied to central nervous system disorders found at birth or infancy and affecting muscle control.

Cervical spine degeneration: The deterioration of the quality of the seven segments of spinal tissue between the base of the skull and the thoracic spine.

Chondrosarcoma: A malignant neoplasm of cartilage.

Club feet: Turning of the heel inward with increased plantar flexion (the toedown motion of the foot at the ankle).

Compliant fixation system: A novel means for securing massive prostheses to bone that uses a spring-type mechanism to avoid long stems, bone cement, and problems of stress shielding and osteolysis.

Decompressions: In relation to the spine, this procedure is carried out to relieve the pressure on the spinal cord or nerve roots. The pressure may result from fracture fragments, disc fragments, tumors, or infections.

Degenerative disc disease: Gradual or rapid deterioration of the chemical composition and physical properties of the disc space.

Desensitization: Treatment of hypersensitivity and pain secondary to nerve injury, partial nerve injury, nerve compression, and soft-tissue injuries.

Discectomy: The excision of intervertebral disc material that may be described as herniated, implying "bulging" or "rupture" through the ligaments.

Dupuytren's contracture: A hereditary thickening of the tough tissue, called fascia, that lies just below the skin of the palm resulting in flexion deformities of the finger.

Edema control: Methods and devices used to minimize persistent swelling in the hand or upper extremity.

EMG (electromyogram): A test to evaluate nerve and muscle function.

Femur: Thighbone.

Fibrous dysplasia: A progressive and usually lethal process in which multiple muscles form bone.

Flatfoot: Condition in which one or both arches have flattened out.

Ganglion cysts: Noncancerous, fluid-filled cysts are common masses or lumps in the hand and usually found on the back of the wrist.

Guillain-Barré syndrome: Viral disorder involving the spinal cord, peripheral nerves, and nerve roots.

HAGL lesion: Humeral avulsion of the glenohumeral ligament.

Hammertoe: A permanent sideways bend in the middle toe joint.

Herniated disc: Fibrous extrusion of semifluid nucleus pulposus through a ruptured intervertebral disc; damage results from pressure on the spinal cord or nerve roots.

Hill-Sachs lesion: Bony defect in the humeral head caused by a shoulder dislocation.

Hip dysplasia: Failure of normal bony modeling of the hip socket.

Joint mobilization: Use of specific passive procedures to restore accessory movements, to stretch joint capsules and ligaments, and to reduce pain and muscle guarding of stiff joints.

Kinematics: That phase of mechanics which deals with the possible motions of a material body.

Kyphosis: Any forward-bending area or deformity in the spine.

Labral lesions: A fibrocartilaginous supporting structure which surrounds the glenoid bone in the shoulder.

Leg length inequity: One leg is shorter than the other.

Ligaments: Connect the bones and keep joints stable.

Little leaguer's elbow: Overuse injury to the lateral aspect of the elbow (capitellum).

Little leaguer's shoulder: Separation of the proximal humeral growth plate.

Locomotor system: The musculoskeletal system movement or the ability to move from one place to another.

Malunion: State of healing of the bone in which bone unites but in an abnormal position and/or alignment.

Morton's neuroma: A pinched nerve usually causing pain between the third and fourth toes.

Multidirectional instability: Shoulder laxity in multiple directions which causes pain or dysfunction.

Myelogram: A specific X-ray study that uses an injection of a dye or contrast material into the spinal canal to allow careful evaluation of the spinal canal and nerve roots.

Nerve block Injection of lidocaine or other medication around a nerve to determine if a particular nerve is causing pain, and to relieve pain.

Neuromuscular re-education: Used in cases of postoperative care of surgical repair of nerve injuries. Involves the retraining of reinnervated muscles.

Nonunion: State of healing of the bone in which there is no healing.

Orthopedic surgery (or orthopedics): The medical specialty devoted to the diagnosis, treatment, rehabilitation, and prevention of injuries and diseases of the body's musculoskeletal system.

Osteoarthritis: Generally, a condition caused by wear and tear leading to inflammation of the joint, causing swelling, pain, and stiffness.

Osteomyelitis: Inflammation of bone marrow, cortex, tissue, and periosteum; can be caused by any organism, but usually bacteria.

Osteoporosis (porous bone): A condition that develops when bone is no longer replaced as quickly as it is removed.

Osteosarcoma: Sarcoma in which cancer cells make bone.

Osteotomy: Surgical procedure that changes the alignment of bone with or without removal of a portion of that bone.

PCL: Posterior cruciate ligament.

Peripheral nerve disorders: Problems involving numbness, tingling, and weakness in the upper extremity.

Phonophoresis: Therapeutic application of ultrasound with a topical drug, most commonly corticosteroid.

Post-polio syndrome: A syndrome of increasing weakness, fatigue, and pain appearing decades after an acute infection of poliomyelitis.

Posterior/anterior spinal fusions: A procedure for fusing two or more spinal segments with or without removal of an intervertebral disc.

Prosthetics: The science that deals with functional and/or cosmetic restoration for all or part of a missing limb.

Reflexive sympathetic dystrophy: A diseased state of an extremity that is characterized by very severe pain, swelling, stiffness, and discoloration.

RICE treatment: Rest, ice, compression, and elevation.

Rotator cuff disease: Inflammation or rupture of one or more of the tendons that lie deep in the shoulder and bridge the glenohumeral joint.

Rotator cuff tendonitis: Inflammation of the rotator cuff and associated bursal sac.

Scoliosis: Side-to-side curve in the back, a lateral and rotational deviation of the spine from the normally straight vertical line of the spine.

SLAP lesion: Superior labral lesion in the shoulder.

Soft tissue: Generally, the ligaments, tendons, and muscles in the musculoskeletal system.

Spina bifida: Congenital absence of a large portion of the posterior spine, usually in the lumbosacral region.

Spondylolisthesis: Displacement of a vertebral body on the one below.

Sprain: A partial or complete tear of a ligament.

Strain: A partial or complete tear of a muscle or tendon.

Stress fractures: A bone injury caused by overuse.

Synovium: A fibrous envelope that produces a fluid to help to reduce friction and wear in a joint.

Tendon: The extension of muscle into a firm, fibrous cord that attaches into a bone or other firm structure.

Tendonitis: Inflammation of a tendon.

Tennis elbow: Stress tendinitis on the lateral epicondyle.

Torn anterior cruciate ligament: Tear in one or both of the two deep ligaments within the knee that are crossed.

Torn medial collateral ligament: A tear in the strong fibrous ligament on the medial side of the knee connecting the femur with the tibia.

Torn meniscus: A tear in the crescent-shaped fibrocartilaginous disc between the two joint surfaces.

Torn rotator cuff: A tear in one or more of the tendons that lie deep in the shoulder and bridge the glenohumeral joint.

Torsion: A type of load that is applied by a couple of forces that are parallel and directed opposite to each other about the long axis of a structure.

Trigger finger: Catching or locking of a finger.

Glossario dei termini urologici

Artificial sphincter: Sometimes complicated cases of incontinence require implantation of a device known as an artificial urinary sphincter.

Assisted reproductive technologies (ART): The new forms of fertility treatment incorporate many methods of sperm retrieval and preparation. Once the sperm have been processed to ensure optimal fertilizing potential, they are used in a variety of procedures that aid the process of conception. These procedures include artificial insemination (AI), in vitro fertilization (IVF), and sperm microinjection techniques.

Behavioral techniques: Different methods to help "retrain" the bladder and get rid of the urgency to urinate (see biofeedback, bladder training, electrical stimulation, habit training, pelvic muscle exercises, prompted voiding).

Benign prostatic hyperplasia: A condition in which the prostate becomes enlarged as part of the aging process.

Benign tumor: A tumor that is not cancerous.

Bilateral: A term describing a condition that affects both sides of the body or two paired organs, such as the kidneys.

Biofeedback: A procedure that uses electrodes to help people gain aware-ness and control of their pelvic muscles.

Bladder: A hollow muscular balloon-shaped organ that stores urine until it is excreted from the body.

Bladder training: A behavioral technique that teaches the patient to resist or inhibit the urge to urinate, and to urinate according to a schedule rather than urinating at the urge.

Brachytherapy: Involves the placement of tiny radioactive pellets into the prostate gland.

Catheter: A tube passed through the body for draining fluids or injecting them into body cavities.

Catheterization: Insertion of a slender tube through the urethra or through the anterior abdominal wall into the bladder, urinary reservoir, or urinary conduit to allow urine drainage.

Chancre: A hard, syphilitic primary ulcer, the first sign of syphilis, appearing approximately 2–3 weeks after infection.

Chemolysis: Certain types of kidney stones can be dissolved with the application of chemicals.

Cryotherapy: During an operation probes are placed in the prostate. The probes are then frozen thereby killing the prostatic cells.

Cystocele: A herniation of the bladder into the vagina.

Cystectomy: Surgical removal of the bladder.

Cystoscopy: A flexible scope is inserted into the urethra and then into the bladder to determine abnormalities in the bladder and lower urinary tract.

Electrohydraulic lithotripsy (EHL): This technique uses a special probe to break up small stones with shock waves generated by electricity.

Enterocele: Herniation of the small bowel into the vagina.

Extracorporeal shock wave lithotripsy (ESWL): Extracorporeal shock wave lithotripsy uses highly focused impulses projected from outside the body to pulverize kidney stones.

Habit training: A behavioral technique that calls for scheduled toileting at regular intervals on a planned basis.

Hormonal therapy: Involves the use of anti-androgens. An androgen is a male hormone needed for the production of testosterone.

Hydrocele: A painless swelling of the scrotum, caused by a collection of fluid around the testicle; commonly occurs in middle-aged men.

Hypermobility: A condition characterized in which the pelvic floor muscles can no longer provide the necessary support to the urethra and bladder neck.

Hyperplasia: Excessive growth of normal cells of an organ.

Intrinsic sphincter deficiency (ISD): Weakening of the urethra sphincter muscles.

Kegel exercises: Exercises to strengthen the muscles of the pelvic floor, which leads to more control and prevents leakage.

Kidney stone: A hard mass composed of substances from the urine that form in the kidneys.

Laparoscopy: Surgery using a laparoscope to visualize internal organs through a small incision.

Laparoscopic lymph node dissection: If a perineal prostatectomy is contemplated, then prior to the operation the pelvic lymph nodes are sampled via three small incisions made in the abdomen.

Lithotripsy: A procedure done to break up stones in the urinary tract using ultrasonic shock waves, so that the fragments can be easily passed from the body.

Menopause: The period that marks the permanent cessation of menstrual activity, usually occurring between the ages of 40 and 58.

Metastasis: The spreading of a cancerous tumor to another part of the body.

Mixed incontinence: Having both stress and urge incontinence.

Nephrectomy: Removal of an entire kidney.

Open nephrolithotomy: The most invasive procedure for removing kidney stones.

Orchiectomy: The surgical removal of one or both of the testicles.

Orchitis: Inflammation of a testicle.

Overactive bladder: A condition characterized by involuntary bladder muscle contractions during the bladder-filling phase which the patient cannot suppress.

Overflow UI: Leakage of small amounts of urine from a bladder that is always full.

Percutaneous nephrolithotomy (PCN): In PCN, the surgeon or urologist makes a 1-cm incision under local anesthesia in the patient's back, through which an instrument called a nephroscope is passed directly into the kidney and, if necessary, the ureter. Smaller stones may be manually extracted. Large ones may need to be broken up with ultrasonic, electrohydraulic, or laser-tipped probes before they can be extracted. A tube may be inserted into the kidney for drainage.

Pelvic muscle exercises: Pelvic muscle exercises are intended to improve pelvic muscle tone and prevent leakage for sufferers of stress urinary incontinence.

Also called Kegel exercises (see Biofeedback).

Post-void residual (PVR) volume: A diagnostic test which measures how much urine remains in the bladder after urination.

Prostate: A muscular, walnut-sized gland that surrounds part of the urethra.

Prostatectomy: Surgical removal of the prostate.

Radical retropubic prostatectomy: Removal of prostate tissue through an abdominal incision.

Perineal prostatectomy: A perineal incision is utilized for prostatectomy.

Prostatic stent: Inserted through a cystoscope, it is a wire device that expands after placement thus pushing prostate tissue away from passageway allowing for easier urination.

Prostatitis: Inflammation of the prostate, Pyelonephritis: Inflammation of the kidney, usually due to a bacterial infection.

Pyuria: The presence of pus in the urine; usually an indication of kidney or urinary tract infection.

Rectocele: A herniation of the rectum into the vagina.

Sexually transmitted disease (STD): Infections that are most commonly spread through sexual intercourse or genital contact.

Sling procedures: Surgical methods for treating urinary incontinence involving the placement of a sling, made either of tissue obtained from the person undergoing the sling procedure or a synthetic material. The sling is anchored to the retropubic and/or abdominal structures.

Sphincter: A ring of muscle fibers located around an opening in the body that regulates the passage of substances.

Stress urinary incontinence/urinary incontinence: The involuntary loss of urine during periods of increased abdominal pressure. Such events include laughing, sneezing, coughing, or lifting heavy objects.

Suprapubic/retropubic prostatectomy: This involves the removal of obstructing prostatic tissue through a suprapubic incision (a cut below the belly button).

Testosterone: The sex hormone that stimulates development of male sex characteristics and bone and muscle growth; produced by the testicles and in small amounts by the ovaries.

Transient urinary incontinence: Temporary episodes of urinary incontinence that are gone when the cause of the episode is identified and treated.

Glossario dei termini relativi alla chirurgia vascolare

Aorta: The main artery in the body from which all of the other arteries arise. It begins at the heart and extends down through the chest and abdomen and finally branches in the lower abdomen into the arteries that go to the legs.

Aneurysm: A balloon-like dilation of a portion of an artery that is a weak point along the course of the vessel, which may lead to rupture or clotting.

Atherosclerosis: Sometimes referred to as "hardening of the arteries." This condition represents an accumulation of fats and cholesterol in the inner lining of an artery that can build up to such a degree that the artery becomes narrowed or completely blocked.

Balloon angioplasty: A technique in which a thin catheter, which has an inflatable balloon on its tip, is inserted into an artery.

Bypass: An operation in which blood is re-routed around a blocked portion of an artery using a graft.

Carotid artery: An artery in the neck that carries blood to the brain.

Claudication: Leg pain caused by inadequate blood flow to the exercising leg muscles.

Compression stockings: Stockings worn to decrease leg swelling and relieve pain associated with conditions such as chronic venous insufficiency and varicose veins.

Coumadin: A pill form of an anticoagulant (blood thinner).

CT scan: An X-ray technique allowing visualization of the internal organs.

Diabetes mellitus: A condition associated with abnormal glucose metabolism and complications such as arterial insufficiency, kidney failure, and visual loss.

Duplex scan: A scan using ultrasound waves that allow visualization of blood vessels and organs.

Endovascular surgery: Correction of conditions affecting arteries and veins by approaching the lesion from within the blood vessel using catheters, balloons, and stents rather than by making an incision into the blood vessel.

Endograft: A fabric-covered metallic stent that is placed inside an aneurysm to prevent rupture.

Femoral artery: The blood vessel that carries oxygen-rich blood from the heart and lungs into the leg.

Femoral vein: The blood vessel that carries blood out of the leg and back to the heart and lungs.

Femoropopliteal or tibial bypass: A surgical bypass created in the leg to carry blood around a blockage in the leg arteries.

Gangrene: Death of tissue due to lack of adequate circulation.

Intestinal angina: Pain in the abdomen that occurs after eating. It is caused by inadequate circulation to the small intestine.

Ischemia: Inadequate arterial blood flow to a portion of the body. For example: leg ischemia, brain ischemia, cardiac ischemia.

Lymphedema: Swelling of an extremity (arm or leg) due to blockage of the normal flow of lymph from an extremity.

MRA: Magnetic resonance angiography. A technique used to visualize blood vessels in a noninvasive manner.

Occlusion: Complete blockage.

Plaque: A deposit of fats and cholesterol within the lining of an artery. Usually referred to as atherosclerotic plaque.

Prosthetic graft: An artificial tube that can be manufactured using synthetic fabric-like material.

Pseudoaneurysm: An opening in an artery which may lead to rupture. It is caused by an injury to the blood vessel.

Sclerotherapy: A technique of injecting a solution into varicose veins or spider veins, which causes the vein to close and shrink.

Stenosis: Narrowing.

Stroke: Death of a portion of brain tissue due to inadequate blood flow.

Thrombolysis: A technique in which drugs are used to dissolve blood clots.

Thrombophlebitis: A condition in which a blood clot forms in the veins.

Transient ischemic attack (TIA): A temporary weakness or numbness of a portion of the body (e.g., an arm or leg) usually lasting just a few minutes, which is due to a temporary interruption of the arterial blood flow to the brain.

Varicose veins: Dilated, tortuous veins of the lower extremities that are caused by incompetence of the valves within the vein.

Capitolo 12

Inglese chirurgico per specialità

In questo capitolo potrete leggere le descrizioni di interventi relativi a differenti specialità chirurgiche. Come potrete supporre, questo non è un libro "how to do it", ma queste descrizioni vi aiuteranno a prepararvi prima di frequentare un ospedale anglofono.

Cardiac Surgery

Aortic Valve Replacement

The patient lies face up on the table under general anesthesia. A midline incision and sternotomy are made and a pericardial well is created. The patient is cannulated via the aorta and a single atrial venous cannula. Most commonly, retrograde cardioplegic solution is used and a left ventricular vent is placed via the right superior pulmonary vein to maintain a dry operative field. The dose of heparin is calculated in relation to the patient's weight. After cross-clamping the aorta and starting extracorporeal circulation, the surgeon performs a transverse aortotomy approximately 1 cm above the take-off of the right coronary artery, slightly above the level of the sinotubular ridge. The incision is extended threequarters of the way around the aorta, leaving the posterior one-quarter of the aorta intact and allowing excellent visualization of the native aortic valve and annulus. The leaflets of the aortic valve are excised to the level of the annulus and the annulus is thoroughly debrided of any calcium. Braided 2–0 sutures with pledgets are used. Beginning at the noncoronary commissure, the annulus is encircled with interrupted mattress sutures extending from the aortic to the ven-

R. Ribes, P. J. Aranda, J. Giba, *Inglese per chirurghi*,
© Springer-Verlag Italia 2012

tricular surface. After placement, the suture bundles are divided into two equal portions and two individual sutures are placed into the sewing ring the prosthesis at the level of the pivot guards, orienting the pivot guard toward the ostia of the left and right coronary arteries. Next, each half of the suture bundles is implanted in the sewing ring and the prosthesis is seated. The pivot guard sutures are tied first followed by the sutures beginning at the left coronary cusp extending to the mid-portion of the right coronary cusp. Lastly, the sutures of the noncoronary cusp are secured, seating the valve appropriately. In a small aortic root, if a valve cannot be seated, paravalvular leak can be prevented by ensuring the unseated area of the valve is in the noncoronary cusp. Leaflet motion should always be checked and the surgeon must be sure that the coronary arteries are not obstructed. The aortotomy is closed with a double layer of polypropylene over-and-over sutures. The patient is placed in the Trendelenburg position and the heart is filled with blood and vented; finally, the cross-clamp is removed. Once the heart starts beating, volume and temperature are recovered slowly to get off-pump. Meanwhile, the surgeon places the pacemaker wires and drainage
tubes. Furthermore, the cannulae and vent are removed and exhaustive hemostasis is required before closing. The first step is to close the pericardium with a few individual sutures, secondly the sternum is approximated with bone wires, and finally the wound is closed by planes.

Cardiochirurgia

Sostituzione valvolare aortica

Il paziente giace supino sul tavolo operatorio, in anestesia generale. Vengono eseguite un'incisione toracica mediana e una sternotomia, poi viene confezionata un'apertura pericardica. Il paziente viene incannulato attraverso l'aorta e una singola cannula venosa atriale. Più frequentemente si utilizza una soluzione cardioplegica retrograda e viene posizionato un deflussore ventricolare sinistro attraverso la vena polmonare superiore destra al fine di mantenere il campo operatorio asciutto.
La dose di eparina è calcolata in rapporto al peso del paziente. Dopo aver clampato l'aorta e aver iniziato la circolazione extracorporea, il

chirurgo esegue un'aortotomia trasversa circa 1 cm al di sopra dello sbocco dell'arteria coronaria destra, leggermente al di sopra del livello della giunzione sinotubulare.

L'incisione dell'aorta viene estesa per tre quarti della circonferenza aortica, lasciando il quarto posteriore della circonferenza aortica intatto e permettendo una visione eccellente della valvola aortica nativa e dell'ostio. I lembi valvolari vengono escissi a livello dell'ostio, che viene accuratamente liberato da ogni calcificazione. Sono utilizzati fili intrecciati 2-0 con pledget. A cominciare dalla commissura non coronarica, l'ostio viene circondato con suture da materassaio tra le superfici ventricolare e aortica. Dopo il loro posizionamento, ciascuna sutura viene divisa in due porzioni uguali e due suture singole sono piazzate nell'anello cucito della protesi a livello dei perni di sicurezza, orientandoli verso gli osti delle coronarie destra e sinistra. Successivamente ciascuna metà di ogni sutura viene impiantata nell'anello cucito e la protesi viene posizionata. Per prime vengono annodate le suture del perno di sicurezza, seguite dalle suture in corrispondenza della cuspide coronarica sinistra andando verso la porzione media della cuspide coronarica destra. Infine vengono annodate le suture della cuspide non coronarica, alloggiando correttamente la valvola. Nel caso di una radice aortica piccola, nella quale non sia possibile alloggiare una valvola, le perdite ematiche paravalvolari possono essere evitate assicurandosi che l'area della valvola non alloggiata si trovi nella cuspide non coronarica. Il movimento del lembo valvolare dovrebbe sempre essere controllato e il chirurgo deve essere sicuro che le arterie coronarie non siano ostruite. L'aortotomia viene chiusa con un doppio strato di polipropilene. Il paziente viene posto in posizione di Trendelemburg e il cuore viene riempito di sangue e svuotato; infine viene rimosso il clamp aortico. Una volta che il cuore inizia a battere, il volume e la temperatura vengono lentamente ripristinati per far ripartire la pompa cardiaca. Nel frattempo, il chirurgo posiziona i cavetti del pacemaker e i tubi di drenaggio. Inoltre vengono rimosse le cannule e il deflusso; è indispensabile un'emostasi accurata prima di chiudere. Il primo passo consiste nel chiudere il pericardio con alcune suture singole, successivamente lo sterno viene chiuso con suture ossee e infine la ferita viene chiusa per piani.

General and Abdominal Surgery

Standard Laparoscopic Cholecystectomy

Cholelithiasis and acute cholecystitis are the indications for this intervention. The patient lies in the Trendelemburg position under general anesthesia. The surgeon stands between the patient's open legs and the assistant stands to the left of the patient. The first step is to induce pneumoperitoneum with a Verres needle or with a mini-laparotomy through the umbilicus. Then the first laparoscope trocar with the optic system is placed above the umbilicus, and the camera is used to place the other laparoscope trocars, sparing the superficial vessels. One of the trocars is inserted in an infrasternal position and the rest are situated in the right abdominal wall under the liver and in the left abdominal wall under the ribs. The optical instrument and the left laparoscope are directed by the assistant, and the other is directed by the surgeon. With the endo-grasper instrument the assistant grips the gallbladder fundus, elevating it and keeping it elevated. The surgeon uses another endo-grasp through the right trocar to grasp Hartmann's pouch and move the gallbladder to look for cystic vessels in Calot's triangle. Through the infrasternal trocar the surgeon introduces the endo-dissect instrument to look for the cystic tract. When the cystic tract is found, the endo-clip instrument is introduced through the infrasternal trocar to clip the cystic duct as near as possible to the gallbladder. After two distal clips and one proximal clip have been placed, the surgeon cuts
between them using the endo-shear instrument (scissors). The same steps are taken to locate and clamp the cystic artery. It is necessary to take care with the common bile duct because it is also situated in Calot's triangle. The next step is to dissect the gallbladder from the liver bed using the monopolar electrocautery hook through the infrasternal trocar, helped by the endo-graspers situated on the right with continued upward traction. The gallbladder is dissected from the clipped cystic artery to the fundus. When the gallbladder has been detached, it is removed with the endo-grasper, endo-clinch instrument, or butterfl y-catcher instrument through the orifice of the trocar. The abdominal cavity is examined and irrigated with saline solution. Saline, blood, and smoke can be aspirated by one of the laparoscopes during the intervention. Finally, the air exits through the orifices, which are then sutured by flats.

Chirurgia generale e addominale

Colecistectomia laparoscopica standard

La colelitiasi e la colecistite acuta rappresentano le indicazione per questo intervento. Il paziente giace in posizione di Trendelemburg, in anestesia generale. Il chirurgo si posiziona tra le gambe aperte del paziente e l'aiuto si trova alla sinistra del paziente. Il primo passo consiste nell'induzione dello pneumoperitoneo con un ago di Verres o con una minilaparotomia attraverso l'ombelico. Successivamente viene posizionato al di sopra dell'ombelico il primo trocar laparoscopico attraverso il quale viene introdotta l'ottica; si utilizza la telecamera per posizionare gli altri trocar laparoscopici, risparmiando i vasi superficiali. Uno dei trocar viene posizionato in posizione sottoxifoidea e gli altri vengono posizionati nella parete addominale destra al di sotto del fegato e nella parete addominale sinistra al di sotto delle costole. L'ottica e il ferro laparoscopico introdotto attraverso il trocar sinistro sono utilizzati dall'aiuto, gli altri dall'operatore. Grazie alla pinza laparoscopica, l'aiuto afferra il fondo della colecisti, sollevandola e tenendola in questa posizione. L'operatore utilizza un'altra pinza laparoscopica attraverso il trocar destro per afferrare l'infundibolo e spostare la colecisti alla ricerca di dotto e arteria cistica nel triangolo di Calot. Attraverso il trocar sottoxifoideo l'operatore introduce il dissettore laparoscopico per identificare il dotto cistico. Quando questo viene trovato, l'endoclip viene introdotta attraverso il trocar sottoxifoideo per posizionare una clip sul dotto cistico il più vicino possibile alla colecisti. Dopo che sono state posizionate due clip distali e una prossimale, l'operatore seziona il cistico tra di loro utilizzando forbici laparoscopiche. Si eseguono le stesse procedure per localizzare e chiudere l'arteria cistica. È necessario prestare attenzione al dotto epatico comune in quanto localizzato anch'esso in corrispondenza del triangolo di Calot. Il passo successivo consiste nel dissecare la colecisti dal letto epatico usando l'uncino a coagulazione monopolare attraverso il trocar sottoxifoideo, con l'aiuto della pinza laparoscopica posizionata a destra, mediante una trazione continua verso l'alto. La colecisti viene dissecata a partire dall'arteria cistica chiusa con clip e sezionata fino al fondo. Quando la colecisti è stata staccata, essa viene rimossa per mezzo di una pinza laparoscopica, di un grasper laparoscopico o di un sacchetto attraverso l'orifizio del trocar. La cavità addominale viene esaminata e lavata con soluzione fisiologica. La soluzione fisiologica, il sangue e il fumo possono essere aspirati durante l'intervento da uno dei laparoscopi. Infine l'aria esce dai tramiti parietali, che vengono suturati per piani.

Gynecology and Obstetrics

Cesarean Section

Under epidural anesthesia, the patient lies face up on the table. The first step is to make an abdominal incision above the pubis with a cold scalpel. Then we use an electric scalpel to open the incision to the muscular fascia and to ensure hemostasis. The assistant retracts the tissue using two Farabeuf retractors to expose the fascia to the surgeon, who makes a small incision with the electric scalpel. With two pairs of Allis forceps, we grasp the borders of the incision to separate and elevate them. With Metzenbaum scissors, the fascia is cut lengthwise, the muscles are retracted, and the peritoneum is reached. We use Kelly's forceps to separate the peritoneum and then make a small incision with Metzenbaum scissors to get into the abdominal cavity. Now we put the Balfour valves into the abdominal cavity to work better and we look for the uterus. The peritoneal fold must be dissected up and down to free the uterus. A transversal incision about 2 cm long is then made with a cold scalpel in the uterine isthmus, which is the thinnest part of the uterus and the part with the fewest vessels. This must be done carefully to avoid injury to the baby, and we widen the gap with our fingers. The fetal membranes are opened with curved Kelly scissors to allow the amniotic fluid to be suctioned out with a Yankauer suction tip. The placenta is retracted with the fingers, the Balfour valves are withdrawn, and the baby is extracted from the uterus with Velasco forceps. We clean the baby, first with a Nelaton catheter connected to an aspiration system and then with a white compress. The umbilical cord is clamped with two curved Rochester clamps and cut with Metzenbaum scissors. Now we can extract the whole placenta from the uterus. The uterine cavity is checked to ensure that it is clean, and it can also be cleaned with a white compress. A blood sample is aspirated from the umbilical cord for analysis. Finally, we close the uterus in two planes with hemostatic sutures, and then we close the peritoneum. It is important to review the fallopian tubes, ovaries, and pelvic cavity and to clean the cavity with sterile water. We then close the abdominal wall by layers.

Ginecologia e ostetricia

Taglio cesareo

La paziente giace in posizione supina, in anestesia peridurale. Il primo passo consiste nell'eseguire un'incisione cutanea sovrapubica con bisturi a lama fredda. Successivamente utilizziamo un bisturi elettrico per approfondire l'incisione fino alla fascia muscolare e per garantire l'emostasi. L'aiuto retrae i tessuti utilizzando due divaricatori di Farabeuf per esporre la fascia all'operatore, che esegue una piccola incisione con il bisturi elettrico. Con due paia di pinze di Allis afferriamo i bordi per separarli ed elevarli. Con forbici di Metzenbaum la fascia viene sezionata longitudinalmente, i muscoli vengono divaricati e si raggiunge il peritoneo. Utilizziamo pinze di Kelly per isolare il peritoneo e successivamente eseguiamo una piccola incisione con forbici di Metzenbaum per accedere alla cavità peritoneale. A questo punto posizioniamo delle valve di Balfour all'interno della cavità peritoneale per lavorare meglio e ci poniamo alla ricerca dell'utero. Il peritoneo deve essere dissecato verso l'alto e il basso per liberare l'utero. Con bisturi a lama fredda si esegue un'incisione traversa lunga circa 2 cm sull'istmo uterino, che è la porzione più sottile e meno ricca di vasi dell'utero. Questa manovra deve essere eseguita con attenzione per evitare danni al bambino; poi allarghiamo l'apertura con le nostre dita. Le membrane fetali vengono aperte con forbici curve di Kelly per permettere l'aspirazione del liquido amniotico con la cannula da aspirazione di Yankauer. La placenta viene retratta con le dita, le valve di Balfour sono rimosse e il bambino viene estratto dall'utero con il forcipe di Velasco. Laviamo il bambino dapprima con un catetere Nelaton connesso con un sistema di aspirazione e poi con garze bianche. Il cordone ombelicale viene clampato con due pinze curve di Rochster e sezionato con forbici di Metzenbaum. A questo punto possiamo estrarre tutta la placenta dall'utero. La cavità uterina viene controllata per assicurarsi che sia pulita e può anche essere pulita con una garza bianca. Si aspira una provetta di sangue dal cordone ombelicale per eseguire degli esami ematochimici. Infine chiudiamo l'utero in due piani con suture emostatiche e poi chiudiamo il peritoneo. È importante riesaminare le tube di Falloppio, le ovaie la cavità pelvica e pulire la cavità con acqua sterile. Infine chiudiamo la parete addominale per piani.

Eye Surgery

Cataract Surgery Technique

There are two primary techniques for removing a cataract:

- Extracapsular cataract extraction (ECCE), which requires a large incision (up to 10–12 mm in length) in the sclera and removes the hard center of the cloudy lens in one piece.
- Phacoemulsification (phaco surgery), which requires a smaller incision in either the sclera or clear cornea (5.53.2 mm or less) on the side of the cornea. Most cataract surgery today is done by phacoemulsification, which is also called small-incision cataract surgery.

Phacoemulsification Technique

Either local or topical anesthesia is used in most cases. The type of anesthesia that the surgeon chooses will depend on the technique used and the condition of the eye. The lens is divided into three different portions: the center part, called the nucleus; the outer part, called the cortex; and a thin transparent membrane, called the lens capsule, that surrounds the nucleus and the cortex. We start with a small (about 3 mm) incision in the temporal part of the sclera with an ophthalmic scalpel. Then we make a second, somewhat larger (5.5–6 mm) incision at a position corresponding to between 10 and 11 o'clock. We then inject viscoelastic material to protect the anterior endothelium and to configure the anterior capsule. We use the Pezzola point to emulsify the cataract, remove the softer cortex from the eye, and try to polish up the capsule in the back; we try to ensure that as few cells as possible are left in the capsule. In most cases, the artificial posterior chamber intraocular lens (IOL) is then inserted through the second incision to compensate for the focusing power that was lost with the removal of the natural lens. Then the viscoelastic material is aspirated. Finally, we inject antibiotics and steroids through the incisions. There is no need to close the small incision in the sclera because it is a self-closing section.

Chirurgia dell'occhio

Tecnica della chirurgia della cataratta

Esistono due tecniche principali per rimuovere la cataratta:

- Estrazione extracapsulare della cataratta (ECCE), che richiede un'incisione ampia (lunghezza maggiore di 10-12 mm) della sclera e rimuove la porzione centrale dura del cristallino opaco in un unico pezzo.

- Facoemulsificazione (chirurgia FACO) che richiede un'incisione più piccola sia nella sclera che nella cornea trasparente, sul lato corneale, (5.5-3.2 mm o meno). La maggior parte degli interventi per cataratta al giorno d'oggi sono eseguiti mediante facoemulsificazione, anche chiamata chirurgia mininvasiva della cataratta.

Tecnica della facoemulsificazione

Nella maggior parte dei casi viene utilizzata l'anestesia locale o topica. Il tipo di anestesia scelta dal chirurgo dipenderà dalla tecnica utilizzata e dalle condizioni dell'occhio. Il cristallino è diviso in 3 porzioni diverse: la parte centrale, chiamata nucleo, la parte esterna, chiamata corteccia e una sottile membrana trasparente, chiamata capsula del cristallino, che circonda il nucleo e la corteccia. Iniziamo con una piccola incisione (circa 3 mm) nella porzione temporale della sclera con un bisturi oftalmico. Dopodiché eseguiamo una seconda incisione, un po' più ampia (5.5-6 mm), in una posizione compresa tra le ore 10 e 11. Successivamente iniettiamo materiale viscoelastico per proteggere l'endotelio anteriore e configurare la capsula anteriore. Usiamo la punta di Pezzola per emulsificare la cataratta, rimuovere la corteccia dall'occhio e tentare di ripulire la capsula nella porzione posteriore. Cerchiamo di assicurarci che vengano lasciate nella capsula meno cellule possibile. Nella maggior parte dei casi il cristallino artificiale (artificial posterior chamber intraocular lens; IOL) viene inserito attraverso la seconda incisione per compensare il potere di messa a fuoco perduto con la rimozione del cristallino. Successivamente il materiale viscoelastico viene aspirato. Infine iniettiamo antibiotici e corticosteroidi attraverso le incisioni. Non c'è bisogno di suturare la piccola incisione nella sclera perché si chiuderà spontaneamente.

Neurosurgery

Ventriculo-Peritoneal Shunting in the United Kingdom

(See the numbered notes below for an explanation of some the particularly British features of this description.)

The patient was anaesthetised [1] in less than ten minutes following the usual routine in the anaesthetic room: Dr Gupta [2], probably the oldest Staff Grade anaesthetist [3] in the hospital, accessed one of the large forearm veins, introduced the brown venflon, and fixed it with a piece of Mepore dressing. The propofol injection was then given and in a few seconds Mr Evans was snoring loudly. When it was clear that the "white stuff" was surfing his blood, Dr McIntyre quickly passed the laryngoscope with the help of a very efficient Dr Gupta, who pressed the cricoid just enough to assist him in the manoeuvre [4]; the endotracheal tube was down the throat in a second and was subsequently secured with tape and two laps of band in order to avoid undesired displacement. He always liked to listen to each lung for half a minute at that time to make sure there was no unilateral intubation. Once the setting was counterchecked, the patient was transferred next door where the operating theatre [5] was ready for action. Mr Evans was moved to the operating table under the theatre lamps by one of the theatre staff nurses, SN Maureen Finley, and Mike, the huge theatre porter [6]. Mr Norris [7], the Consultant Neurosurgeon [8] in charge of the case, started to position the patient adequately for the procedure. He liked to be extremely quick in performing ventriculo-peritoneal [9] shunts; this was one of his many secrets so as to avoid infection, and over the years he had designed a particularly precise ritual that he followed meticulously. The hospital gown was removed and a large foam roll was placed under the right side of the patient's naked body, tilting him enough to conveniently expose the right side of his anatomy. Then, using the Mayfield horseshoe, the head was placed comfortably rotated to the left so the patient's occipital area was accessible almost in its entirety; this step was especially important as the intraventricular catheter should penetrate the occipital horn of the lateral ventricle almost from the midline. Once Mr Norris was satisfied with the correct body position, he looked at his new Specialist Registrar [10], a ginger-haired Irish woman called Miss Murphy, who immediately took over whilst the boss disappeared to the coffee room. The targeted posterolateral [11] aspect of the head was neatly shaved and each single hair along the trajectory from the ear to the right iliac fossa was made redundant. Following this, a considerable amount of Betadine non-alcoholic solution was used to systematically disinfect the skin from top to bottom, twice. While the Povidone was left to dry and kill the remaining bugs by burning evaporation, Miss Murphy proceeded to the scrub room in order to disinfect herself. Using the chlorhexidine-impregnated nail brushes, she carefully cleaned her arms, hands and delicate fingers, paying special attention to the nails. Not until the scheme was repeated three times was she pleased and returned to the theatre where Mary Coombs, the Senior Theatre Sister [12], awaited her to start draping the patient.

A set of two large drapes was laid alongside to leave uncovered just a narrow line through which the peritoneal catheter would undermine Mr Evans' skin. Following this, two short drapes were used to isolate a small occipital area barely big enough to cut the scalp. Now, a large and sticky steridrape was used to fix the whole operative field and ensure perfect asepsis during the procedure. The instrument table was efficiently arranged and the surgeons approached the main table at this stage so the operation could commence.

Two light handles were inserted in the lamp knobs so the surgeons could touch them and adjust the illumination at their wish. Miss Murphy was helped into her operating gown and two six-and-a-half gloves were given to her. Once properly dressed and tied up, she looked at the scrub room where Mr Norris had just entered and was washing his hands. With a gesture, he asked his SpR [13] to start the operation. "Knife and two swabs, please," asked the Irish woman. Sister Mary handed over the knife and two wet swabs, and Miss Murphy incised the previously selected abdominal area with a perfect 2-in. paramedian incision to the right side of the belly button. The knife was handed back and a little amount of fat protruded through the surgical wound; helping herself with the swabs, the first fascial layer was found. "Clips, please"; Sister Mary put two small straight clips near Miss Murphy's hands before she finished requesting them. The fascia was skillfully pinched. "Knife, please"; the scalpel was back in Miss Murphy's right hand even before she could ask for it and the fascia was cut to find a red muscle layer. "Non-toothed forceps, please," requested the SpR. Using the non-toothed straight forceps, a few muscle fibres were split and a pale blue fascia appeared at the bottom of the incision; this was again clipped and cut in the same fashion and the last obstacle was then negotiated before finding the peritoneum. "Another two clips and the knife, please," said Miss Murphy. The peritoneum was dexterously snapped and a small 2-mm cut was performed with the scalpel; the omentum tried to escape: "This is it; we're in. Betadine swab to cover please, Sister." At this stage, Mr Norris was already sitting at the head of the patient ready to start the "top end" of the procedure. "Knife, Mary," he requested dryly. He performed a classic "hockey stick" incision in the right occipital area and expertly dissected the scalp skin layer to expose the periosteum. "Self-retainers and a cut Betadine swab, Mary"; a couple of self-retainer clips were handed and he placed them within the cut to leave the wound open, surrounded by a Betadine swab. "Craniotome, Mary," he mechanically ordered after a very quick "cross-cut" of the periosteum. A shiny "Midas Rex Legend" was diligently produced and Mr Norris proceeded to make a clean burr hole in the patient's bone while Miss Murphy irrigated the area with normal saline through a 20-ml syringe. "Keep the bone dust, Mary." Sister Mary collected the small pieces of bone with a Volkmann's spoon and kept them in the red lid of one of the pathology bottles. "Adson's, Mary"; the Adson's periosteum elevator was presented and the consultant lifted the inner table of the bone at the bottom of that pristine burr hole to expose the dura mater, which appeared in its usual bluish grey colour [14]. "Bipolar, Mary"; the yellow bipolar diathermy forceps was delicately put in Mr Norris's right hand and Miss Murphy made sure that the pedal was nearby. "On, Miss Murphy," said Mr Norris, and his registrar pushed the pedal with her tiny right foot so the boss could coagulate the dural surface. The bipolar machine spoke: "forty-five", was heard. Once the dura was coagulated enough, Mr Norris requested the tunneller [15]. "Go ahead, Miss Murphy: bottom to top, as usual." Miss Murphy took the tunneller, a long thin metal reusable stick which she passed through the abdominal wound, dramatically undermining the skin of the abdomen, reaching the thorax and jumping over the clavicle to appear just a few millimetres [16] under the skin of the neck, where there was a bit of a struggle to keep going. "C'mon, girl: push harder ... for God's sake!" moaned the consultant. Then, after a last sweaty effort, the tip of the tunneller was seen through the head incision. "It's okay. Give me the peritoneal catheter, Mary. In 80 mg of Gentamycine wash to prime it, I expect," said Mr Norris. Precisely, a kidney-shaped pot containing a normal saline plus 80 mg of Gentamycine mix was organised to soak and prime the peritoneal catheter and the valve, already swimming around. "Two nontoothed, hurry up"; a couple of straight forceps were handed to Mr Norris, who used them to pass the peritoneal tube through the hollow tunneller without touching it with his fingers, and the tunneller was subsequently removed, cunningly leaving catheter as the only tenant under Mr Evans' skin. "Dural knife and hook, Mary." A 15-mm blade and a dural hook were carefully offered and Mr Norris proceeded to cross-cut the dura, proficiently lifted with the help of the tiny silver hook. "Coag, Miss Murphy," said the boss and the Reg obediently burned the four corners of the dural incision, leaving a squared diamond opening through which some cerebro-spinal fluid (CSF) fl owed and it was possible to contemplate a very healthy-looking pulsating brain. "Ventricular catheter, primed in Genta with introducer, Mary." The next step, undoubtedly the most critical of the whole procedure was about to take place. Placing his left thumb in the middle of the forehead, just above the glabella, and his left finger before the external auditive meatus, the man visualised the entire ventricular system layout in his imagination and firmly pushed the intraventricular catheter forward, stopping himself when the ninth centimetre [17] had just disappeared within the brain substance. Magically, colourless [18], medium-pressure cerebro-spinal [19] fluid started to exit from the ventricle depth. "Bulldog, Mary," requested Mr Norris; a tiny silver self-retaining clip was placed at the tip of the catheter temporarily stopping the waste of more CSF. "Give me the valve primed in that stuff, Mary, and a 1/0 silk tie to secure it," said Mr Norris looking at sister Mary. "Prepare yourself to cut the tube when and where I say," he ordered Miss Murphy, who followed the whole procedure as if her own life depended on it (and it probably did at that stage of her training!). Sister Mary handed a Medtronic 1.5 delta valve immersed and primed in the antibiotic solution, and Mr Norris indicated the exact point where the intraventricular catheter was about to be cut by the assisting SpR. "Now," he ordered; Miss Murphy shortened the tube with the Mayo scissors just the right amount to allow Mr Norris to assemble the valve at the end of it. Before he could finish pushing the cranial valve end inside the white tube, Miss Murphy already had the black silk tie ready to secure the critical junction with a double knot, making impossible any movement in the future. The same procedure was repeated to bring together the peritoneal end of the sophisticated device, neatly finishing the cranial end of the operation. Both the consultant and the registrar looked at the end of the peritoneal catheter, which was left resting on the Betadine-soaked big swab on the patient's abdomen, awaiting the CSF to appear there. In a few seconds, clear CSF fl owed indicating that the diversion had been successfully achieved. "I'll close the head, Mary. Go for it. Sister, call for the next patient," said the boss. Whilst he sutured the subcutaneous layer of the scalp with the bright blue 2/0 vicryl thread,

Miss Murphy played with the holding clips left at the beginning of the operation indicating the way in Mr Evan's tummy, to widely open the peritoneum and introduce the free end of the peritoneal catheter. Once this was achieved, she started to close the layers with the same suture that her boss was using for the scalp. She was barely starting to do this when Mr Norris requested the 3/0 nylon for the skin as he always liked to perform a continuous locked suturing for the skin scar. So did Miss Murphy a few minutes later, once the peritoneum and the inner fascial layer were hermetically closed sequentially. "Perfect: thirty-nine minutes, skin to skin. This is a new record, isn't it, Sister?" asked Mr Norris. "Indeed, John: congratulations," answered Sister Mary proudly. Mr Evans was uncovered at this stage and only two beautifully sutured incisions accounted for the operation performed there. Dr Gupta took over whilst [20] Miss Murphy sat down to write in the theatre logbook. Mr Norris was already in the coffee room having his tea.

"Mr Evans! Mr Evans! Operation is finished, Sir. Breathe for me, please, sir," said Dr Gupta in his warm Southern Indian accent. Mr Evans started to wake up. Sister Mary collected all the dirty utensils and trays whilst shouting outside the door: "Mike! Bring the bed sweetie pie. It's over."

1. anaesthetised = anesthetized.
2. Dr Gupta: note the absence of a period (.) after abbreviations like "Dr" and "Mr"
3. anaesthetist = anesthesiologist. In the UK, an anaesthetist is a physician, whereas in the USA an anesthetist is a technician who only administers anesthesia under an anesthesiologist's supervision.
4. manoeuvre = maneuver
5. operating theatre = operating room
6. porter = orderly
7. Mr Norris: In the UK, surgeons are referred to and addressed as Mister rather than Doctor
8. Consultant Neurosurgeon: In the UK, a consultant is a full specialist
9. ventriculo-peritoneal = ventriculoperitoneal, usually hyphenated in the UK
10. Specialist Registrar = a resident
11. postero-lateral = posterolateral
12. Sister = Nurse
13. SpR = Specialist registrar = resident
14. blueish grey colour = bluish gray color

15. tunneller = tunneler
16. millimetres = millimeters
17. centimeter = centimeter
18. colourless = colorless
19. cerebro-spinal = cerebrospinal
20. whilst = while

Neurochirurgia

Shunt ventricolo-peritoneale nel Regno Unito

Il paziente venne addormentato nella sala anestesiologica in meno di 10 minuti seguendo la solita routine: il Dr Gupta, probabilmente l'anestesista più anziano dello staff dell'ospedale, incannulò una delle grosse vene dell'avambraccio, introdusse un venflon marrone e lo fissò con una porzione di medicazione Mepore. Dopodichè fu eseguita la somministrazione di propofol e in pochi secondi Mr Evans stava russando rumorosamente. Quando fu chiaro che il "liquido bianco" era in circolo, il Dr McIntyre inserì rapidamente il laringoscopio, con l'aiuto di un efficiente dr Gupta, che esercitò una pressione sulla cricoide appena sufficiente ad aiutarlo nella manovra; il tubo endotracheale fu posizionato in gola in un secondo e fu fermato con il nastro adesivo in due giri allo scopo di evitare dislocazioni indesiderate. A quel punto auscultava ciascun polmone per almeno mezzo minuto per essere sicuro che non vi fosse intubazione unilaterale. Una volta ricontrollato l'impianto, il paziente fu spostato alla porta successiva, oltre la quale era pronta la sala operatoria.

Mr Evans fu spostato sul tavolo operatorio sotto la lampada scialitica da una delle infermiere di sala, SN Maureen Finley e da Mike, l'enorme portantino di sala. Mr Norris, lo specialista neurochirurgo responsabile del caso, iniziò a posizionare adeguatamente il paziente per l'intervento. Voleva essere rapido nell'esecuzione degli shunt ventricolo-peritoneali; questo era uno dei suoi numerosi segreti per evitare l'infezione e col passare degli anni aveva progettato un preciso rituale che seguiva meticolosamente. Il camice ospedaliero fu rimosso e un rotolo di gommapiuma venne posizionato sotto il lato destro del corpo nudo del paziente, inclinandolo abbastanza da esporre il lato destro della sua anatomia. Dopodichè, utilizzando il fissatore a ferro di cavallo di

Mayfield, la testa venne immobilizzata, comodamente ruotata a sinistra, in modo che l'area occipitale del paziente fosse quasi interamente
accessibile; questa fase era particolarmente importante perchè il catetere intraventricolare doveva penetrare il corno occipitale del ventricolo
laterale quasi sulla linea mediana. Una volta che Mr Norris fu soddi-
sfatto della corretta posizione del paziente, guardò il suo nuovo specializzando, una donna dai capelli rossicci di nome Miss Murphy, che
immediatamente prese il suo posto mentre il capo si dileguò nella stan-
za del caffé. La regione postero-laterale della testa fu rasata accuratamente e ogni pelo lungo la linea dall'orecchio alla fossa iliaca destra fu
eliminato. Successivamente, fu utilizzata una grossa quantità di soluzione di betadine non alcolico per disinfettare sistematicamente la cute
per due volte dalla testa ai piedi. Mentre il povidone veniva lasciato ad
asciugare per evaporazione e ad annientare i germi residui, Miss
Murphy si recò nella sala lavaggio per disinfettarsi. Utilizzando le
spazzolette per unghie impregnate di clorexidina, si lavò accuratamente le braccia, le mani e le dita, prestando particolare attenzione alle
unghie. Si sentì soddisfatta solo quando la procedura di lavaggio venne
ripetuta tre volte; quindi ritornò in sala operatoria dove Mary Coombs,
l'infermiera di sala più anziana, l'aspettava per iniziare a coprire il
paziente. Due larghi telini protettivi furono stesi sul fianco del paziente, lasciando scoperta solo una sottile linea attraverso la quale il catetere peritoneale sarebbe entrato nel sottocute di Mr Evans.
Successivamente furono utilizzati due piccoli telini per isolare una piccola area occipitale sufficiente a sezionare il cuoio capelluto. A questo
punto, si utilizzò un largo steridrape adesivo per fissare l'intero campo
operatorio e garantire l'asepsi perfetta durante l'intervento. Il tavolo dei
ferri operatori fu preparato in maniera efficiente e i chirurghi si avvicina-
rono al tavolo operatorio, in modo che l'intervento potesse cominciare.
Sulla manopola della lampada scialitica furono inseriti due manicotti,
cosicché i chirurghi potessero toccarli e modificare la direzione della
luce come preferivano. Miss Murphy fu aiutata a indossare il suo camice chirurgico e le furono consegnati due paia di guanti misura 6 e $\frac{1}{2}$.
Una volta che ebbe indossato il camice operatorio, guardò nella sala
lavaggio; Mr Norris era appena entrato e si stava lavando le mani. Con
un gesto egli le chiese di iniziare di intervento.
"Un bisturi e due tamponi, per favore", chiese la donna irlandese.
L'infermiera Mary le consegnò il bisturi e due tamponi umidi e Miss
Murphy incise l'area addominale, precedentemente selezionata, con
una perfetta incisione paramediana di due pollici di lunghezza, sul lato
destro dell'ombelico. Il bisturi venne restituito e una piccola quantità di

grasso protruse dalla ferita chirurgica; aiutandosi con i due tamponi, fu identificato il primo piano fasciale. "Pinze, per favore"; l'infermiera Mary avvicinò due piccole pinze rette alle mani di Miss Murphy prima ancora che questa finisse di chiederle.

La fascia fu abilmente pizzicata. "Bisturi, per favore"; il bisturi tornò nella mano destra di Miss Murphy ancora prima che lei potesse chiederlo e la fascia fu incisa per scoprire uno strato muscolare. "pinze senzadenti, per favore", richiese la specializzanda. Utilizzando le pinze rette senza denti, furono separate alcune fibre muscolari e apparve nella parte più profonda della ferita una pallida fascia blu; questa fu nuovamente afferrata e incisa allo stesso modo e così fu superato l'ultimo ostacolo prima di raggiungere il peritoneo. "Altre due pinze e il bisturi, per favore", disse Miss Murphy. Il peritoneo fu aperto con destrezza e fu praticata un'incisione di 2 mm con il bisturi; l'omento cercò di scappare: "ci siamo; siamo dentro. Garza imbevuta di betadine per coprire, per favore."

A questo punto Mr Norris era già seduto alla testa del paziente pronto a iniziare la parte cruciale dell'intervento. "Bisturi, Mary", chiese freddamente. Eseguì una classica incisione a mazza da hockey nella regione occipitale destra e abilmente dissecò il cuoio capelluto per esporre il periostio. "Retrattori autostatici e tampone con betadine, Mary"; gli fu passata una coppia di pinze divaricatrici autostatiche e lui le posizionò dentro l'incisione per tenere la ferita aperta, circondata dal tampone betadinato. "Craniotomo, Mary," ordinò meccanicamente dopo aver effettuato una rapida incisione del periostio. Gli fu diligentemente porto uno scintillante "Midas Rex Legend" e Mr Norris procedette a praticare un foro pulito nell'osso del paziente mentre Miss Murphy irrigava l'area con soluzione salina mediante siringa da 20 ml. "Prenda la polvere ossea, Mary." L'infermiera recuperò i piccoli pezzi di osso con un cucchiaio di Volkmann e li mise nel coperchio rosso di una provetta per anatomia patologica. "Adson, Mary"; gli fu dato l'elevatore Adson e il chirurgo sollevò lo strato più profondo dell'osso al fondo del foro originario per esporre la dura madre, che si presentò con il suo consueto colore grigio-bluastro. "Bipolare, Mary"; la pinza bipolare gialla fu delicatamente posizionata nella mano destra di Mr Norris e Miss Murphy si accertò che il pedale fosse vicino. "Prema, Miss Murphy," disse Mr Norris e la sua specializzanda pigiò il pedale con il suo piccolo piede destro cosicchè il suo superiore potesse coagulare la superficie durale. L'apparecchiatura bipolare disse: "quarantacinque". Una volta che la dura fu coagulata a sufficienza, Mr Norris chiese il tunnellizzatore. "Vada avanti, Miss Murphy: dal basso verso l'alto, come al

solito." Miss Murphy prese il tunnellizzatore, un lungo e sottile baston-
cino metallico riutilizzabile, che passò attraverso la ferita addominale,
creando un tunnel sottocutaneo nell'addome, raggiungendo il torace e
passando sulla clavicola, per comparire solo pochi millimetri sotto la
cute del collo, dove incontrò un po' di fatica per andare avanti. "Avanti,
ragazza: spingi più forte... Per l'amor di Dio!" si lamentò l'operatore.
Dopo un ultimo faticoso sforzo, comparì la punta del tunnellizzatore
attraverso l'incisione sul capo. "Va bene. Mi dia il catetere peritoneale,
Mary. Lo immerga in una vaschetta con 80 mg di gentamicina per pre-
pararlo, io aspetto," disse Mr Norris. Per la precisione fu preparata una
vaschetta reniforme contenente normale soluzione salina con 80 mg di
gentamicina, per mettere a bagno e preparare il catetere peritoneale e la
valvola, già immersa. "Due pinze senza denti, rapidamente"; due pinze
rette furono passate a Mr Norris, che le usò per far passare il catetere
peritoneale attraverso la cavità del tunnellizzatore senza toccarlo con le
dita; successivamente il tunnellizzatore fu rimosso abilmente lasciando
il catetere peritoneale inserito sotto la cute di Mr Evans. "Bisturi durale e uncino, Mary." Gli furono dati una lama da 15 mm e un uncino
durale e Mr Norris incise la dura madre, efficacemente sollevata dal
piccolo uncino durale. "Coaguli, Miss Murphy," disse il capo e il medico interno obbedientemente bruciò i quattro angoli dell' incisione
lasciando una losanga quadrata attraverso la quale fuoriuscì del liquido
cerebro-spinale e fu possibile osservare il cervello pulsante in apparen-
te buona salute.
"Catetere ventricolare, preparato in genta, con introduttore, Mary." Il
passo successivo, indubbiamente il più critico dell'intero intervento
stava per arrivare. Posizionando il suo pollice sinistro in mezzo alla
fronte, appena sopra la glabella, e il suo dito sinistro sul davanti del
meato uditivo esterno, l'uomo visualizzò nella sua immaginazione lo
schema dell'intero sistema ventricolare e con fermezza spinse il catetere intraventricolare, fermandosi quando il nono centimetro scomparve
sotto la materia cerebrale. Magicamente, del liquido cerebrospinale trasparente, a pressione media, cominciò a defluire dal ventricolo.
"Bulldog, Mary," chiese Mr Norris; fu posizionata una piccola pinza
autostatica argentea sulla punta del catetere, per bloccare la perdita di
liquido cerebrospinale. "Mi dia la valvola preparata in quella soluzione
e un filo di seta 1/0 per fissarla," disse Mr Norris guardando l'infermiera. "Si prepari a tagliare il tubo quando e dove le dico," ordinò a Miss
Murphy, che seguiva tutta la procedura come se la sua stessa vita dipen-
desse da essa (e probabilmente era così, nella fase del suo training!).
L'infermiera gli passò una valvola Medtronic 1.5 delta immersa e pre-

parata nella soluzione antibiotica e Mr Norris indicò l'esatto punto dove il catetere stava per essere tagliato dal medico interno. "Ora," ordinò; Miss Murphy accorciò il tubo con le forbici di Mayo della lunghezza giusta per permettere a Mr Norris di assemblare la valvola alla sua estremità. Prima che lui potesse finire di spingere la porzione terminale della valvola craniale dentro il tubo bianco, Miss Murphy disponeva già del filo di seta pronto per assicurare la giunzione critica con un doppio nodo, rendendo impossibile ogni movimento futuro. Fu eseguita la stessa procedura per collegare il catetere peritoneale e il sofisticato apparecchio, terminando perfettamente la parte cranica dell'intervento. Sia l'operatore che l'aiuto guardarono l'estremità del catetere peritoneale che era stata lasciata a riposo in un grosso tampone intriso di betadine sulla pancia del paziente, aspettando che il liquido cerebrospinale comparisse al suo interno. Dopo qualche secondo il liquido cerebrospinale comparve, indicando che la derivazione era stata eseguita con successo. "Chiuderò la testa, Mary. Avanti. Chiami il prossimo paziente," disse il capo. Mentre suturava lo strato sottocutaneo del cuoio capelluto con il filo di vicryl blu chiaro 2/0, Miss Murphy giocherellava con le pinze lasciate all'inizio dell'intervento a indicare la direzione per l'interno dell'addome di Mr Evans, per aprire ampiamente il peritoneo e introdurre l'estremo libero del catetere peritoneale. Fatto ciò, cominciò a chiudere gli strati con le stesse suture che il suo capo usava per chiudere il cuoio capelluto. Aveva appena cominciato quando Mr Norris chiese il Nylon 3/0 per la cute, poiché preferiva sempre eseguire una sutura continua per la ferita cutanea. Lo stesso fece Miss Murphy qualche minuto dopo che il peritoneo e gli strati fasciali più profondi furono chiusi ermeticamente in maniera sequenziale. "Perfetto: trentanove minuti, da cute a cute. É un nuovo record, no?"Chiese Mr Norris. "Certo, John: congratulazioni," rispose Mary con orgoglio. A questo punto Mr Evans fu scoperto e solo due magnifiche cicatrici testimoniavano l'intervento eseguito. Il Dr Gupta subentrò mentre Miss Murphy si sedette per scrivere nel registro operatorio. Mr Norris era già in sala pausa, con il suo tè.

"Mr Evans! Mr Evans! L'intervento è finito. Respiri, per favore," disse Mr Gupta nel suo cordiale accento indiano. Mr Evans iniziò a svegliarsi. L'infermiera Mary recuperò tutti i ferri operatori sporchi e le vaschette, gridando fuori dalla porta: "Mike! Porta il letto, zuccherino. È finita."

Thoracic Surgery

Video-Assisted Lobectomy

Video-assisted lobectomy to remove a bronchogenic carcinoma is a surgical technique introduced by Roviaro in 1991. Under general anesthesia with selective intubation, the patient lies laterally with a small pillow under the chest to open the intercostals spaces. One 10-mm trocar is introduced through the fourth or fifth intercostal space in the medial shoulder blade line. Here we introduce the 0° optic and examine the thoracic cavity. If there are no lesions in the pleural cavity, we can introduce the second trocar, also through the fourth or fi fth intercostal space, along the posterior armpit line. When we do not have a histological diagnosis, we introduce a third trocar in the auscultatory triangle and we try to remove the tumor, assisted by the videothoracoscopy. When the diagnosis of carcinoma is confirmed, we make a minithoracotomy about 6 cm long around the third trocar incision. We dissect the fascia between the serratus anterior and deltoid muscles and 1 or 2 cm of the posterior edge of the latissimus dorsis muscle. Then we use a small rib spreader to open the intercostal space no more than 2 cm. The surgeon is situated to the back of the patient and can work with direct vision through the thoracotomy or by the video images on the monitor, but the assistant may only look at the monitor. To remove the tumor we use conventional instruments like DeBakey forceps and electric scalpel; alternatively, the harmonic scalpel with forceps head (AutoSonix-UntraShear) may be used to dissect the vessels and to look for the mediastinal nodes. The biggest vessels are clipped with EndoGIA 30 and the smallest with endoclips or with ligature. The lobar bronchus is sutured with EndoGIA 30. The next step is to look for mediastinal and hilar nodes; and we can be helped by the optic systems introduced through the trocar incisions or directly through the thoracotomy. Finally, we leave two drainage tubes inside the thoracic cavity through the trocar incision and close the thoracotomy by layers.

Chirurgia toracica

Lobectomia video-assistita

La lobectomia video-assistita per asportare un carcinoma broncogeno è una tecnica introdotta da Roviaro nel 1991. In anestesia generale con intubazione selettiva, il paziente giace in decubito laterale con un cuscino sottile sotto il torace per aprire gli spazi intercostali. Un trocar da 10 mm viene introdotto attraverso il quarto o quinto spazio intercostale nella linea scapolare media. Qui introduciamo l'ottica da 0° ed esaminiamo la cavità toracica. Se non ci sono lesioni nella cavità pleurica possiamo introdurre il secondo trocar, anch'esso attraverso il quarto o quinto spazio intercostale, lungo la linea ascellare posteriore. Quando non disponiamo di una diagnosi istologica, introduciamo un terzo trocar nel triangolo auscultatorio e proviamo ad asportare il tumore, con l'aiuto della video-toracoscopia. Quando la diagnosi di carcinoma è confermata, eseguiamo una minitoracotomia di circa 6 cm intorno all'incisione del terzo trocar. Dissechiamo la fascia tra i muscoli dentato anteriore e il deltoide e 1 o 2 cm del bordo posteriore del muscolo gran dorsale. Dopodichè utilizziamo un piccolo divaricatore per aprire lo spazio intercostale non più di 2 cm. Il chirurgo si pone dietro il dorso del paziente e può lavorare con una visione diretta attraverso la toracotomia o le immagini video sul monitor, ma l'aiuto può vedere solo il monitor. Per rimuovere il tumore utilizziamo strumenti convenzionali come pinze di DeBakey e bisturi elettrico; in alternativa si può utilizzare l' harmonic scalpel (autosonix-ultrashear) per dissecare i vasi e per cercare i linfonodi mediastinici. I vasi più voluminosi sono chiusi con Endogia 30. Il passo successivo è ricercare i linfonodi mediastinici e ilari; a questo scopo può esserci d'aiuto l'ottica introdotta attraverso i tramiti dei trocar o direttamente attraverso la toracotomia. Infine lasciamo due tubi di drenaggio nella cavità toracica attraverso i tramiti dei trocar e chiudiamo la toracotomia per piani.

Urology

Transurethral Prostate Resection (TURP) with Local Anesthesia

The indication for this technique depends on the general surgical risk of the patient, scored with the ASA. Local anesthesia begins with intraurethral lidocaine gel, while clamping the urethra with peneane forceps. Then, bupivacaine with a vasoconstrictor is injected transrectally into each lobe of the prostate with a Franzen needle. After that, mepivacaine is infiltrated suprapubically into the urinary bladder wall. After anesthesia, the operation may go on following the usual technique. A conventional resector is used to get into the urinary bladder, the bladder is dilated by sufflation of air through a cystoscope, and a suprapubic tube is placed. We start the operation with a 1-cm suprapubic incision using a cold scalpel to introduce a Reuter trocar. We introduce a 7 F ureteral catheter through the Reuter trocar, then the trocar is removed and we introduce an Amplatz tube to get inside the urinary bladder. All the procedures are supervised by endoscopic control. The catheter is removed to introduce a 90-cm-long polyvinyl tube through which the resected fragments are suctioned out to a fi lter. When the urinary bladder is empty, each prostate lobe is infiltrated with bupivacaine and a vasoconstrictor drug, and then they are pricked with an Orandi needle, located inside the resector.

The resection of each lobe is facilitated by the absence of bleeding and the high flow produced by the suprapubic drainage. The fragments are suctioned automatically by the Amplatz tube, and thus the resection system is not necessary for aspiration and the risk of a bloody field is lowered.

Urologia

Resezione prostatica transuretrale in anestesia locale

L'indicazione per questa tecnica dipende dal rischio operatorio del paziente, quantificato secondo la classificazione ASA. L'anestesia locale inizia con l'applicazione di gel di lidocaina intrauretrale, mentre l'uretra viene chiusa con una pinza peniena. Successivamente viene iniettata per via transrettale in ciascun lobo prostatico una soluzione di bupivacaina con vasocostrittore mediante un ago di Franzen. Dopodichè viene iniettata della mepivacaina in regione sovrapubica nella parete della vescica. Dopo l'anestesia, l'intervento può proseguire seguendo la tecnica standard. Viene utilizzato un resettore classico per entrare nella vescica; essa viene dilatata mediante insufflazione di aria attraverso un cistoscopio, poi viene posizionato un tubo sovrapubico. Iniziamo l'intervento con un'incisione sovrapubica di 1 cm utilizzando un bisturi a lama fredda, per introdurre un trocar di Reuter. Attraverso il trocar di Reuter introduciamo un catetere ureterale 7F, poi il trocar viene rimosso e si introduce un tubo di Amplatz per accedere all'interno della vescica. Tutte le procedure avvengono sotto controllo endoscopico. Il catetere viene rimosso per introdurre un tubo in polivinile di 90 cm attraverso il quale i frammenti vengono aspirati. Quando la vescica è vuota, ciascun lobo prostatico viene infiltrato con bupivacaina e con un farmaco vasocostrittore; successivamente vengono punti con un ago di Orandi, presente all'interno del resettore. L'exeresi di ciascun lobo è facilitata dall'assenza di sanguinamento e dall'alto flusso prodotto dal drenaggio sovrapubico. I frammenti sono aspirati automaticamente dal tubo di Amplatz, così il sistema di resezione non è necessario per l'aspirazione e il rischio di avere un campo operatorio emorragico è diminuito.

Vascular Surgery

Femoro-femoral Bypass

Under epidural anesthesia, the patient lies face up on the surgery table. The surgeon and the assistant begin the inguinal dissection on each side to find the femoral arteries. The incision is made with a cold scalpel, under the inguinal ligament, following the direction of the femoral artery and directed to the belly bottom, about 10 cm long. Aided by Adson retractors, DeBakey forceps, coagulation scalpels, and Metzenbaum scissors, the surgeons dissect the femoral arteries. When they have found the femoral artery, they use the Baby Mixter forceps to pass a few vessel loops around the common femoral artery, proximal and distal to the site of the bypass. It is also important to pass a vessel loop around the internal femoral artery to make a bloodless suture. The next step is to open the donor artery with the cold scalpel, with a small incision along the artery; bleeding is prevented by clamping the artery with the vessel loops fixed with serrated straight hemostats (Halsted-Mosquito). Before clamping, the surgeons inject heparinized physiological saline directly through the incision.

A Dacron graft is used as a bridge between the femoral arteries. The first joint is made in the healthy one, with a continuous double-needle prolene suture. Later, the vessel loops are released, the suture is checked, and the Dacron graft is clamped close to the arterial suture.

Furthermore, it is necessary to bypass the fatty suprapubic tissues to pass the other side of the graft to the opposite groin. To do this, the surgeons use Kocher forceps to make the tunnel carefully.

When the end of the graft is on the other side, they make a new artery-graft anastomosis in the same way, often directing the tip of the anastomosis to the origin of the deep femoral artery. Subsequently, the loops are released and the blood flow is tested. Finally, hemostasis is achieved with the coagulation scalpel and the lymph nodes are ligated with silk sutures to improve wound healing. Bilateral wounds are closed by planes.

Chirurgia vascolare

Bypass femoro-femorale

Il paziente giace supino sul tavolo operatorio, in anestesia epidurale. Il primo operatore e l'aiuto iniziano la dissezione inguinale da ciascun lato per raggiungere le arterie femorali. L'incisione, di circa 10 cm di lunghezza, viene eseguita con un bisturi a lama fredda, sotto il legamento inguinale, seguendo la direzione dell'arteria femorale e andando verso ombelico. Con l'aiuto dei retrattori di Adson, delle pinze di DeBakey, del bisturi elettrico e delle forbici di Metzenbaum, gli operatori isolano le arterie femorali. Una volta rilevata l'arteria femorale, usano il dissettore sottile per passare dei lacci vascolari intorno all'arteria femorale comune, prossimalmente e distalmente alla sede del bypass. È inoltre importante passare un laccio vascolare intorno all'arteria femorale interna al fine di eseguire una sutura non emorragica. Il passo successivo consiste nell'aprire l'arteria sana con un bisturi a lama fredda, mediante una piccola incisione lungo l'arteria; viene evitato il sanguinamento occludendo l'arteria con i lacci fissati con pinze emostatiche rette (halsted-mosquito). Prima di clampare, l'operatore inietta nel vaso soluzione fisiologica eparinizzata attraverso l'incisione. Come ponte tra le arterie femorali viene usata una protesi in Dacron. La prima anastomosi è quella sull'arteria sana, con una sutura continua con prolene doppio ago. Successivamente i lacci vascolari vengono rilasciati, la sutura viene controllata e la protesi in Dacron viene clampata vicino all'anastomosi arteriosa.

È inoltre necessario superare il tessuto adiposo sovrapubico per passare l'altro estremo del nuovo vaso nel lato opposto. Per fare ciò, l'operatore utilizza pinze di Kocher allo scopo di creare il tunnel in modo accurato. Quando l'estremità della protesi vascolare è dalla parte opposta, gli operatori eseguono nella stessa maniera una nuova anastomosi tra protesi e arteria, spesso dirigendo la punta della protesi verso l'origine dell'arteria femorale. Quindi i lacci vascolari vengono rilasciati e il flusso ematico viene verificato. Infine l'emostasi è ottenuta mediante bisturi elettrico e i linfonodi vengono legati con suture in seta per migliorare la guarigione della ferita chirurgica. Le ferite da ambo i lati vengono chiuse per piani.

Capitolo 13

Raccogliere un'anamnesi

L'anamnesi raccolta dai chirurghi spesso non è approfondita come quella raccolta dagli internisti. Ritengo comunque che sia sufficientemente esaustiva, anche se è ragionevole orientare la conversazione verso la nostra area di interesse. I migliori chirurghi sono stati spesso definiti come "medici con la capacità di operare, ma prima di tutto medici".

Capacità comunicative

Un buon rapporto tra il medico e il paziente è fondamentale per raccogliere un'anamnesi accurata. Nelle pagine seguenti presenteremo numerose key sentences che vi potranno essere di aiuto interrogando un paziente.

1. Saluti e presentazioni:
   - Good morning, Mr. Lee. Come and sit down. I'm Dr. Vida.
   - Good afternoon, Mrs. Lafontaine. Take a seat, please.

2. Invito a descrivere i sintomi:
   - Well now, what seems to be the problem?
   - Well, how can I help you?
   - Would you please tell me how can I help you?
   - Your GP says you've been having trouble with your right shoulder. Tell me about it.
   - My colleague Dr. Sanders says your left knee has been aching lately. Is that correct?

3. Istruzioni per svestirsi:
   - Would you mind taking off all your clothes except your underwear?

> Would you please take off all your clothes except your underwear and bra? (women)
> You should take off your underwear, too.
> Please take your shoes and your socks off. I need to check your pulses.
> Lie on the examination table and cover yourself with the sheet.
> Lie on the examination table with your shoes and socks off, please.
> Roll your sleeve up, please; I'm going to examine your elbow.

4. Istruzioni per la posizione da assumere sul lettino:
> Lie down, please (supine position).
> Lie face down, please (prone position).
> Please turn over and lie on your back again.
> Roll over onto your right side.
> Sit up and bend your knees.
> Lean forward.
> Get off the examination table.
> Stand up, please.
> Lie on your back with your knees bent and your legs wide apart.
> Lie on your stomach and relax.
> Let yourself go loose.

5. Istruzioni per rivestirsi:
> You may get dressed now. Take your time; we are not in a hurry.
> Please get dressed. I will tell you what I think in a minute.

6. Non è necessario alcun trattamento:
> There is nothing wrong with you.
> This will clear up on its own.
> There does not seem to be anything wrong with your shoulder, but I will order an X-ray.

7. È necessario un trattamento:
> I am sorry to say that the only way to solve your problem is having an operation.
> If you agree with the operation we can schedule it for the first week of September.

La cartella clinica

Nella tabella 13.1 è mostrata una tipica cartella clinica. Come si può vedere, nel caso non ne siate al corrente, una cartella clinica è scritta quasi interamente in abbreviazioni mediche.

Prendete una cartella clinica, fotocopiatela ed esaminatela accuratamente; prima lo fate, meglio è.

Raccogliere un'anamnesi

Poiché diamo per scontato che il livello del vostro inglese vi permette di comprendere la maggior parte delle possibili domande da porre ai pazienti e siamo consapevoli che ogni specializzazione possiede il proprio assortimento di domande tipiche, questa sezione non si propone come il solito manuale. Il suo unico scopo è quello di fungere da esempio allo scopo di incoraggiarvi a creare una lista di frasi e osservazioni. Nella tabella 13.2 vi forniamo una lista di frasi che i pazienti usano comunemente per descrivere i propri sintomi e il significato delle loro frasi.

Tabella 13.1. Cartella clinica tipica.

Surname (1st):   Hall   First name: Kevin
Age 32   Sex: M   Marital status: M
Occupation: Truck driver
Present complaint: Frontal headaches 3/12 (a). Worse in a.m. "Dull" (b), "throbbing" (c). Relieved by lying down. Also c/o (d) progressive deafness.
O/E (e)
General condition: Obese, H 165 cm,   W 85 kg
ENT (f):   Wax (g) + +, both sides
RS (h):   NAD (i)
CVS (j)   p (k) 80/min reg, BP (m) 180/120, HS (n) Normal
GIS (o)
GUS (p)
CNS (q)   Fundi (r) normal
Intermediate past history: weight gain
Points of note: none
Investigations (s):   Urine -ve (t) for sugar and albumin
Retinoscopy
Diagnosis: Hypertension
Management:
Date 26.3.08   Signature: Peter Weiss, MD

a. 3/12: for 3 months (similarly, 6/52, 6 weeks and 4/7 4 days)
b. Dull: "A dull sort of ache." Not felt distinctly. Not sharp
c. Throbbing: Pounding or beating strongly
d. c/o: Complains of
e. O/E: on examination
f. ENT: Ear, nose, and throat
g. Wax: Wax within the external auditory canal
h. RS: Respiratory system
i. NAD: Nothing abnormal detected, also non-apparent distress
j. CVS: Cardiovascular system
k. P: Pulse
l. reg: Regular (other: SR sinus rhythm)
m. BP: Blood pressure
n. HS: Heart sounds
o. GIS: Gastrointestinal system
p. GUS: Genitourinary system
q. CNS: central nervous system
r. Fundi: Equivalent to "found"
s. Investigations tests.
t. 've: negative (+ve positive)

Tabella 13.2. Frasi comunemente utilizzate dai pazienti.

Quando un paziente dice...	Il medico capisce...
I can't breathe	Dyspnea
Everything is spinning	Vertigo
It's itchy	Pruritus
I can't eat or I've lost my appetite	Anorexia
It stings when I pee	Dysuria
I don't feel like doing anything	Asthenia
Headache	Cephalgia
My nose is dripping/running	Rhinorrhea
I have vaginal dripping/discharge	Leukorrhea
I'm having a period	Menstruation
My hair is falling out	Alopecia
I can't remember a thing	Amnesia
My skin looks yellow	Jaundice
I can't move (a limb)	Paralysis
I can't see anything	Blindness
Bad breath	Halitosis
I have a cavity	Caries
It hurts when I swallow	Odynophagia
I can't swallow	Dysphagia
I cough up blood	Hemoptysis
I've got a burning sensation/heartburn	Pyrosis
I'm always running to the bathroom	Polyuria
I'm always thirsty	Polydipsia
My ankle is swollen	Edema
My urine is dark	Choluria
My stool is white	Acholia
I can't sleep	Insomnia
I can't go pee	Anuria
Toothache	Odontalgia
Bruise	Hematoma

Domande e ordini

1. Per iniziare l'anamnesi:
   - Well now, how can I help you?
   - What brings you here today?
   - What can I do for you?
   - Tell me about your problem.
   - Your doctor says you have been having trouble with your left knee…
   - Well, Mr. Goye, what's the trouble?
   - How long has this problem been bothering you?
   - How long have you had it/them?
   - Did it start all of a sudden?
   - How many days have you been indisposed?
   - What do you think the reason is?
   - Do you think there is any explanation?

2. Domande generali e ordini:
   - How many times?
   - How much?
   - How often?
   - How old are you?
   - Have you had a fever?
   - Have you had any nose bleeding?
   - Have you lost weight lately?
   - Open your mouth, please.
   - Please remove your clothing.
   - Raise your arm.
   - Raise it higher.
   - Say it once again
   - Swallow, please.
   - Take a deep breath.
   - Breathe normally.
   - Grasp my hand.
   - Try again.
   - Bear down as if you were to have a bowel movement (Valsalva's maneuver).
   - Please lie face down (prone position).
   - Please turn over and lie on your back.
   - Roll over onto your right/left side.
   - Bend your knees.
   - Keep your right knee bent.

 – Lean forward.
 – Get off the examination table and stand up.
 – Walk across the room.
 – You can get dressed now. Don't hurry. Take your time.

Sintomi comuni per ambiti:

Dolore
Domande:
 – Which part of your (head, arm, face, chest, ...) is affected?
 – Where does it hurt?
 – Where is it sore?
 – Can you describe the pain?
 – What is the pain like?
 – Is your pain severe?
 – What kind of pain is it?
 – Is there anything that reduces the pain?
 – Does anything make it worse?
 – Does anything relieve the pain?
 – Does lying down help the pain?

Frasi per descrivere le caratteristiche del dolore:
 – A dull sort of pain.
 – A feeling of pressure.
 – Very sharp, like a knife.
 – A burning pain.
 – A gnawing kind of pain.
 – A sharp, stabbing pain.
 – Raw.
 – The pain's gone.
 – A sharp pain.
 – I ache all over.
 – I'm in a lot of pain.
 – I've got a very sore arm.

Febbre
 – I think I have a temperature.
 – I think I'm running a fever.
 – High fever.
 – High temperature.

- When do you have the highest temperature?
- Do you shiver?
- Were you cold last night?
- When does your temperature come down?

Malessere
- I feel queasy.
- I feel sick.
- I think I'm going to vomit.
- I thing I'm going to throw up.
- My head is swimming.
- I feel dizzy.
- He's feeling giddy.
- She's feeling faint.

Debolezza
- I feel weak.
- I'm tired.
- I'm not in the mood for....
- Are you hungry?
- I've lost weight.
- Do you still feel very weak?

Sonno
- Do you feel sleepy?
- Do you sleep deeply?
- I wake up too early.
- Do you snore?

Vista
- I can't see properly.
- Everything is fuzzy.
- I can't see with my left eye.
- My eye is itchy.
- My eye is stinging.
- What's happened to your eye?

Altro
- Have you had a cough?
- Do you pass any blood?
- Do you have a discharge?
- My foot has gone to sleep.

Parole chiave riguardanti sintomi e segni

Sintomi generali
- Malaise: malessere
- Anorexia: anoressia
- Weakness: debolezza
- Vomiting: vomito
- Mialgia: mialgia
- Muscle pain: dolore muscolare
- Weight loss: perdita di peso
- Drowsiness: sonnolenza
- Night sweats: sudorazioni notturne
- Chills: sensazione di freddo
- Numbness: intorpidimento
- Tingling: formicolio
- Fever: febbre
- Costipation: costipazione
- Regular movements: evacuazioni regolari
- Diarrea: diarrea

Tegumenti
- Rash: esantema
- Lump: nodulo
- Pruritus: prurito
- Itch: prurito
- Scar: cicatrice
- Bruising: contusione
- Moles: nei
- Swelling: tumefazione
- Puffiness: gonfiore, edema
- Tingle: formicolio

Apparato respiratorio
- Cough: tosse
- Productive/dry cough: tosse produttiva/secca
- Hemoptysis: emottisi
- Cold: raffreddore, corizza
- Runny nose: naso che cola
- Sore throat: mal di gola
- Dyspnea: dispnea
- Out of puff: senza fiato

- Chest pain: dolore toracico
- Orthopnea (dispnea in posizione supina): ortopnea

Apparato cardiocircolatorio:
- chest pain: dolore toracico
- pain behind the breastbone: dolore retrosternale
- Intermittent claudication: cladicatio intermittent
- Cramps: crampi
- Palpitations: palpitazioni
- Angina: angina
- Tachicardia: tachicardia
- Cyanosis: cianosi

Apparato gastroenterico
- Abdominal pain: dolore addominale
- Nausea: nausea
- Vomitus: vomito
- Diarrea: diarrea
- Costipation: costipazione
- Flatulence: flatulenza

Apparato genitourinario
- Polyuria: poliuria
- Disuria: disuria
- Pollakiuria: pollachiuria
- Tenesmus: tenesmo
- Leukorrhea: leucorrea
- Menorrhagia: menorragia
- Dysmenorrhea: dismenorrea
- Impotence: impotenza
- Frigidity: frigidità
- Menstrual cramps: dolori mestruali

Sistema nervoso
- Tremor: tremore
- Rigidity: rigidità
- Seizure: attacco
- Paralysis: paralisi
- Palsy: paralisi
- Paresthesia: parestesia
- Reflex: riflesso
- Ataxia: atassia

- Incontinence: incontinenza
- Jumbled speech: linguaggio confuso
- Knee jerk: riflesso patellare

Esami speciali e analisi di laboratorio

Biochimica
   Prothrombin
   Fibrinogen
   Erythrocyte sedimentation rate (ESR)
   Glucose
   Urea
   Creatinine
   Ion
   Amylase
   Calcium
   Phosphate
   Aspartate aminotransferase (AST) = serum glutamic oxaloacetic transaminase (SGOT)
   Alanine aminotransferase (ALT) = serum glutamate pyruvate transaminase (SGPT)
   Alkaline phosphatase
   Urate
   Triglycerides
   Creatinine kinase
   LDH (lactate dehydrogenase)
   Iron
   Proteins
   Albumin

Emocromo
   Red blood cells (RBC) = erythrocytes
   Hemoglobin
   Hematocrit
   Mean cell volume
   Leukocytes
   Neutrophils
   Eosinophils
   Basophils
   Platelets
   Capillary blood sampling

Diagnostica strumentale
  Radiography
  Echography
  Arteriography
  Mammography
  Barium enema
  Double contrast enema
  Urography
  Magnetic resonance (MR)
  Magnetic resonance angiography (MRA)
  Computed tomography (CT)
  Computed tomography angiography (CTA)
  Endoscopy
  Bronchoscopy
  Nuclear medicine
  Spirometry
  Ergometry

Capitolo 14

Scrivere un atto operatorio, descrivere una tecnica chirurgica, dettare un atto

Che siate ginecologi, chirurghi generali o cardiochirurghi, se lavorate in un ospedale all'estero, dovrete scrivere l'atto operatorio in inglese. Alcuni centri dispongono di un database in sala operatoria nel quale è necessario solo selezionare le caselle appropriate per le condizioni del paziente e descrivere la tecnica chirurgica.

Comunque la maggior parte dei centri dispone di un foglio di carta per scrivere l'atto operatorio o di un microfono per dettarlo.

Come nella vostra lingua originaria, dovrete descrivere tutto in una maniera strutturata.

Questo è l'esempio di un modulo standard che potreste trovare.

Patient name

History number

Date: mm/dd/yy

Surgeon

First Assistant

Second Assistant

Anesthesia: Local Regional Epidural General

Anesthesiologist:

Antibiotic Prophylaxis: Yes No Name:

Patient's Disease or Main Condition:

Postoperative Diagnosis:

R. Ribes, P.J. Aranda, J. Giba, *Inglese per chirurghi*,
© Springer-Verlag Italia 2012

Intervention Performed:

Brief Summary of the Operation:

Description of the Operation:

Potete scrivere facilmente e in maniera decente una relazione, seguendo queste linee guida:

1. Posizione del paziente:

Supine Left lateral Right lateral Prone

2. Incisione eseguita:

Laparotomy: lateral McBurney median infraumbilical supraumbilical
infrasupraumbilical (or xifopubic) Chevron (left and right subcostal).

Gynecology: Pfannenstiel Inguinal fossa Episiotomy.

Heart surgery/Thoracic surgery: median sternotomy thoracotomy
(name the ntercostals space) thoracophrenolaparotomy.

Neurosurgery: craniotomy.

3. Riscontri intraoperatori:

In questa sezione dovete descrivere tutto quello che vedete e che attrae
la vostra attenzione. Per esempio:

After median laparotomy, numerous adhesions were freed up with the
electrocautery. A serous collection was found in the paracolic fossa and
in the Douglas pouch. No macroscopic lesions were found in the liver
or the spleen. The gallbladder was not present (previous excision).
A broad inflammatory area was found in the left Eustachian tube and a
diagnosis of ectopic pregnancy was made.

4. Tecnica chirurgica:

È il momento di descriver tutte le fasi dell'intervento che avete eseguito, per esempio:
opening hollow organs, resecting masses, ligating vessels, making anastomoses (normally end-to-end, end-to-side), implanting any kind of
prosthesis.

È importante anche segnalare ciò che non avete fatto, che si presume avreste dovuto fare e perché non l'avete fatto.

Dovete anche evidenziare altri eventuali gesti chirurgici, cioè quelle piccole operazioni extra eseguite al termine dell'operazione che ha condotto il paziente in sala operatoria, come ad esempio l'esecuzione di un'appendicectomia al termine di una gastrectomia.

Normalmente, dovrete anche segnalare il tipo di sutura o il tipo di materiale utilizzato.

5. Cateteri o tubi di drenaggio lasciati in sede.

Molti interventi richiedono il posizionamento di uno o più drenaggi lasciati in sede. Questi drenaggi possono essere aperti e funzionare per capillarità (Penrose-like), oppure per suzione grazie a un contenitore chiuso a pressione negativa (Jackson-Pratt, Redon, ...), o ancora per suzione grazie a un contenitore aperto o impermeabile (Argyle, Blake, Pleur-evac, ...).

6. Tecnica di chiusura:

Descrivete la modalità di sutura. Potreste aver effettuato una chiusura "en-bloc", nella quale tutti gli strati della parete sono inclusi in un'unica sutura continua (tecnica utilizzata talvolta in chirurgia addominale), oppure descrivere la tecnica di sutura e il materiale utilizzato per ogni strato. Per esempio:

The peritoneum was approximated with a running suture of 3/0 Dexon®; afterwards, the linea alba was closed with a running 2/0 Maxon® suture. The subcutaneous layer was approximated with a running 2/0 Dexon® suture and finally the skin was closed with staples.

Dovete essere concisi senza tuttavia tralasciare eventuali dettagli che potrebbero essere importanti. La vostra relazione potrebbe essere molto utile a voi e ai vostri colleghi per altri interventi o reinterventi, talvolta anche dopo molti anni. Questo documento è legalmente obbligatorio e potrebbe, in futuro, essere utilizzato in tribunale. Quindi, la soluzione è essere concisi includendo più dettagli importanti possibile.

Capitolo 15

Scrivere una lettera di dimissione

Secondo la legge vigente nella maggior parte dei paesi, al momento di lasciare l'ospedale, i pazienti devono essere muniti di una lettera di dimissione. Questo documento è spesso considerato un flagello per il chirurgo, poiché consiste in un tedioso lavoro d'ufficio che rompe l'esaltazione della "vera chirurgia". Per tale motivo è spesso compilata in maniera inaccurata.

Esistono molte ragioni per cui è importante compilare correttamente una lettera di dimissione:

1. Essa rappresenterà la vostra lettera di presentazione agli altri medici.
2. La prognosi a lungo termine del vostro paziente, dopo un intervento, dipende dal fatto che questi segua le raccomandazioni fornite alla dimissione.
3. Aiuterà voi o i vostri colleghi a curare il paziente in futuro (specialmente in caso di reinterventi).
4. Come ultima cosa, ma non meno importante, essa ha una grande importanza dal punto di vista legale.

È importante ricordare che è obbligatorio darne copia a qualsiasi paziente (o tutore legale) che trascorra almeno una notte in ospedale o in clinica.

Come minimo, una lettera di dimissione deve:

1. Essere scritta a macchina o a mano, per poter essere facilmente lettae.
2. Identificare l'ospedale e il dipartimento, includendo nome, indirizzo e numero di telefono. Deve riportare per intero il nome del medico e la sua firma.

R. Ribes, P. J. Aranda, J. Giba, *Inglese per chirurghi*,
© Springer-Verlag Italia 2012

3. Identificare chiaramente il paziente mediante la numerazione anam-
nestica, il numero di accesso, il nome, la data di nascita e il sesso.
Deve anche fornire l'indirizzo del paziente.
4. Mostrare la data del ricovero e della dimissione.

Al giorno d'oggi le lettere di dimissione sono di solito elaborate al
computer sulla base di modelli che automaticamente includono tutte le
suddette informazioni, cosicchè vi sarà richiesto solo di controllare
quelle informazioni e di fornire i dati successivi:

Reason for the admission:
Enunciate ogni segno, sintomo, o situazione che ha portato al ricovero
del paziente e alla degenza ospedaliera (e.g., chest pain, fever, poly-
trauma, etc.).

Allergies and medications:
Elencate le allergie note del paziente, specialmente quelle ai farmaci.
Definite i trattamenti medici in corso e quelli pregressi.

Family history:
Annotate le malattie più importanti da cui sono affetti i familiari del
paziente.

Past medical history:
Includete le malattie, le abitudini voluttuarie, i fattori di rischio cardio-
vascolare, gli interventi chirurgici e le possibili complicanze chirurgiche pregresse.

Current symptoms and complaints:
Fate riferimento prevalentemente ai sintomi del paziente.

Physical examination:
Fate riferimento ai segni evidenti all'esame fisico del paziente.

Diagnostic tests:
Fornite informazioni riguardanti gli esami *eseguiti* (blood tests, ultraso-
nography, etc.) e i loro risultati.

Surgical or obstetric procedures:
Descrivete brevemente l'intervento eseguito. In caso di parto, specificate peso, altezza e stato di salute di ogni bambino.

Other significant procedures:
Dichiarate tutti i trattamenti specialistici richiesti durante la degenza (e.g., colonoscopy, angiography, biopsy, etc.).

Evolution:
Riassumete brevemente l'evoluzione durante il ricovero, facendo riferimento a eventuali complicanze. In caso di morte, descrivete i risultati dell'autopsia in un paragrafo dedicato.

Reason for discharge:
Specificate se la dimissione è stata volontaria o conseguente ai trattamenti e al miglioramento delle condizioni cliniche, alla morte, o al trasferimento presso un altro centro per la diagnosi o il trattamento.

Main diagnosis:
Provate a dichiarare una sola diagnosi. Evitate di riportare le complicanze durante il ricovero, evitate gli acronimi, le abbreviazioni, o il nome delle procedure eseguite.

Other diagnoses:
Dedicate questo paragrafo alle altre situazioni menzionate nel paragrafo precedente.

Therapeutic recommendations:
Cominciate con le raccomandazioni generali (regarding diet, habits, etc.), proseguite con le raccomandazioni riguardanti la cura della ferita chirurgica. Indicate i trattamenti medici e la data per le visite ambulatoriali di follow-up.

Capitolo 16

Scrivere una lettera per richiedere uno stage

La prima fase nell'organizzazione di uno stage in un centro riconosciuto pubblicamente nella vostra specialità è rappresentato da una lettera di autorizzazione.

Che stiate programmando di andarci a lavorare, di chiedere una borsa di studio post-universitaria o di fare una visita informale in un centro di eccellenza, dovrete mettervi in contatto con l'ospedale e ottenere la loro approvazione. Tenete a mente che molto probabilmente loro non sanno niente di voi; potrebbero aver sentito parlare del vostro primario, se è ben conosciuto nel campo, e potrebbero sapere qualcosa del vostro paese o anche della vostra città, ma questo è quanto. Con una sola lettera, dovrete superare eventuali fraintendimenti riguardo alle vostre abilità, intenzioni, o anche alla città dalla quale provenite.

Al giorno d'oggi, il concetto di "lettera" in quanto tale appartiene al passato. La maggior parte, se non tutti i chirurghi rinomati nel mondo controllano regolarmente la loro e-mail. L'e-mail fornisce un accesso istantaneo a qualsiasi parte del mondo ed è gratuita. Di conseguenza, vi suggeriamo di controllare l'indirizzo e-mail del capo del dipartimento che volete visitare. Non perdete tempo a cercare di mettervi in contatto con qualcuno che lavora lì o con la segretaria del capo dipartimento. Potreste rimanere stupiti scoprendo che la maggior parte dei vostri "idoli chirurgici" sono in realtà persone piacevoli e molto disponibili nell'incontrare professionisti provenienti da tutto il mondo per far vedere loro stessi e il proprio team all'opera.

Certamente, se siete abbastanza fortunati da avere un "padrino", il vostro capo o qualcuno che ha realmente un rapporto di amicizia personale con il direttore del dipartimento che vorreste visitare, non esitate a servirvene. In questo caso, il vostro contatto dovrà chiamare o mandare una e-mail alla persona in questione parlandogli di voi. Se così sarà, avrete un grosso vantaggio (ammesso che il rapporto di amicizia tra i capi di dipartimento sia buono come sembra!).

R. Ribes, P.J. Aranda, J. Giba, *Inglese per chirurghi*,
© Springer-Verlag Italia 2012

Ma torniamo alla situazione classica. Voi siete specializzandi in chirurgia e il vostro ospedale vi consente di passare 3 mesi in un centro internazionale. Vi piace molto la chirurgia laparoscopica e sapete, grazie alle vostre ricerche, che il posto dove andare si trova in Wisconsin. Se non avete delle conoscenze personali ad aiutarvi, la prima cosa da fare sarà procurarvi l'indirizzo e-mail del capo dipartimento. Ancora una volta Internet vi sarà di aiuto – potrete trovarlo in un articolo, tra i contatti registrati nella pagina web di una società scientifica, o nel sito web dell'ospedale.

Vi mostriamo un modello di lettera:

Your hospital data
Your telephone
Your fax
Your e-mail
June 6, 2009

Dr. ....
His/her address
E-mail
Dear Dr. ....,

My name is .... I am a fourth-year surgeon-in-training currently working at ....Hospital, in (City), (Country).

I am well aware of your achievements in (e.g., minimally invasive surgery) and it would be a great honor for me to visit your center.

The purpose of my stay is to gain hands-on training/to pay an informal visit/ learn more about your center. I am interested in spending X months with your team. The period from (January to March) would fit very nicely with this year's schedule, but I am open to any other period that you might suggest.

Of course, I will cover all my travel expenses and do not expect any remuneration.

I look forward to your answer and hope to be able to start the preparations as soon as possible.

Yours sincerely,
........., MD
...........Hospital

In generale, dovreste presentarvi brevemente. Dopodichè, dichiarate le vostre intenzioni: sia facendo richiesta di una visita informale, sia inoltrando una domanda per un posto vacante, o per una borsa di studio post-universitaria. Siate precisi riguardo al periodo in cui vorreste iniziare la vostra esperienza e a quanto tempo desiderate rimanere, ma ricordate sempre di essere aperti riguardo eventuali alternative. È anche importante dichiarare che non state richiedendo una borsa di studio dall'ospedale ospite (se effettivamente non la state chiedendo!).

È abbastanza frequente che alla vostra richiesta risponda un assistente personale o una segretaria. Se così fosse, vi aiuteranno sicuramente a preparare i documenti necessari e probabilmente continuerete il resto della corrispondenza mediante loro.

Tenete a mente che la maggior parte dei centri europei ospitano chirurghi europei abbastanza facilmente e, a patto che voi passiate un certo periodo di tempo da loro, vi sarà permesso di aiutare in sala operatoria o anche di operare alcuni pazienti fornendo dei documenti facili da reperire. Se state programmando di andare negli USA, sarete facilmente accettati come "external observer"; tuttavia, se avete intenzione di partecipare a degli interventi chirurgici, dovrete programmare la vostra permanenza con ampio anticipo ed essere pronti a fornire una grande quantità di documenti. La mole di documenti aumenta ancora di più se state programmando di fare richiesta per un "fellowship", per un regolare tirocinio specialistico o per un posto di lavoro permanente. Alcune compagnie online offrono posti di lavoro per medici provenienti da tutto il mondo, compresi i cosiddetti lavori interinali. Questi impieghi consistono in posizioni vacanti, a breve termine, all'interno degli ospedali; di solito coprono tutte le vostre spese e pagano abbastanza bene. Dovreste considerare questa occasione anche come un modo per migliorare il vostro inglese.

Ad ogni modo, se state pianificando di svolgere un lavoro clinico, c'è il rischio che vi sia richiesto almeno di avere un check-up medico (principalmente per accertarsi che non abbiate malattie infettive) presso il centro dove andrete; vi potrebbe anche essere richiesto di avere un'assicurazione per coprire possibili responsabilità civili o altre questioni legali.

Internet vi fornirà il 90% delle informazioni di cui avrete bisogno per capire cosa fare in ogni paese.

Capitolo 17

Scrivere un curriculum vitae internazionale

A un certo punto della vostra carriera vi sarà richiesto di inviare il vostro curriculum vitae (CV). Se fate domanda per un lavoro, una borsa di studio, una carica di fellow, o anche solo uno stage informale, la maggior parte delle istituzioni vi chiederanno di mandarne uno. Scrivere un CV è una cosa seria: rappresenta la vostra lettera di presentazione e il datore di lavoro spesso eseguirà una prima selezione sulla base dei CV ricevuti. Si suppone che i CV siano scritti in una maniera particolare, sulla base di un modello accettato a livello internazionale. I CV devono essere facili da leggere e devono mantenere un ordine chiaro.

Ci sono tre concetti da tenere a mente: Curriculum Vitae, Résumé e Cover Letter.

Quando inviate il vostro CV, è importante allegare una Cover Letter indipendente. La Cover Letter vi presenterà; essa rappresenta spesso un importante strumento per attrarre l'attenzione del datore di lavoro e avere un colloquio di lavoro. Un CV è una presentazione più formale del vostro bagaglio culturale, delle vostre imprese professionali, pubblicazioni, comunicazioni, programmi di ricerca ed esperienze di insegnamento. Può essere più lungo di due pagine. Negli USA, un CV è utilizzato principalmente per fare domanda per un posto di lavoro in ambito internazionale, universitario, pedagogico, scientifico o di ricerca, oppure quando si richiede una borsa di studio o un posto di fellow. Un Résumé è una breve compilazione della vostra educazione, capacità e storia professionale. Non dovrebbe essere più lungo di una o due pagine (non aspettatevi che chi lo legga gli dedichi più di un minuto). Probabilmente vi sarà richiesto un Résumé se state pianificando di visitare un ospedale, in modo da sapere da dove venite.

In ogni caso, deve essere esauriente. Ricordate: se non menzionate nulla, non avete fatto nulla.

R. Ribes, P. J. Aranda, J. Giba, *Inglese per chirurghi*,
© Springer-Verlag Italia 2012

Ecco alcuni consigli:

- Includere una fototessera non è obbligatorio, ma è consigliabile.
- Scegliete la giusta dimensione dei caratteri: provate ad adattare il testo di modo che entri in una sola pagina.
- Evidenziate il titolo dei paragrafi in grassetto e lasciate uno spazio aggiuntivo tra i paragrafi.
- Tenete lo stesso margine a destra e a sinistra.
- Controllate sempre con il computer l'ortografia del vostro CV e, meglio ancora, mostratelo a qualcuno che conosce l'inglese meglio di voi.
- Non date niente per scontato. Spiegate ogni cosa in maniera chiara e concisa.
- Non usate mai abbreviazioni, a meno che non sia assolutamente indispensabile. Se le utilizzate, spiegate il loro significato.
- Non è necessario firmare il vostro CV.

Covering Letter

È quasi sempre una buona idea allegare una Cover Letter al vostro CV, specialmente se siete un chirurgo sconosciuto che sta facendo domanda per un posto di lavoro. Questa lettera indirizzerà il vostro CV alla persona voluta (cercate di scoprire il suo nome, o inviatela direttamente al capo di dipartimento). Dovrebbe anche essere in grado di attrarre l'attenzione del datore di lavoro e di renderlo interessato a leggere le informazioni allegate. Dovrete anche dichiarare il motivo per cui volete lavorare in quell'ospedale e perché pensate di essere la persona giusta per quel posto. All'interno della vostra lettera concentratevi su quegli aspetti specifici che considerate più importanti e che potrebbero essere trascurati inviando semplicemente il CV.

Cover Letter Template

Contact Information
Your address
Your city, state, zip code
Your phone number
Your e-mail address

Employer Contact Information
Name
Title
Company
Address
City, state, zip code

Salutation:
Dear Dr.

Introduction of cover letter
Il corpo della vostra cover letter serve a far capire al vostro principale per che tipo di lavoro state facendo domanda, perché dovrebbe scegliere proprio voi per un colloquio e cosa farete seguire alla vostra cover letter.

First paragraph
Presentatevi brevemente (My name is....., I am a surgeon in training currently working at.....). Dopodiché fate sapere al vostro principale per che posizione state facendo domanda e qual è il vostro campo di interesse.

Middle paragraphs
Cercate di "farvi un po' di pubblicità", cosicché il vostro datore di lavoro sappia perché pensate di essere qualificati per quel determinato lavoro e sottolineate quei punti del vostro CV che sono particolarmente correlati al lavoro per cui state facendo domanda.

Final statement
Ringraziate il lettore per aver preso in considerazione il vostro CV e proponete un incontro privato.

Complimentary close
Respectfully yours/Yours sincerely/Kind regards (especially if you know them).

Signature

Firma scritta a mano (nel caso di una lettera cartacea).

Firma battuta a macchina (nel caso di una e-mail).

Curriculum Vitae

Quello che segue è un esempio di Curriculum Vitae formale.

Curriculum Vitae Format

Your Contact Information

Name

Address

Telephone

Cell phone

E-mail

Personal Information

Date of birth

Place of birth

Citizenship

Visa status

Gender

Optional Personal Information

Marital status

Spouse's name

Children

Certified Education

Elencate in ordine cronologico inverso. Includete date, specializzazione, dettagli riguardanti i titoli, tirocini e certificazioni.

Post-doctoral Training

Graduate School

University

High School

Employment History
Elencate in ordine cronologico inverso, includendo dettagli relativi l'impiego in questione e date. Work History
Academic Positions
Research and Training

Professional Qualifications
Certifications and Accreditations
Computer Skills
Languages you speak and level of expertise.

Awards

Communications

Publications

Books

Professional Memberships

Interests

Résumé

Spesso, specialmente nel caso in cui siate interessati solo a visitare un ospedale come osservatore esterno, vi sarà richiesto solo un résumé. Potrete utilizzare questo modello.

Résumé Format

Your Contact Information
First name, last name
Street address
City, state, zip
Phone (cell/home)
E-mail address

Education
In questa sezione elencate l'università frequentata, i titoli ottenuti, i premi e le onorificenze vinte.
College, Degree
Awards, Honors

Experience
Questa sezione racconta punto per punto la vostra storia lavorativa. Elencate le strutture ospedaliere per le quali avete lavorato in ordine cronologico inverso, le date di impiego, i ruoli occupati e una lista delle vostre responsabilità e dei traguardi raggiunti.
Hospital 1, City, State, Dates Worked. Job Title
Hospital 2, City, State, Dates Worked. Job Title
Se avete visitato o svolto una parte del vostro tirocinio in diversi ospedali, non dimenticate di menzionarlo.

Skills
Includete eventuali abilità correlate all'impiego per il quale state facendo una domanda di lavoro. Se siete in grado di eseguire interventi chirurgici non routinari in tutti gli ospedali, segnalatelo.

Research
Author of more than .... communications at national/international congresses.
Author of ... articles in national/international publications and ... books.
Currently involved in ... lines of investigations.

Awards (indicate only if relevant)

References available upon request
Ancora una volta, servitevi dei vostri contatti e buona fortuna! Non rimanete frustrati in caso di mancata accettazione. Il nostro è un campo molto competitivo, ma fortunatamente è abbastanza vasto per trovare qualcuno disposto ad accogliervi nel proprio dipartimento.

Capitolo 18

Strumenti chirurgici

Quando lavorerete in un ospedale straniero probabilmente avrete la vostra occasione di "fare sul serio", ovvero potrete finalmente partecipare alla chirurgia pratica. Quel giorno, probabilmente vi accorgerete che l'inglese che avete imparato fino a quel momento non è sufficiente perché vi manca la conoscenza delle parole fondamentali per quella situazione, comprese le parole per indicare gli strumenti chirurgici.
Come chiederete lo strumento per tagliare, afferrare, aspirare...?
Fortunatamente, molti strumenti chirurgici portano il nome del loro ideatore, così in qualche modo probabilmente riuscirete a sopravvivere. In questo capitolo cercheremo di aiutarvi a costruire un vocabolario di base che vi renda capaci di cominciare a lavorare. Per prima cosa, vi descriveremo alcuni degli strumenti più comuni utilizzati nella maggior parte delle specialità; poi selezioneremo un po' di strumenti specifici per ogni singola specialità. Comunque, principalmente, abbiamo raggruppato gli strumenti per tipo piuttosto che per specialità (per esempio, tissue forceps, scissors, etc.).
Come potete immaginare, esistono cataloghi di strumenti chirurgici di 1000 pagine, molti per ogni fornitore, ma questo elenco sarà sufficiente, molto probabilmente, per la maggior parte delle specialità chirurgiche.

R. Ribes, P. J. Aranda, J. Giba, *Inglese per chirurghi*,
© Springer-Verlag Italia 2012

Strumenti diagnostici di base

Anche se non prettamente chirurgici, è più che probabile che usiate uno

STETHOSCOPE

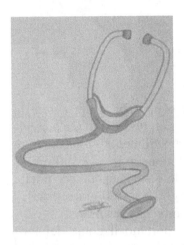

O un PERCUSSION HAMMER: TAYLOR

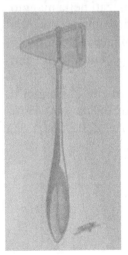

Senza dubbio avrete bisogno anche di un camice chirurgico, "gown" (che può essere linen, paper, o plastic).

A un certo punto avrete bisogno di materiale per suturare.

I fili di sutura possono essere "braided" o "monofilament", "absorbable" o "non-absorbable". Il termine *braid* fa riferimento a tutti i fili di sutura creati intrecciando o avvolgendo tre o più fili di uno o più materiali con una sovrapposizione diagonale.

I fili di sutura più comuni sono in acido poliglicoico (suture sintetiche assorbibili), catgut cromico e liscio, seta intrecciata, nylon monofilamento, polipropilene monofilamento, poliestere intrecciato, fili metallici monofilamento senza stagno.

Comunque, i fili di sutura prendono spesso il nome del marchio di fabbrica: Prolene, Dexon, Monocryl, etc.

In tempi recenti, le colle topiche in cianoacrilato sono state usate in combinazione o in alternativa alle suture per chiudere le ferite. Le colle rimangono allo stato liquido finché sono a contatto con l'acqua o con sostanze che contengono acqua, dopodiché polimerizzano e formano un film flessibile che salda lo strato sottostante. Lo strato adesivo agisce come una barriera al passaggio dei microbi finché il film adesivo rimane intatto. I limiti degli adesivi tissutali sono rappresentati dall'uso in vicinanza degli occhi e da un curva di addestramento all'uso piuttosto lenta.

Gli aghi possono essere:

•	Tapered point
○	Blunt point
▲	Cutting edge
▼	Reverse cutting edge
▾	Micro-point reverse cutting
⊗	Micro-point curved spatula

- Taper (la sezione dell'ago è rotonda e si assottiglia armonicamente a un'estremità)
- Cutting (la sezione dell'ago è triangolare e presenta un bordo affilato e tagliente rivolto all'interno)

- Reverse cutting (il bordo tagliente è rivolto all'esterno)
- Trocar point or tapercut (la sezione dell'ago è rotonda, ma l'ago termina con una piccola punta triangolare tagliente)
- Blunt points (punte smusse), per cucire tessuti friabili.
- Side cutting or spatula points (aghi piatti in coda e in punta con un bordo tagliente al centro della parete interna ed esterna) per la chirurgia oculistica.

Anche le forme degli aghi possono cambiare. Possono essere a mezza circonferenza, a 3/8, a 1/4, a 5/8, retti o a J.

Tipi di suture di base

Le suture possono essere classificate in base al tipo. Possono essere a punti staccati o continue (anche note come *running sutures*).
Sentirete parlare di suture semplici (simple), a materasso (mattress), continue autobloccanti (continuous docking), intradermiche (subcuticular), o a borsa di tabacco (purse-string, usate quando si esegue un'appendicectomia, per esempio).
Sentirete parlare anche di tecniche di sutura diritte o a rovescio (forehand or backhand).
Le suture maggiormente utilizzate per chiudere la cute sono le cosiddette *vertical mattress* (eseguite con uno strato superficiale e uno profondo) e *horizontal mattress:*

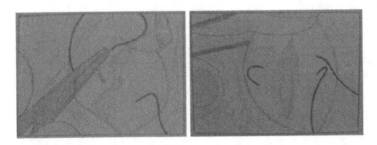

La posizione dell'ago nel porta-aghi si chiama *stance.*
La cute sarà spesso chiusa con una suturatrice a punti metallici. Per rimuovere i punti utilizzerete un apposito "remover".

Strumenti chirurgici di base

La prima cosa di cui avrete bisogno è un bisturi (KNIFE o SCALPEL). La seconda: un elettrobisturi (ELECTROCAUTERY, o semplicemente cautery). Ci sono altri tipi di bisturi, come l'"harmonic scalpel."

Forbici (Scissors)

I tipi più comuni sono MAYO SCISSORS,

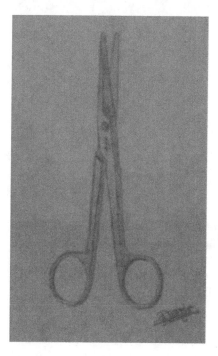

MICRO-SCISSORS, e abbastanza frequentemente le METZENBAUM
(o "Metzs"):

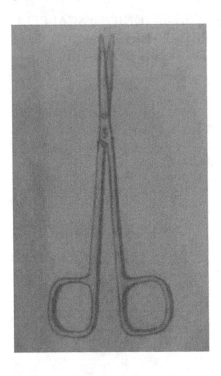

Pinze chirurgiche e da dissezione_(Dissecting and tissue forceps)

Alcune pinze usate frequentemente sono: MICRO-SUTURE TYING
FORCEPS, ADSON, STANDARD, o DE BAKEY (vedi sotto).

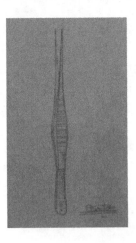

HEMOSTATIC FORCEPS, BULLDOG CLAMPS, VESSEL CLIPS, e APPROXIMATORS

BULLDOG CLAMP (piccolo, con meccanismo a molla), DE BAKEY BABY MOSQUITO (vedi sotto):

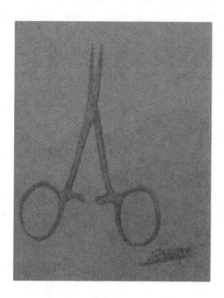

BENGOLEA (più lunghe, leggermente curve, talvolta a punta arrotondata), PEAN, o KOCHER (vedi sotto):

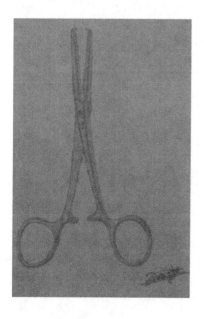

Pinze da dissezione e da legatura (Dissecting and Ligature Forceps)

Le pinze da dissezione/legatura comunemente utilizzate sono le MIX-TER e le BABYMIXTER (vedi sotto):

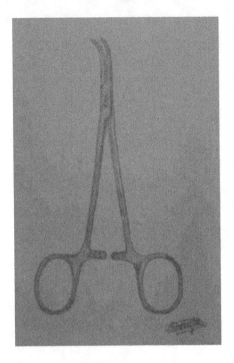

Porta-aghi (Needle Holders)

Questo nome è facile da ricordare (ha un senso). Alcuni nomi sono: CASTROVIEJO (utilizzato per suture fini) o il CONVERSE.

Divaricatori (Wound Retractors)

Possono essere del tipo che si tiene a mano (Hand-held, come il palpebrale Desmarres) o auto statici (self-retained).
HAND-HELD
Per esempio, il FARABEUF:

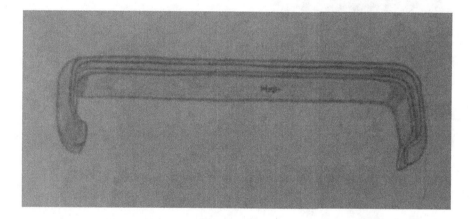

Così come il ROUX o l' HARRINGTON:

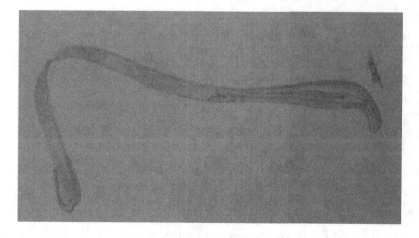

Dovreste conoscere bene anche l'ALLISON e gli ABDOMINAL
RETRACTORS:

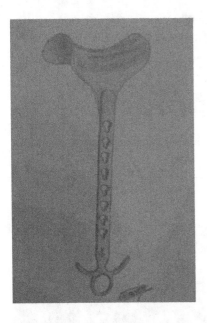

Divaricatori autostatici (Self-retaining Retractors)

In ogni tipo di chirurgia è molto usato il divaricatore di ADSON:

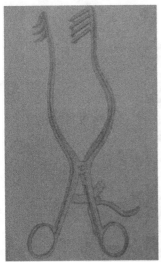

Anche il GOSSET dovrebbe esservi familiare.

Strumenti chirurgici specifici

Chirurgia addominale

Strumenti per l'intestino e il retto

- INTESTINAL and TISSUE GRASPING FORCEPS
Fondamentale è la pinza di ALLIS:

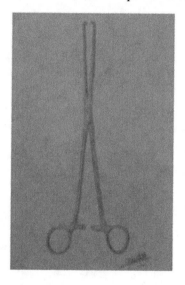

Altri nomi che sentirete: BABCOCK, DUVAL, ROCHER, INTESTI-NAL CLAMPS ...
Anche la cosiddetta MILLING:

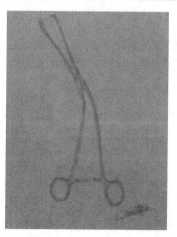

Strumenti genito-urinari

Alcuni nomi sono: KIDNEY CLAMP, KIDNEY STONE FORCEPS, MILLING (per la prostatectomia) tra molti altri.

In ginecologia userete spesso alcuni dei seguenti:
VAGINAL SPECULA (CUSCO), UTERINE PROBES (MAYO), UTERINE DRESSING FORCEPS (BOZEMANN), POLYPUS e OVUM FORCEPS (DOYEN) (vedi sotto)

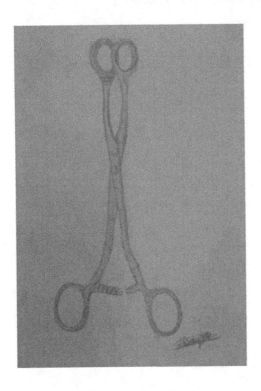

UTERINE-ELEVATING FORCEPS (COLLIN) o UTERINE CURETTES (come le cosiddette BLAKE) sono altri strumenti molto usati in questo tipo di chirurgia.

Ostetricia

VACUUM EXTRACTORS e FORCEPS sono alcuni dei nomi.

Chirurgia cardiovascolare e toracica

Sentirete parlare di: VEIN STRIPPERS, VASCULAR SPATULAS, e
MÜLLER VASCULAR CLAMPS, tra gli altri.
Alcuni VASCULAR CLAMPS sono:

DE BAKEY:

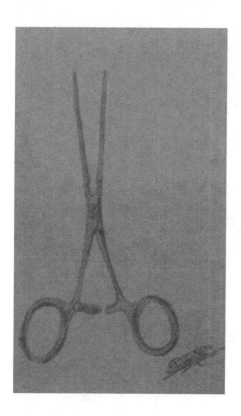

Il CASTANEDA o il classico SATINSKY

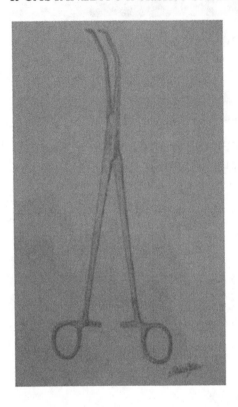

Divaricatori (Retractors)

Alcuni sono il FINOCHIETTO THORACIC RETRACTOR, il MORSE STERNUM RETRACTOR:

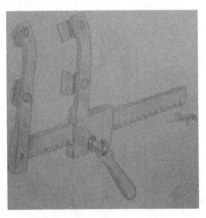

O il MINI MAMMARIA RETRACTOR

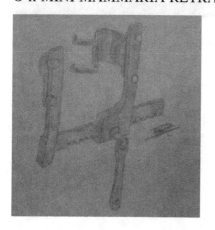

Anche il COOLEY atrium retractor:

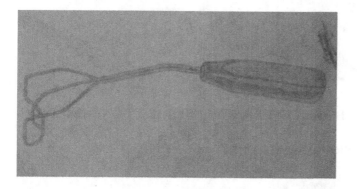

Cannule da aspirazione

Sono utilizzate in tutte le chirurgie:
La DE BAKEY o la YANKAUER (vedi sotto):

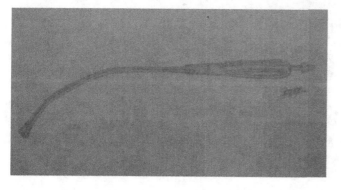

Strumenti per i traumi

LISTON (usato spesso per le amputazioni)

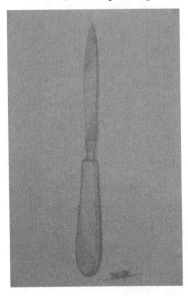

Altri nomi sono: BONE LEVERS, RASPATORIES, BONE-HOLDING
FORCEPS,
BONE RONGEURS (come il LUER):

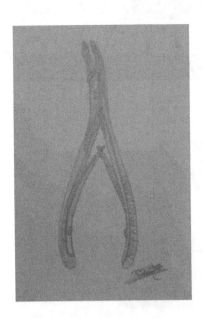

MENISCUS KNIVES, OSTEOTOMES (come il MALLETS MEAD o il COTTLE) fanno anch'essi parte dello strumentario del traumatologo. Infine, ricordate che questa è solo una guida rapida e superficiale agli strumenti chirurgici e serve solo per darvi un'idea dello strumentario classico. Quindi, vi consigliamo di leggere alcuni libri sull'argomento prima di operare in una sala operatoria dove si parla inglese.

Capitolo 19

Gestione di un dipartimento chirurgico

Gli interventi chirurgici rappresentano una parte significativa delle entrate di un ospedale e spesso una parte ancora maggiore del suo margine di contribuzione. Comunque sta diventando progressivamente più difficile aumentare i profitti in un ambiente sempre più competitivo. Molti ospedali pubblici sono orientati verso una medicina finalizzata al denaro più che agli interessi dei pazienti. Ciò significa che anche se non siete a capo del vostro dipartimento, è molto probabile che la vostra struttura esiga che voi conosciate il sistema economico dell'ospedale; inoltre, sarete "invitati" a perseguire gli obiettivi economici dell'ospedale e a uniformarvi alle sue regole.

Al giorno d'oggi, gestire un reparto chirurgico include diverse aree di responsabilità. Le principali sono quelle relative a:

- Miglioramento degli interventi chirurgici
- Relazioni ospedaliere
- Pianificazione dell'attività
- Assunzione del personale
- Selezione e implementazione di nuove tecnologie
- Pianificazione del marketing
- Assicurazione della redditività
- Controllo della qualità
- Politica di bilancio
- Soddisfazione del paziente
- Controllo della sicurezza

Il direttore di un dipartimento chirurgico deve essere un professionista completo e vario, versatile, tecnicamente competente, dotato di senso pratico nel campo degli affari, finalizzato al servizio del cliente, con molti anni di esperienza, certificazioni professionali e titoli maggiori.

R. Ribes, P. J. Aranda, J. Giba, *Inglese per chirurghi*,
© Springer-Verlag Italia 2012

Sarà responsabile dell'agevole funzionamento del dipartimento chirurgico per 24 ore al giorno per 7 giorni alla settimana e riceverà ben poco in cambio di ciò.

Il direttore del dipartimento chirurgico è responsabile di tutti i problemi correlati alle aree sopra elencate. Il suo obiettivo finale è di assicurare il continuo miglioramento del dipartimento chirurgico. Il suo ruolo è quello di imporre delle linee guida per raggiungere tali obiettivi e creare le strutture necessarie per adempiere alla missione del dipartimento.

Frasi usate comunemente

- We can't hire another physician's assistant... sorry, you will have to wait to increase your activity (Hospital VP for ancillary services).
- What do you mean your productivity is only 30% of the Surgical Society mean? (Hospital VP to Surgery Chair, when asked for funding).
- I believe we have tripled our volume since I arrived (any newly appointed Section Chief).
- One of my staff surgeons is leaving and we have had an increase in minimally invasive cases... I need to hire two new staff members (the same Section Chief).
- We are working harder in our section than anywhere else, and don't believe RVUs is a fair system to assess workload (any surgeon).
- With the reports you dictate it is impossible to bill! (coder).
- It takes at least 4 months to get payer approval for a new surgeon; don't let her operate until I tell you (billing office manager to the Chair).

Grandi domande, semplici risposte

Q: We installed a PACS 4 years ago: why are we still printing film? (Hospital COO = Chief Operating Officer).

A: PACS implementation does not eliminate the films in the OR, those requested by referring physicians, or patient copies.

Solution: Start distributing images in CD format or through the intranet.

Q: Do HIPAA regulations represent a risk for my business?

A: No. Even though HIPAA has been in force since 1996 and is therefore mandatory and includes penalties for failure to comply, surgical managers' concerns are limited to the enforcement of privacy and security rules to protect patients' sensitive personal information. Therefore, every practice must enforce and comply with HIPAA regulations, but they do not represent a risk if information is managed appropriately.

Q: How come some surgical centers manage to serve 150 patients per day and maintain a high level of patient satisfaction while others are able to serve only 75 patients with the same level of infrastructure?

A: It is all about the revenue cycle. Improvements in scheduling and registration, patient communication, staffing resources, documentation and the billing process, and reporting will ultimately produce increased productivity and profitability.

Glossario

Access: Time (days or hours) from intervention request to completion of the operation. It is a key measure when deciding to expand services.

Balanced scorecard: The balanced scorecard is a management system that enables organizations to clarify their vision and strategy and translate them into action. It provides feedback around both the internal business processes and external outcomes in order to continuously improve strategic performance and results.

Benchmarking: The process of setting goals, where these goals are chosen by comparisons with other providers, drawn from the best practices within the organization or industry. The benchmarking process identifies the best performance in the industry for a particular process or outcome, determines how that performance is achieved, and applies the lessons learned to improve performance.

Billings: Gross billed charges entered into the billing system for each CPT code.

Capitation: Method of payment for health services in which a physician or hospital is paid a fixed amount for each person served regardless of the actual number or nature of services provided.

Case-mix index (CMI): The average DRG weight for all cases paid under PPS. The CMI is a measure of the relative costliness of the patients treated in each hospital or group of hospitals (*see also* DRG).

Charge: The amount asked for a service by a health-care provider. It is contracted with the cost, which is the amount the provider incurs in furnishing the service.

Charge lag: The number of days it takes to enter a service charge in the billing system from the date of the service.

CFTE imputed: A measure of clinical activity of an individual physician or group of physicians relative to the benchmark value for a given specialty. This is computed by dividing the actual RVUs (work or total) generated by the benchmark value selected in the report (mean, median, 75th percentile, etc.).

CFTE reported: The percentage of time spent in billable clinical activity, as reported by the participant. Participants must provide these data in order to calculate other measures. *Note*: if you see patients and a bill is not entered into the billing system from which data are submitted to the FPSC, you should reduce the reported CFTE by the appropriate amount.

CFTE imputed/reported: The ratio of the imputed CFTE to the reported CFTE. This ratio measures the relative productivity of providers. In other words, it tells what an individual provider or group of providers is producing compared to what is expected.

Clinical full-time equivalent (CFTE): The percent of full-time activity a provider spends in billable, clinical activity. Percent clinical effort cannot exceed 100%.

Cost: The value of opportunity forgone as a result of engaging resources in an activity. Note that there can be a cost without the exchange of money ($/RVU).

In considering the production process, costs may be differentiated as follows:

- *Average costs*: equivalent to the average cost per unit; i.e., the total costs divided by the total number of units of production.

- *Fixed costs*: those costs which, within a short time span, do not vary with the quantity of production; e.g., heating and lighting.

- *Incremental cost*: the extra costs associated with an expansion in activity of a given service.

- *Marginal cost*: the cost of producing one extra unit of a service.

- *Variable costs*: those costs which vary with the level of production and are proportional to quantities produced.

In considering health problems, costs may be differentiated as follows:

- *Direct costs*: those costs borne by the health-care system, community, and patients' families in addressing the illness.

- *Indirect costs*: mainly productivity losses to society caused by the health problem or disease.

Cost-effectiveness analysis (CEA): An economic evaluation in which the costs and consequences of alternative interventions are expressed per unit of health outcome. CEA is used to determine technical efficiency; i.e., comparison of costs and consequences of competing interventions for a given patient group within a given budget.

CPT family: A grouping of CPT codes related to a common category of procedure (e.g., surgery, evaluation, and management).

CPT range: A subset of codes within a CPT family that defines a particular grouping of related procedures (e.g., surgery–musculoskeletal).

Current procedural terminology (CPT): The coding system for physicians' services developed by the CPT Editorial Panel of the American Medical Association; basis of the HCFA Common Procedure Coding System.

Current procedural terminology code (CPT code): A systematic listing and coding of procedures and services performed by physicians. Each procedure or service is identified with a five-digit CPT code to simplify the reporting and billing of services.

Dashboard: An at-a-glance snapshot of the economic reality of the numbers inside a department. The purpose of the dashboard is to provide a tool that gives anyone the capacity to see in graphical "whole pictures" the relationships between the financial statement fragments you currently use.

Diagnosis-related groups (DRGs): A system for determining case mix, used for payment under Medicare's PPS and by some other payers. The

DRG system classifies patients into groups based on the principal diagnosis, type of surgical procedure, presence or absence of significant comorbidities or complications, and other relevant criteria. DRGs are intended to categorize patients into groups that are clinically meaningful and homogeneous with respect to resource use. Medicare's PPS uses almost 500 mutually exclusive DRGs, each of which is assigned a relative weight that compares its costliness with the average for all DRGs.

Effectiveness: The net health benefits provided by a medical service or technology for typical patients in community practice settings.

Efficiency: Making the best use of available resources; i.e., getting good value for resources.

Examination volume: Number of procedures performed by time unit, e.g., appendectomies per year.

Fee-for-service: The traditional method for financing health services; pays physicians and hospitals for each service they provide.

Fee schedule: A list of predetermined payment rates for medical services.

Fiscal year: A 12-month period for which an organization plans the use of its funds. FYs are referred to by the calendar year in which they end; for example, the Federal FY2006 began October 2005.

Full-time equivalent (FTE): A way to measure a worker's *productivity* and/or involvement in a project. An FTE of 1.0 means that the person is equivalent to a full-time worker. An FTE of 0.5 may signal that the worker is only half-time, or that his projected output is only half of what one might expect.

Health maintenance organization (HMO): A managed care plan that integrates financing and delivery of a comprehensive set of health-care services to an enrolled population. HMOs may contract with, directly employ, or own participating health-care providers.

Health technology assessment: Evaluation of biomedical technology in relation to cost, efficacy, utilization, etc., and its future impact on social, ethical, and legal systems.

HIPAA (Health Insurance Portability and Accountability Act): The Administrative Simplification provisions of the Health Insurance Portability and Accountability Act of 1996 (HIPAA, title II) require the

Department of Health and Human Services (HHS) to establish national standards for electronic health-care transactions and national identifiers for providers, health plans, and employers. It also addresses the security and privacy of health data. Adopting these standards will improve the efficiency and effectiveness of the nation's health-care system by encouraging the widespread use of electronic data interchange in healthcare.

Hospital costs: The expenses incurred by a hospital in providing care. The hospital costs attributed to a particular patient care episode include the direct costs plus an appropriate proportion of the overhead for administration, personnel, building maintenance, equipment, etc.

Hospital inpatient prospective payment system (PPS): Medicare's method of paying acute-care hospitals for inpatient care. Prospective per case payment rates are set at a level intended to cover operating costs for treating a typical inpatient in a given DRG. Payments for each hospital are adjusted for differences in area wages, teaching activity, care to the poor, and other factors.

Indicator: A measure of a specific component of a health improvement strategy. An indicator can reflect an activity implemented to address a particular health issue or it might reflect outcomes from activities already implemented.

Limiting charge: The maximum amount that a nonparticipating physician is permitted to charge a Medicare beneficiary for a service: in effect, a limit on balance billing. Since 1993 the limiting charge has been set at 115% of the Medicare allowed charge.

Managed care organization (MCO): Any organization that is accountable for the health of an enrolled group of people. In contrast to organizations that provide services at a discount but do not attempt to coordinate care, MCOs actually have responsibility for the health of enrollees and, as a consequence, seek improvements in both the results and cost-effectiveness of the services provided.

Management performance indicators: indicators utilized for management of departmental activities to improve performance.

Outcome: The consequence of a medical intervention on a patient.

Outcome evaluation: Outcome evaluation is used to obtain descriptive data on a project and to document short-term results. Task-focused results are those that describe the output of the activity (e.g., the number of public inquiries received as a result of a public service announcement).

Outliers: Cases with extremely long lengths of stay (day outliers) or extraordinarily high costs (cost outliers) compared with others classified in the same diagnosis-related group.

Peer review organization (PRO): An organization that contracts with HCFA to investigate the quality of healthcare furnished to Medicare beneficiaries and to educate beneficiaries and providers. PROs also conduct limited review of medical records and claim to evaluate the appropriateness of care provided.

Per diem payments: Fixed daily payments that do not vary with the level of services used by the patient. This method generally is used to pay institutional providers, such as hospitals and nursing facilities.

Performance measure: A specific measure of how well a health plan does in providing health services to its enrolled population. Can be used as a measure of quality. Examples include mammography rate, or percentage of enrollees indicating satisfaction with care.

Performance standard: The target rate of expenditure growth set by the Volume Performance Standard system.

Practice expense relative value unit (practice expense RVU): A unit of measure used to express the amount of practice overhead costs of a service relative to other services.

Productivity: The ratio of outputs (goods and services produced) to inputs (resources used in production). Increased productivity implies that the hospital or health-care organization is either producing more output with the same resources or the same output with fewer resources.

Prospective payment: A method of paying health-care providers in which rates are established in advance. Providers are paid these rates regardless of the costs they actually incur.

Relative value unit (RVU): A non-monetary unit of measure used to express the time, complexity, and cost of performing a given service relative to those of performing other procedures.

RVU to FTE ratio: A clinical productivity measure. It represents the average output of each physician, and can be used as a workload measure.

Report turnaround: Time interval between the completion of a study and the production of the final report.

Revenue: The inflow of assets that results from sales of goods and services and earnings from dividends, interest, and rent.

In $/RVU: Represents the corresponding income for each worked unit.

Spider graphs/charts: A technique or tool to combine analyses of a market's level of managed care evolution with an internal readiness review. It involves three steps: market assessment, internal analysis, and gap analysis. Components of the graph include: network formation, managed care penetration, utilization levels, reimbursement, excess inpatient capacity, geographic distribution, commercial premium, physician integration, managed care characteristics, employer and purchaser base, outcomes management, strategic alignment, organization and governance, access to markets, delivery systems, medical management, finance, performance management, and information technology.

Standard: Something set up and established by authority as a rule for the measure of quantity, weight, extent, value, or quality.

Transcription time: Time measure from completion of a procedure to the final report.

Technology adoption patterns: Organizational characteristic method of providing new technologies; e.g., innovators are considered those hospitals that develop their own technologies or that make them available to the public at an early stage.

Total relative value unit (total RVU): The value consists of three components: the physician work involved (work RVU), practice overhead costs (practice expense RVUs), and malpractice expense (malpractice RVUs). RVUs are used as the basis for reimbursement of physicians' services by Medicare and by many other third party players.

Utilization management (UM): The process of evaluating the necessity, appropriateness, and efficiency of health-care services against established guidelines and criteria. Evaluation of the necessity, appropriateness, and efficiency of the use of health-care services, procedures, and facilities.

Utilization review (UR): The review of services delivered to evaluate appropriateness, necessity, and quality. The review can be performed on a prospective, concurrent, or retrospective basis.

Work relative value unit (work RVU): A unit of measure used to express the amount of effort (time, intensity of effort, technical skills) required of a provider in performing a given service relative to other services.

Riferimenti bibliografici

Academy for Healthcare Management (2001) Managed healthcare: an introduction, 3rd edn. Academy for Healthcare Management, Washington, DC

AcademyHealth (2004) Glossary of terms commonly used in health care. AcademyHealth, Washington, DC

American Association of Health Plans (1996) Capitation: questions and answers. American Association of Health Plans, Washington, DC

American Medical Association (1993) Advocacy brief: health reform glossary. American Medical Association, Chicago, IL

Batstone G, Edwards M (1996) Achieving clinical effectiveness: just another initiative or a real change in working practice? J Clin Effect 1(1):19–21

Cofer J (1985) Legislative currents: Prospective Payment Assessment Commission (ProPAC). J Am Med Rec Assoc 56(3):28

Dorland's Illustrated Medical Dictionary, 28th edn (1994). W.B. Saunders, Philadelphia, PA

Drummond MF, O'Brien B, Stoddart GL, Torrance GW (1997) Methods for the economic evaluation of health care programmes, 2nd edn. Oxford University Press, Oxford

Kelly MP, Bacon GT, Mitchell JA (1994) Glossary of managed care terms. J Ambul Care Manage 17(1):70–76

Mar Queisser RL (1995) Carve-out bundled-service contracts: a new type of CBC? Northwest Physician Magazine, Spring, pp 26–27

Medicare Payment Advisory Commission (1998) Medicare Payment Policy. Report to the Congress. Medicare Payment Advisory Commission, Washington, DC

National Library of Medicine (1994) HSTAR Fact Sheet. National Library of Medicine, Bethesda, MD

National Library of Medicine. Medical Subject Headings. Available at: http:// www.nlm.nih.gov

National Library of Medicine. PubMed Tutorial Glossary. Available at: http:// www.nlm.nih.gov

New Jersey Hospital Association (2006) Glossary of healthcare terms and abbreviations. New Jersey Hospital Association, Princeton, NJ. Available at: http:// www.njha.com/publications/pubcatalog/glossary.pdf

Office of Technology Assessment (1993) Benefit design: clinical preventive services. Office of Technology Assessment, Washington, DC

Pam Pohly Associates (2006) Glossary of terms in managed health care. Pam Pohly Associates, Hays, KS. Available at: http://www.pohly.com

Physician Payment Review Commission (1996) Annual Report to the Congress. Physician Payment Review Commission, Washington, DC

Pickett JP et al. (eds) (2000) The American heritage dictionary of the English language, 4th edn. Houghton Miffl in Company, Boston, MA

Player S (1998) Activity-based analyses lead to better decision making. Healthc Financ Manage 52(8):66–70

Prospective Payment Assessment Commission (ProPAC) (1996) Medicare and the American Health Care System. Report to the Congress, June 1996. Prospective Payment Assessment Commission, Washington, DC

Rhea JC, Ott JS, Shafritz JM (1988) The facts on file dictionary of health care management. Facts on File Publications, New York

Rossi PH, Freeman HE (1993) Evaluation: a systematic approach. Sage, Newbury Park

Scott DL (2003) Wall Street words: an A to Z guide to investment terms for today's investor. Houghton Miffl in Company, Boston, MA

Timmreck TC (1997) Health services cyclopedic dictionary: a compendium of health-care and public health terminology. Jones & Bartlett, Sudbury, MA

Tufts Managed Care Institute (1996) Managed care at a glance: common terms, 6. Tufts Managed Care Institute, Boston, MA

Turnock J (2001) Public health, what it is and how it works. Aspen, Gaithersburg, MD

US Congressional Budget Office (1988) Including capital expenses in the prospective payment system. Congress of the United States, Washington, DC

Washington State Department of Health (1994) Public Health Improvement Plan: a progress report. Olympia, WA

World Bank (2001) Health systems development. Health Economics. World Bank, Washington, DC

Zarnke KB, Levine MA, O'Brien BJ (1997) Cost-benefit analyses in the healthcare literature: don't judge a study by its label. J Clin Epidemiol 50(7):813–822

http://www.fi nancialscoreboard.com/dashboard.html

http://www.cms.hhs.gov/HIPAAGenInfo

Capitolo 20

Guida a una conversazione chirurgica

In questo capitolo troverete alcune tipiche conversazioni che si possono avere con i pazienti all'interno dell'ospedale. Troverete anche alcuni trucchi ed esempi che vi potranno aiutare a cavarvela nelle situazioni più comuni che vi capiteranno lavorando in un ospedale anglofono o semplicemente visitandolo.

Informare il paziente. Consegnare il modulo per il consenso informato

Nella maggior parte dei paesi, il chirurgo è responsabile dell'informazione del paziente riguardo all'intervento proposto. Questa informazione deve essere fornita almeno 24 ore prima dell'intervento, eccezion fatta per le emergenze. L'informazione deve essere adattata al livello di istruzione del paziente o dei suoi familiari per essere certi che abbiano capito. L'informazione deve essere esauriente e coprire tutte le possibili complicanze. La maggior parte delle specialità dispongono di consensi già pronti, forniti da differenti associazioni mediche. Oltre a un consenso scritto con la descrizione dell'intervento e la ragione per cui è necessario eseguirlo, i benefici attesi e i possibili rischi (consenso che deve essere firmato dal chirurgo e dal paziente o dal suo tutore legale), il chirurgo deve fornire un'informazione orale.

È obbligatorio per i chirurghi rispondere alle domande del paziente e informarlo dettagliatamente. Questa "chiacchierata" preoperatoria è molto importante, non solo per ragioni legali, ma anche per rassicurare il paziente e garantire un buon rapporto medico-paziente.

Il consenso informato rappresenta qualcosa di più di una semplice firma. È un processo di comunicazione tra il paziente e il suo medico, che risulta nell'autorizzazione o nell'accordo del paziente a sottoporsi a un parti-

R. Ribes, P. J. Aranda, J. Giba, *Inglese per chirurghi*,
© Springer-Verlag Italia 2012

colare intervento medico. In questo processo, Voi, come medici propo-
nenti o esecutori di un dato trattamento o procedura, dovete discutere con
il vostro paziente:

- La diagnosi, se nota
- Le caratteristiche e gli obiettivi del trattamento proposto
- I rischi e i benefici del trattamento proposto
- Le alternative (indipendentemente dal loro costo e dal grado di coper-
  tura da parte dell'assicurazione sanitaria)
- I rischi e i benefici dei trattamenti alternativi
- I rischi e i benefici dell'astensione da un trattamento

Vi forniamo l'esempio di un paziente ospedalizzato che necessita a breve
di un intervento chirurgico:

Doctor: Mr. Smith, good morning. I hope I did not wake you up.

Patient: Good morning, Doctor. What news do you have for me?

Doctor: Well, Mr. Smith, we have been discussing your case in our morning meeting. We have the results of all your tests. Unfortunately, we think
that you have a "growth" in your colon, and it does not look very good.
The reason why you have felt so tired lately is because you are slowly
losing blood through your stools, and that is why you required a blood
transfusion recently.

Patient: But is it "bad," Doctor?

Doctor: Well, as I told you it does not look very good. However, we are
lucky that we caught it relatively early and it has not gone very far.
Therefore, we recommend you have it removed. If we do the operation
now, the chances of it spreading to other parts of your body will be minimal.

Patient: Is it a serious operation, Doctor?

Doctor: In your case, we can remove the tumor by open, standard surgery, or via laparoscopic surgery. There are no other real treatment
options. Lap surgery makes the operation longer but the scars will be
minimized, normally offering a faster recovery. However, unfortunately,
in both cases we will have to do a "colostomy"; that means that, for a
period of time you will have to wear a plastic bag on your belly to receive
your stools. If everything goes well, we will re-connect your colon a few
months later, so that you will be able to go to the toilet normally.

Patient: Yes, I have heard about that.

Doctor: This is a "big" operation, and there are some risks that you should know about. First, there are the possibilities of bleeding, infection, wound opening, and heart problems after the operation. However, you are still a young man and quite fit, so, these perioperative risks are relatively low.

Patient: When will the second operation take place?

Doctor: Once we have checked that your liver is clean and that the tumor is gone during follow up, we will talk about this operation, but you should know that it may take months to years. This situation will affect your quality of life; however, it is the best solution we can offer to cure your disease or at least keep you tumorfree as long as possible.

Patient: When will the operation be?

Doctor: If you agree with the procedure, we could schedule it for next Wednesday. After the operation, you normally spend 10–14 days in the ward to get you used to the new situation.

Patient: OK, I guess I have no other choice.

Doctor: I think it is your best option. This is a written form that explains all the details about the procedure and the possible risks and benefits. I will leave it here for you and your family. Read it and please sign it and give to your nurse when you are finished.

Thank you. See you later, Mr. Smith.

Patient: Thank you. See you tomorrow, Doctor.

Visitare il paziente in reparto

Visitare i pazienti in ospedale durante la degenza postoperatoria è un dovere assoluto per la maggior parte dei chirurghi.
Ecco una tipica conversazione mattutina tra medico e paziente ricoverato:

Doctor: Good morning, Ms. Hübler.

Patient: Good morning.

Doctor: How do you feel today? Did you sleep well?

Patient: I think I am doing quite OK. The wound is a bit sore and tonight I could not sleep very much.

Nurse: She had a peak of temperature at around 2:00 am, but it resolved with 1 gram of acetaminophen and it has not recurred.

Doctor: OK. Let me listen to your chest (with a stethoscope). Have you had any coughing?

Patient: No, not really.

Doctor: The urinary catheter is still in; we will take it out now. *To the nurse*: Please send a urine sample to the laboratory to look for white cells. The wound looks quite nice. The operation was only a couple of days ago and it is normal to be a bit uncomfortable.

Patient: Thank you, Doctor.

Doctor: Thank you. Take it easy, we will order an X-ray and a blood test, but everything seems to be OK. See you tomorrow.

Nurse: Shall we review the treatment?

Doctor: Of course. Please leave an order to take a blood culture if the temperature rises again. We will also take the central line out, but leave the peripheral catheter in situ until we have the results of the WCC (white cell count).

Let's check the treatment.

Parlare in una riunione clinico-chirurgica

La maggior parte dei dipartimenti chirurgici tengono un breve incontro mattutino dedicato a:

- Discutere l'evoluzione clinica dei pazienti ricoverati ("morning rounds").

- Passare in rassegna un argomento chirurgico (di solito una breve presentazione da parte di uno specializzando), anche nota come "scientific sessions."

- Analizzare la mortalità e la morbilità. In questi incontri vengono presentati dei casi sfortunati e si discute mettendo in evidenza eventuali tranelli e per imparare da essi.

- Clinico-surgical sessions: in questi incontri gli specialisti di diverse aree cliniche presentano possibili candidati alla chirurgia e vengono prese decisioni a riguardo in maniera coordinata.

Se vi capiterà di partecipare attivamente a uno di questi incontri, probabilmente avrete bisogno di usare una di queste frasi:

- Dr. McCulough, will you please show us the CT images again, I would like to double-check the liver slices.
- Dr. Kinsdale, how long has the patient had these symptoms? Is she symptomatic at the moment?
- According to the pathological findings, I think the patient needs surgery soon; however, is she really fit for such an aggressive operation? Has she had a cardiological check-up?
- Is the patient willing to accept the risks of the operation? Does he have family support to take care of him after the operation?
- I think we need to know more about the patient. According to the guidelines, a heart cath should be performed before the operation to rule out ischemic heart disease.
- We think that the patient should be placed on the waiting list: he needs surgery but he can wait.
- What is his bed number? Please transfer the patient to our ward and we will schedule the operation for next Monday.

Conversazioni in ambulatorio

I pazienti che vengono a un appuntamento nel vostro studio generalmente rientrano in una di queste tre categorie:

1. Nuovi pazienti. Generalmente riferitivi da un medico generalista.
2. Visite postoperatorie.
3. Pazienti in Follow-up.

Vi riportiamo una tipica conversazione con un paziente abituale dell'ambulatorio:

Doctor: Will you please send in the next patient?

Nurse: Of course. Next patient, please.

Patient: Good morning.

Doctor: Good morning, Mr. Wang. Please take a seat.

OK, so how have you felt these past months?/How are you doing?

Patient: Fortunately, I feel much better now than I felt last January.

Doctor: Yes, I can see in your history that the last time I saw you your back was hurting almost all the time. We ruled out significant pathology with the MRI, though. So, are you taking any medication at the moment?

Patient: Right now, I am not taking any, at least not on a regular basis. I still need some of these painkillers every now and then. I have felt quite a lot of improvement with the exercises you recommended to me last time. I am back to work and the physiotherapist is working closely with me.

Doctor: I am glad to hear that. Will you please take your shirt off? Let me see, does it hurt here, here, here... OK. Tell me if it hurts when I raise your legs, ... OK. You may get dressed.

Patient: So ...

Doctor: Mr. Wang, thankfully, I think you are doing much better. The osteoarthritis in your spine does not seem to be progressing and your exercising is helping you a lot. As far as we are concerned, I think your family physician can follow you up perfectly, and at least for the moment you will not need an operation. Therefore, I will discharge you from this office.

Patient: That sounds great, Doctor. Thank you for your advice. I live quite far from the hospital and I will appreciate going to my GP down the street.

Turno di guardia

Tipicamente, uno specialista in chirurgia in servizio deve svolgere I seguenti compiti:

1. Valutare i pazienti in pronto soccorso
2. Informare i familiari
3. Preparare la sala operatoria in caso di intervento

Ecco un esempio:

Cell phone rings.

Surgeon: This is Dr. Wolfe speaking.

Emergency room (ER) doctor: Is that vascular surgery?

Surgeon: Yes, what do you have for me?

ER doctor: I'm calling you about a 55-year-old man, smoker, who came to the ER about 20 minutes ago. He reports acute abdominal pain that started some 4 hours ago. He collapsed because of the pain, though he recovered by himself. I'm calling you because we just got the lab results and his hemoglobin is down to 7. I think he might have a ruptured abdominal aneurysm.

Surgeon: Has he had a CT? Did you palpate a pulsatile abdominal mass?

ER doctor: Not yet, I just ordered it. I think it will be finished in about 30 minutes. I did not really palpate anything because the patient is quite obese.

Surgeon: OK, it looks like a possibility. Listen, I will get the OR ready. Please call me once the patient is at the CT unit and we will transfer him immediately. Meanwhile, ask for six packs of red blood cells and try to keep his blood pressure under control, especially with fluids.

ER doctor: Sure.

Surgeon (*new call*): May I speak to the anesthesiologist on duty, please?

Operator: Just a second.

Surgeon: Would you call the cardiovascular nurses as well? Please tell them to get OR number 9 ready, we have an emergent operation—a ruptured aneurysm.

Operator: OK, Dr. Wolfe. Here is the anesthesiologist.

Anesthesiologist: Yes, Dr. Wolfe? What's up?

Surgeon: Who is this?

Anesthesiologist: This is Dr. Holmes speaking.

Surgeon: Good evening, Dr. Holmes. We seem to have a ruptured aneurysm in a 55-year-old patient. The patient is on his way to the CT and I would like to transfer him directly to the OR. At the moment, his BP is still holding.

Anesthesiologist: We were just finishing an operation, no problem. I will send someone to OR 9—give me a call once the CT is finished and we'll escort the patient to the OR.

Surgeon: Thanks, Dr. Holmes. See you in a while.

Capitolo 21

Conversazione: guida alla sopravvivenza

Introduzione

La dimestichezza con la lingua rende sicuri di sé, mentre la mancanza di conoscenza rende insicuri.

Con questo capitolo non intendiamo sostituire le guide alla conversazione, che al contrario vi consigliamo di utilizzare secondo il vostro livello di conoscenza della lingua.

Sarebbe stato sciocco scrivere una guida alla conversazione senza includere delle traduzioni. Allora perché abbiamo scritto questo capitolo? Lo scopo di questo capitolo è fornire una "guida alla sopravvivenza", uno strumento di base che può essere consultato da coloro che conoscono l'inglese a livello medio-alto, ma che possono avere difficoltà a esprimersi con sicurezza in certe situazioni inusuali, come per esempio trovandoci con un collega che ci chiede di accompagnarlo in una gioielleria per comprare un braccialetto a sua moglie.

Tenete presente che è virtualmente impossibile essere spigliati in ogni situazione, anche nella vostra lingua. Trovandomi a parlare in inglese, ho provato imbarazzo e frustrazione solo in tre situazioni: in tintoria, all'aeroporto, e in una terza occasione, al ristorante. Prima di allora mi ero sempre considerato abbastanza spigliato in inglese ma, sotto pressione, i pensieri sono più veloci delle parole, per cui la capacità di esprimersi può essere sopraffatta dall'agitazione. Accettate questo consiglio: a meno che non siate bilingue, evitate di entrare in discussione in una lingua che non sia la vostra.

Molte persone che conoscono l'inglese a un livello medio-alto non portano con sé una guida alla conversazione quando viaggiano, pensando che il loro livello di conoscenza sia molto superiore rispetto a quanti necessitano di una guida per costruire frasi elementari, e si vergognano nel farsi vedere mentre ne consultano una (anche io ci sono passato).

R. Ribes, P. J. Aranda, J. Giba, *Inglese per chirurghi*,
© Springer-Verlag Italia 2012

Questo è un grosso errore, in quanto per coloro che conoscono l'inglese a livello medio-alto, l'uso della lingua ha utilizzi differenti e molto importanti (non appena il mio livello di conoscenza dell'inglese è aumentato, anch' io ho realizzato che il mio uso di queste guide era cambiato; non ne avevo bisogno per la traduzione, eccetto che per poche parole, ma ricercavo solamente una maniera più naturale di dire le cose).

Ritengo che, anche per coloro che sono bilingue, la guida alla conversazione sia estremamente importante nel momento in cui ci si trova in un ambiente non familiare, come ad esempio dal fioraio. Quanti nomi di fiori conoscete nella vostra lingua? Probabilmente meno di dodici. Ogni conversazione ha un proprio gergo e una guida alla conversazione vi può dare dei suggerimenti di cui anche un conoscitore di livello medio-alto può necessitare per essere più spigliato. Quindi, non vergognatevi di portare con voi una guida; è il modo più breve per sfoggiare una conversazione brillante in quelle situazioni non familiari che sporadicamente mettono alla prova il vostro livello di inglese e, cosa più importante, la vostra sicurezza in inglese.

Quando andate a cena, per esempio, ripassate sulla guida le parole chiave e le frasi più frequenti. Farlo non vi richiederà più di dieci minuti e la vostra cena sarà anche migliore, poiché avrete ordinato con grande sicurezza e precisione. Quella che è una semplice raccomandazione per coloro che conoscono l'inglese a livello medio-alto, diventa un obbligo assoluto per chi conosce la lingua a livello medio-basso; questi ultimi, prima di lasciare l'albergo, dovrebbero rivedere la guida per ripetere le frasi necessarie per chiedere ciò che vogliono mangiare o, perlomeno, per evitare di ordinare cose che non avrebbero mai mangiato. Se guardate le facce dei vostri colleghi non appena viene servita la prima portata, potete facilmente capire chi sta mangiando la cosa che desiderava e chi, al contrario, non sa che cosa ha ordinato e, quello che è peggio, che cosa sta in realtà mangiando.

Pensiamo un momento all'incidente che è successo a me mentre mi trovavo al UCSF Medical Center. Ero stato invitato a pranzo in una trattoria (*diner*) vicino all'ospedale e, quando ho chiesto di avere dell'acqua minerale naturale (*still mineral water*), il cameriere mi ha risposto vagamente perplesso che avevano solo quella frizzante (*sparkling*) poiché nessuno aveva mai ordinato una simile delizia e mi ha offerto dell'acqua di rubinetto (*plain water*).

Coloro che hanno raggiunto un certo livello di dimestichezza con l'inglese, sono consci di quante situazioni imbarazzanti hanno dovuto superare in passato per diventare maggiormente spigliati in buona parte delle circostanze in cui ci si può trovare.

Saluti

> Hi.
> Hello.
> Good morning.
> Good afternoon.
> Good evening.
> Good night.
> How are you? (Very) Well, thank you.
> How are you getting on? All right, thank you.
> I am glad to see you.
> Nice to see you (again).
> How do you feel today?
> How is your family?
> Good bye.
> Bye bye.
> See you later.
> See you soon.
> See you tomorrow.
> Give my regards to everybody.
> Give my love to your children.

Presentazioni

> This is Mr./Mrs. . . .
> These are Mister and Misses . . .
> My name is . . .
> What is your name? My name is . . .
> Pleased/Nice to meet you.
> Let me introduce you to . . .
> I'd like to introduce you to . . .
> Have you already met Mr. . . .? Yes, I have.

Dati personali

> What is your name? My name is . . .
> What is your surname/family name? My surname/family name is . . .

> Where are you from? I am from . . .
> Where do you live? I live in . . .
> What is your address? My address is . . .
> What is your email address? My email address is . . .
> What is your phone number? My phone number is . . .
> What is your mobile phone/cellular number? My mobile phone/cellular number is . . .
> How old are you? I am . . .
> Where were you born? I was born in . . .
> What do you do? I am a radiologist.
> What do you do? I do MRI/US/CT/chest . . .

Frasi di cortesia

> Thank you very much. You are welcome (Don't mention it).
> Would you please . . . ? Sure, it is a pleasure.
> Excuse me.
> Pardon.
> Sorry.
> Cheers!
> Congratulations!
> Good luck!
> It doesn't matter!
> May I help you?
> Here you are!
> You are very kind. It is very kind of you.
> Don't worry; that's not what I wanted.
> Sorry to bother/trouble you.
> Don't worry!
> What can I do for you?
> How can I help you?
> Would you like something to drink?
> Would you like a cigarette?
> I would like . . .
> I beg your pardon.
> Have a nice day.

Parlando in una lingua straniera

> Do you speak English/Spanish/French…? I do not speak English/Only a bit/Not a word.
> Do you understand me? Yes, I do. No, I don't.
> Sorry, I do not understand you.
> Could you speak slowly, please?
> How do you write it?
> Could you write it down?
> How do you spell it?
> How do you pronounce it?
> Sorry, what did you say?
> Sorry, my English is not very good.
> Sorry, I didn't get that.
> Could you please repeat that?
> I can't hear you.

Al ristorante

"*The same for me*" è una delle frasi più frequenti che si possono sentire ai tavoli dei ristoranti, in tutto il mondo. La persona che non conosce bene l'inglese lega il proprio destino gastronomico alle persone che parlano meglio, per evitare scomode domande come "*How would you like your meat, sir?*".
Una semplice occhiata alla guida pochi minuti prima della cena, vi garantirà un vocabolario sufficiente per chiedere qualsiasi cosa vogliate. Non permettete che la vostra scarsa dimestichezza rovini una buona opportunità di degustare piatti e vini deliziosi.

Scambi preliminary

> Hello, do you have a table for three people?
> Hi, may I book a table for a party of seven for 6 o'clock?
> What time are you coming, sir?
> Where can we sit?
> Is this chair free?
> Is this table taken?

> Waiter/waitress, I would like to order.
> Could I see the menu?
> Could you bring the menu?
> Can I have the wine list?
> Could you give us a table next to the window?
> Could you give me a table on the mezzanine?
> Could you give us a table near the stage?

Ordinare

> We'd like to order now.
> Could you bring us some bread, please?
> We'd like to have something to drink.
> *Here you are.*
> Could you recommend a local wine?
> Could you recommend one of your specialties?
> Could you suggest something special?
> What are the ingredients of this dish?
> I'll have a steamed lobster, please.
> *How would you like your meat, sir?*
> Rare/medium-rare/medium/well-done.
> Somewhere between rare and medium rare will be OK.
> Is the halibut fresh?
> What is there for dessert?
> *Anything else, sir?*
> No, we are fine, thank you.
> The same for me.
> *Enjoy your meal, sir.*
> *How was everything, sir?*
> The meal was excellent.
> The sirloin was delicious.
> Excuse me, I have spilled something on my tie. Could you help me?

Lamentele

> The dish is cold. Would you please heat it up?
> The meat is underdone. Would you cook it a little more, please?

> Excuse me. This is not what I asked for.
> Could you change this for me?
> The fish is not fresh. I want to see the manager.
> I asked for a sirloin.
> The meal wasn't very good.
> The meat smells off.
> Could you bring the complaints book?
> This wine is off, I think...
> Waiter, this fork is dirty.

Il conto [The check (US)/ The bill (UK)]

> The check, please.
> Would you bring us the check, please?
> All together, please.
> We are paying separately.
> I am afraid there is a mistake; we didn't have this.
> This is for you.
> Keep the change.

Trasporto in città

> I want to go to the Metropolitan Museum.
> Which bus/tram/underground (US subway) line must I take for the Metropolitan?
> Which bus/tram/underground (US subway) line can I take to get to the Metropolitan?
> Where does the number [...] bus stop?
> Does this bus go to ...?
> How much is a single (US one-way) ticket?
> Three tickets, please.
> Where must I get off for ...?
> Is this seat occupied/vacant?
> Where can I get a taxi?
> How much is the fare for ...?
> Take me to [...] Street.
> Do you know where the ...is?

Shopping

Domandare l'orario di apertura dei negozi

> When are you open?
> How late are you open today?
> Are you open on Saturday?

Scambi preliminari

> *Hello sir (UK madam, US ma'am), may I help you?*
> *Can I help you find something?*
> Thank you, I am just looking.
> I just can't make up my mind.
> *Can I help you with something?*
> If I can help you, just let me know.
> *Are you looking for something in particular?*
> I am looking for something for my wife.
> I am looking for something for my husband.
> I am looking for something for my children.
> It is a gift.
> Hi, do you sell . . .?
> I am looking for a . . . Can you help me?
> Would you tell me where the music department is?
> Which floor is the leather goods department on? *On the ground floor (on the mezzanine, on the second floor)*.
> Please would you show me . . . ?
> What kind do you want?
> Where can I find the mirror? There is a mirror over there.
> *The changing rooms are over there.*
> *Only four items are allowed in the dressing room at a time.*
> Is there a public rest room here?
> *Have you decided?*
> *Have you made up your mind?*

Comprare scarpe/vestiti

> Please, can you show me some natural silk ties?
> I want to buy a long-sleeved shirt.
> I want the pair of high-heeled shoes I saw in the window.
> Would you please show me the pair in the window?
> What material is it?
> What material is it made of ? *Cotton, leather, linen, wool, velvet, silk, nylon, acrylic fiber.*
> What size, please?
> *What size do you need?*
> Is this my size?
> Do you think this is my size?
> Where is the fitting room?
> Does it fit you?
> I think it fits well although the collar is a little tight.
> No, it doesn't fit me.
> May I try a larger size?
> I'll try a smaller size. Would you mind bringing it to me?
> I'll take this one.
> How much is it?
> This is too expensive.
> Oh, this is a bargain!
> I like it.
> May I try this on?
> *In which color?* Navy blue, please.
> Do you have anything to go with this?
> I need a belt/a pair of socks/pair of jeans/pair of gloves. . . .
> I need a size 38. (But remember, sizes are different in different countries.)
> I don't know my size. Can you measure me?
> Would you measure my waist, please?
> Do you have a shirt to match this?
> Do you have this in blue/in wool/in a larger size/in a smaller size?
> Do you have something a bit less expensive?
> I'd like to try this on. Where is the fitting room?
> How would you like to pay for this? Cash/credit
> *We don't have that in your size/color.*
> *We are out of that item.*
> It's too tight/loose.
> It's too expensive/cheap.
> I don't like the color.

> Is it in the sale?
> Can I have this gift-wrapped?

Nel negozio di scarpe

> A pair of shoes, boots, sandals, slippers, shoelace, sole, heel, leather, suede, rubber, shoehorn. *What kind of shoes do you want?*
> I want a pair of rubber-soled shoes/high-heeled shoes/leather shoes/ suede slippers/boots.
> I want a pair of lace-up/slip-on shoes good for the rain/for walking.
> *What is your size, please?*
> They are a little tight/too large/too small.
> Would you please show me the pair in the window?
> Can I try a smaller/larger size, please?
> This one fits well.
> I would like some polish cream.
> I need some new laces.
> I need a shoehorn.

All'ufficio postale

> I need some (first class) stamps, please.
> First class, please.
> Airmail, please.
> I would like this to go express mail.
> I would like this recorded/special delivery.
> I need to send this second-day mail (US).
> Second-class for this, please (UK).
> I need to send this parcel post.
> I need to send this by certified mail.
> I need to send this by registered mail.
> Return receipt requested, please.
> How much postage do I need for this?
> How much postage do I need to send this airmail?
> Do you have any envelopes?
> How long will it take to get there? *It should arrive on Monday.*
> *The forms are over there. Please fill out* (UK: *fill in*) *a form and bring it back to me.*

Al teatro (USA: Theater, UK: Theatre)

> *Sorry, we are sold out tonight.*
> *Sorry, these tickets are non-refundable.*
> *Sorry, there are no tickets available.*
> *Would you like to make a reservation for another night?*
> I would like two seats for tonight's performance, please.
> Where are the best seats you have left?
> Do you have anything in the first four rows?
> Do you have matinees?
> How much are the tickets?
> Is it possible to exchange these for another night?
> Do you take a check (UK cheques)/credit cards?
> How long does the show run? *About 2 hours.*
> When does the show close?
> Is there an intermission? *There is an intermission.*
> Where are the restrooms?
> Where is the cloakroom?
> Is there anywhere we can leave our coats?
> Do you sell concessions?
> How soon does the curtain go up?
> *Did you make a reservation?*
> *What name did you reserve the tickets under?*
> *The usher will give you your program.*

In farmacia (US drugstore, UK chemist)

> Prescription, tablet, pill, cream, suppository, laxative, sedative, injection, bandage, sticking plasters (US Band-Aids), cotton wool (US cotton balls), gauze, alcohol, thermometer, sanitary towels, napkins, tampons, toothpaste, toothbrush, paper tissues, duty chemist (US all-night pharmacy).
> Fever, cold, cough, headache, toothache, diarrhea, constipation, sickness, insomnia, sunburn, insect bite.
> I am looking for something for . . .
> Could you give me . . . ?
> Could you give me something for . . . ?
> I need some aspirin/antiseptic/eye drops/foot powder.
> I need razor blades and shaving cream (UK foam).

❭ What are the side effects of this drug?
❭ Will this make me drowsy?
❭ Should I take this with meals?

In profumeria

❭ Soap, shampoo, deodorant, antiperspirant, shower gel, hair spray, sun-tan lotion (UK cream), comb, hairbrush, toothpaste, toothbrush, make-up, cologne water, lipstick, perfume, hair remover, scissors, face lotion, cleansing cream, razor, shaving cream (UK foam).

In libreria/edicola

❭ I would like to buy a book on the history of the city.
❭ Has this book been translated into Japanese?
❭ Do you have Swedish newspapers/magazines/books?
❭ Where can I buy a road map?

Dal fotografo

❭ I want a 36-exposure film for this camera.
❭ I want new batteries for my camera.
❭ Could you develop this film?
❭ Could you develop this film with two prints of each photograph?
❭ How much does developing cost?
❭ When will the photographs be ready?
❭ My camera is not working, would you have a look at it?
❭ Do you take passport (ID) photographs?
❭ I want an enlargement of this one and two copies of this other.
❭ Have you got a 500-megabyte data card to fit this camera?
❭ How much would a 1-gigabyte card be?
❭ How many megapixels is this one?
❭ Does it have an optical zoom?
❭ Can you print the pictures on this CD?

Dal fioraio

> I would like to order a dozen roses.
> I would like a bouquet.
> *You can choose violets and orchids in several colors.*
> Which flowers are the freshest?
> What are these flowers called?
> Do you deliver?
> Could you please send this bouquet to the NH Abascal Hotel manager at 47 Abascal Street before noon?
> Could you please send this card too?

Per pagare

> Where is the cash/ATM machine?
> Is there a CashPoint near here?
> How much is that all together?
> *Will you pay cash or by credit card?*
> *Next in line (UK queue).*
> Could you gift-wrap it for me?
> Can I have a receipt, please?
> Can I have a receipt, please?

Dal parrucchiere/barbiere

Mentre mi trovavo a Boston mi è capitato di dover andare dal barbiere e la mia mancanza di dimestichezza con l'inglese è stata responsabile di un drastico cambiamento della mia immagine per un paio di mesi, tanto che mia moglie non mi ha quasi riconosciuto quando sono andato a prenderla all'aeroporto di Logan, una delle tante volte in cui è venuta a trovarmi nel New England. Vi posso assicurare che non dimenticherò mai più il termine *"sideburns"* (basette); la parrucchiera, una robusta signora afroamericana, me le ha tagliate drasticamente prima che fossi in grado di ricordare il nome di quella parte insignificante della mia peluria facciale. Per la verità, non avevo mai considerato quanto fossero importanti le basette, prima di non averle più.

Se non vi fidate dell'ignoto barbiere o parrucchiera, *"just a trim"* (appena una spuntatina) è un modo educato per evitare un disastro.

Vi suggerisco, prima di andare dal parrucchiere, di rivedere la guida per acquisire confidenza con alcune parole, quali: *scissors, comb, brush, dryer, shampooing, hair style, hair cut, manicure, dyeing, shave, beard, moustache, sideburns* (!) (US), *sideboards* (UK), *fringe, curl,* o *plait*.

Uomini e donne

> How long will I have to wait?
> *Is the water OK?* It is fine/too hot/too cold.
> My hair is greasy/dry.
> I have dandruff.
> I am losing a lot of hair.
> A shampoo and rinse, please.
> *How would you like it?*
> *Are you going for a particular look?*
> I want a (hair) cut like this.
> Just a trim, please.
> *However you want.*
> *Is it OK?*
> That's fine, thank you.
> How much is it?
> How much do I owe you?
> Do you do highlights?
> I would like a tint, please.

Uomini

> I want a shave.
> A razor cut, please.
> Just a trim, please.
> Leave the sideburns as they are (!) (UK: sideboards).
> Trim the moustache.
> Trim my beard and moustache, please.
> Toward the back, without any parting.
> I part my hair on the left/in the middle.

> Leave it long.
> Could you take a little more off the top/the back/the sides?
> *How much do you want me to take off ?*

Donne

> *How do I set your hair?*
> *What hairstyle do you want?*
> I would like my hair dyed/bleached/highlighted.
> *Same color?*
> A little darker/lighter.
> I would like to have a perm (permanent wave).

Automobili

Come sempre, iniziate con le parole. *Clutch, brake, blinkers* (UK: *indicators*), *trunk* (UK: *boot*), *tank, gearbox, windshield* (UK: *windscreen*) *wipers, (steering) wheel, unleaded gas* (UK: *petrol*), ecc. sono parole che devono appartenere al vostro vocabolario come anche altre frasi frequenti, come:

> How far is the nearest gas (petrol) station? Twenty miles from here.
> In what direction? Northeast/Los Angeles.

Dal benzinaio (USA: Gas Station, UK: Petrol Station)

> Fill it up, please.
> Unleaded, please.
> Could you top up the battery, please?
> Could you check the oil, please?
> Could you check the tire pressures, please?
> *Do you want me to check the spare tire too?* Yes, please.
> Pump number 5, please.
> Can I have a receipt, please?

Dal carrozziere

> My car has broken down.
> What do you think is wrong with it?
> Can you mend a puncture (US can you fix a flat)?
> Can you take the car in tow to downtown Boston?
> *I see . . . , kill the engine, please.*
> *Start the engine, please.*
> The car goes to the right and overheats.
> *Have you noticed if it loses water/gas/oil?*
> Yes, it's losing oil.
> *Does it lose speed/power?*
> Yes, and it doesn't start properly.
> I can't get it into reverse.
> The engine makes funny noises.
> Please, repair it as soon as possible.
> I wonder if you can fix it temporarily.
> How long will it take to repair?
> *I am afraid we have to send for spare parts.*
> The car is very heavy on gas (UK petrol).
> I think the right front tire needs changing.
> I guess the valve is broken.
> Is my car ready?
> Have you finished fixing the car?
> Did you fix the car?
> Do you think you can fix it today?
> I think my rear passenger-side tire is flat (UK I've got a puncture rear offside.)
> The spare's flat as well.
> I've run out of gas (UK petrol).

Al parcheggio (US: Parking Garage/Structure, UK: Car Park)

> Do you know where the nearest car park (US parking lot) is?
> Are there any free spaces?
> How much is it per hour?
> Is the car park (US lot) supervised?
> How long can I leave the car here?

Noleggiare una macchina

> I want to rent a car.
> I want to hire a car (UK).
> *For how many days?*
> *Unlimited mileage?*
> What is the cost per mile?
> Is insurance included?
> *You need to leave a deposit.*

Come posso arrivare a . . .?

> How far is Minneapolis?
> *It is not far. About 12 miles from here.*
> Is the road good?
> *It is not bad, although a bit slow.*
> Is there a toll road between here and Berlin?
> How long does it take to get to Key West?
> I am lost. Could you tell me how I can get back to the highway?

Prendere un drink (o due)

Dopo una giornata di duro lavoro, ci sono poche cose più desiderabili di un drink. Purtroppo, anche in una situazione così rilassata si possono verificare imbarazzanti incidenti; spesso c'è una difficile contro-domanda alla semplice richiesta *"can I have a beer?"* come *"would you prefer lager?"* o *"small, medium or large, sir?"*. Quando ero un principiante, odiavo le contro-domande e mi ricordo di essere diventato rosso quando, in un pub di Londra, il barman, invece di darmi la birra che avevo chiesto, ha iniziato a elencare l'intera lista delle birre del pub. *"I have changed my mind; I'll have a Coke instead"* è stata la mia risposta sia all'"aggressione" che all'imbarazzo derivante dalla mia scarsa dimestichezza. *"We don't serve Coke here, sir"*.
Queste situazioni possono rovinare le serate più promettenti. Rivediamo quindi una serie di frasi comuni:

> Two beers please; my friend will pay.
> Two pints of bitter and half a lager, please.
> Where can I find a good place to go for a drink?
> Where can we go for a drink at this time of the evening?
> Do you know any pubs with live music?
> *What can I get you?*
> I'm driving. Just an orange juice, please.
> A glass of wine and two beers, please.
> A gin and tonic.
> A glass of brandy. Would you please warm the glass?
> Scotch, please.
> *Do you want it plain (UK neat), with water, or on the rocks?*
> Make it a double.
> I'll have the same again, please.
> Two cubes of ice and a teaspoon, please.
> This is on me.
> What those ladies are having is on me.

Al telefono

Molti problemi cominciano quando si solleva la cornetta. I suoni della tastiera, della suoneria o del segnale di "occupato" potrebbero essere diversi da paese a paese. Le conversazioni telefoniche sono tra le situazioni più terrificanti per un interlocutore che non parla bene inglese. Il telefono ha altre due difficoltà: la sua immediatezza e l'assenza di immagine ("se potessi vedere questa persona, sarei in grado di capire cosa sta dicendo"). Non vi preoccupate, sono pochi gli scambi preliminari in questo tipo di conversazione.

Le segreterie telefoniche sono un nuovo e ben più difficile problema, la cui trattazione va oltre gli scopi di questa guida alla sopravvivenza. Solo un suggerimento: non riattaccate. Cercate di capire quello che dice la segreteria telefonica e riprovate nel caso non siate in grado di seguire le istruzioni. Molti dottori, non appena sentono l'inconfondibile suono di questi strumenti, riattaccano terrorizzati. La maggior parte dei messaggi sono però facili da capire e meno "meccanici" rispetto a quelli di tanti operatori "umani" (e generalmente "noiosi").

> Where are the public phones, please?
> Where is the nearest phone booth (UK call-box)?

> This telephone is out of order.
> Operator, what do I dial for the USA?
> *Hold on a moment . . . the number "1."*
> Would you get me this number please?
> *Dial straight through.*
> What time does the cheap rate begin?
> Have you got any phone cards, please?
> Can I use your cell/mobile phone, please?
> Do you have a phone book (directory)?
> I'd like to make a reverse charge call to Korea.
> I am trying to use my phone card, but I am not getting through.
> Hello, this is Dr. Vida speaking.
> The line is busy (UK engaged).
> There's no answer.
> It's a bad line.
> I've been cut off.
> I would like the number for Dr. Vida on Green Street.
> What is the area code for Los Angeles?
> I can't get through to this number. Would you dial it for me?
> Can you put me through to Spain?

Situazioni d'emergenza

> I want to report a fire/a robbery/an accident.
> This is an emergency! We need an ambulance/the police.
> Get me the police, and hurry!

In banca

Oggi, la diffusione delle carte di credito rende questo paragrafo virtualmente non necessario, ma per esperienza personale, se le cose vanno veramente male, avrete bisogno di andare in banca.
La disinvoltura scompare in una situazione così stressante; in caso dobbiate risolvere un problema in banca, rivedete non soltanto questa serie di frasi, ma anche l'intera relativa sezione della vostra guida.

> Where can I change money?
> I'd like to change 200 Euros.

> I want to exchange 1,000 Euros into Dollars/Pounds.
> Could I have it in tens, please?
> What's the exchange rate?
> What's the rate of exchange from Euros to Dollars?
> What are the banking hours?
> I want to change this travelers' check (UK cheque).
> Have you received a transfer from Rosario Nadal addressed to Fiona Shaw?
> Can I cash this check that's made out to me (UK bearer cheque)?
> I want to cash this check (UK cheque).
> Do I need my ID to cash this check (UK cheque)?
> *Go to the cash desk.*
> *Go to counter number 5.*
> May I open a current account?
> Where is the nearest cash machine?
> I am afraid you don't seem to be able to solve my problem. Can I see the manager?
> Who is in charge?
> Could you call my bank in France? There must have been a problem with a transfer addressed to myself.

Alla stazione di polizia

> Where is the nearest police station?
> I have come to report a . . .
> My wallet has been stolen.
> Can I call my lawyer (UK solicitor)?
> I have been assaulted.
> My laptop has disappeared from my room.
> I have lost my passport.
> I will not say anything until I have spoken to my lawyer/solicitor.
> I have had a car accident.
> Why have you arrested me? I've done nothing.
> Am I under caution?
> I would like to call my embassy/consulate.

Capitolo 22

Poche parole per una comunicazione efficace

Conoscere molto bene la lingua inglese NON è la sola cosa di cui si ha bisogno per comunicare in maniera efficace. Di fatto, si dice che le persone creino una vostra immagine mentale nei primi 5 secondi in cui vi vedono.

Comunicare è infatti una "forma d'arte". Noi comunichiamo ogni volta che interagiamo con altri. Il modo in cui effettivamente lo facciamo determina in modo definitivo il nostro successo in vari campi. Ricordate che molto spesso non è così importante cosa si dice, ma come lo si dice. Alcuni esempi sono una conversazione al coffee break, con un insegnante, durante un colloquio di lavoro, dopo cena ...

La tipologia più difficile di comunicazione è quella nella quale si cerca di convincere gli altri. Noi "vendiamo" le nostre idee, le nostre abilità professionali, o i nostri prodotti, ma in realtà stiamo "vendendo" noi stessi.

Se state preparando una comunicazione orale per un congresso internazionale, vi suggerisco di riprendervi con una videocamera. Ciò vi darà un riscontro riguardo la vostra pronuncia, il vostro linguaggio del corpo e quali punti si devono rafforzare prima di fare la vostra presentazione al congresso.

Ricordate questi punti chiave:

1. Siate consapevoli di chi è il vostro pubblico. Mentre siete di fronte al pubblico, dovreste focalizzarvi sulle persone di maggiore interesse (il vostro capo, gli organizzatori del congresso......); se possibile, tentate di porvi di fronte a loro. Ciò non significa che non dobbiate guardare gli altri membri del pubblico; dovreste dirigere il vostro sguardo a tutte le aree del pubblico, ma mettendovi di fronte alla parte a cui siete più interessati.

2. Non utilizzate un puntatore laser. In molti congressi ci sono uno - due grandi schermi per il pubblico; usate lo schermo del pc portatile sul

R. Ribes, P. J. Aranda, J. Giba, *Inglese per chirurghi*,
© Springer-Verlag Italia 2012

podio e muovete il mouse per indicare cosa desiderate. Ciò vi permetterà di mantenere un contatto visivo con il vostro pubblico, che sarà quindi più interessato ad ascoltare quello che dite.

3. Utilizzate gli "effetti" di Power Point nelle vostre slides. NON temete di apparire "cool" in un ambiente formale e scientifico. Utilizzare poche parole; farle comparire nelle vostre slides mentre le illustrate renderà la vostra presentazione più intensa e meno monotona.

4. Se il vostro inglese non è fluente, riducete la lunghezza del vostro discorso. Siate molto concisi e utilizzate parole che riuscite a pronunciare facilmente. Ricordate che VOI scegliete cosa dire, solo così non diventerete il vostro peggior nemico. Il pubblico sarà sempre felice di ascoltare una comunicazione breve, coincisa e facilmente comprensibile.

5. Segnalate chiaramente quando iniziate e finite il vostro discorso. È consigliabile iniziare con un'espressione formale del tipo "Mr. Chairman, dear colleagues, thank you for giving me the opportunity to participate in this meeting...". Potete anche presentarvi (specialmente se non lo siete stati in maniera adeguata). Per terminare la vostra presentazione è spesso consigliabile dedicare una slide a un'immagine (relazionata o meno alla chirurgia) e "Thank you for your attention" oppure "I will be glad to answer your questions...".

Ciascuno di noi è diverso. Alcune persone sono "non-speakers" (tipicamente timidi con abilità interpersonali poco sviluppate e poca oppure nessuna esperienza nel parlare di fronte a un pubblico). Altri sono speaker occasionali che si sentono in qualche modo nervosi prima e durante un discorso pubblico, ma accettano la sfida di parlare quando devono farlo. Un terzo gruppo comprende gli speaker volontari che, sebbene non siano tecnicamente perfetti, hanno perso il timore di rendersi ridicoli e parlano tranquillamente in ogni occasione. Infine, alcune persone provano in realtà un gran gusto a parlare in pubblico: viene loro spontaneo e semplicemente gli piace.

Indipendentemente dal tipo di persona che siete, potete gestire il parlare in pubblico e la comunicazione (persino in inglese) se preparate il vostro discorso accuratamente e fate molte prove. Non lasciatevi sfuggire l'occasione di parlare di fronte a una folla (sempre che abbiate qualcosa da dire, ovviamente). Un ottimo posto per iniziare è il vostro ospedale. Provate a fare qualche incontro clinico o di review della letteratura scientifica in inglese; gli interni con molta probabilità vorranno seguirvi in questa attività e gli errori saranno facilmente perdonati e dimenticati fra colleghi.

Ricordate che una comunicazione efficace è per il 50% visiva, per il 30% vocale e solo per il 20% verbale. Ciò significa che raggiungere e convincere il vostro pubblico con il vostro messaggio dipende non solo dall'accuratezza e dall'importanza dei vostri dati scientifici (la parte verbale) ma anche dalla vostra abilità a mantenere l'attenzione del pubblico con la risonanza e l'intonazione della vostra voce (la parte vocale) e dalle immagini e dai video nella vostra presentazione, così come dai gesti, la vostra postura e i vostri abiti (la parte visiva). Ricordate che il vostro messaggio sarà efficace solo se raggiunge l'obbiettivo. Mantenere l'attenzione del pubblico e aprirlo al messaggio che avete intenzione di comunicargli è il solo modo per centrare l'obiettivo.

Il linguaggio del corpo è di somma importanza. Siate consapevoli di come vi presentate di fronte agli altri, della vostra postura e dei vostri gesti. Recentemente ho avuto l'opportunità di assistere alla presentazione di un chirurgo durante un congresso internazionale. Il contenuto scientifico di questa presentazione era probabilmente il migliore della mattinata. Il suo inglese, sebbene non eccellente, era abbastanza buono da trasmettere il suo messaggio. Tuttavia, la presentazione è stata probabilmente la meno efficace dell'intero congresso. Ecco alcuni degli errori che ha fatto:

- Ha letto un foglio durante tutta la presentazione
- Raramente ha guardato il pubblico
- L'intonazione delle voce era totalmente piatta durante gli 8 minuti della presentazione (ciò significa che sembrava fosse durata 60 minuti!!).
- Indossava un abito che era troppo largo per lui, e ha sudato abbondantemente durante tutta la presentazione.
- Le slides contenevano troppe parole, non avevano abbastanza immagini e nessun effetto speciale.
- Il suo messaggio parlato non era coordinato con il suo messaggio visivo: quello che stava leggendo non combaciava con le slides che stavamo tentando di leggere.
- Il suo intervento è finito bruscamente quando ha letto l'ultima frase della sezione "Conclusioni": non ha nemmeno detto "Grazie"......

Sebbene come scienziati e chirurghi non stiate vendendo lavatrici, non potete rischiare di rovinare l'impegno vostro e dei vostri colleghi sbagliando nel comunicare e nel trasmettere le informazioni ad altri colleghi. Asserire che non siete dei "parlatori nati" non vi esonera da questa responsabilità. Dovete capire che anche il modo in cui trasmettete il vostro messaggio è importante, e dovete analizzare e migliorare la vostra dizione il più possibile.

Non dimenticate che la vostra voce trasmette energia; di conseguenza, non leggete mai un discorso (sebbene ogni tanto si possa dare un'occhiata al proprio notebook). Prestate attenzione al timbro della vostra voce e alla sua risonanza. Fate particolarmente attenzione a misurare il vostro discorso e agli intervalli della respirazione. "Er" e "uhm" sono delle "non-parole" che la maggior parte dei relatori usano inconsapevolmente come dei riempitivi. Sembrano così naturali che molti relatori non si rendono conto di usarli e ne abusano. L'unico modo di accorgersi di come queste espressioni intaccano la vostra relazione, è di registrarvi o di dire a qualcuno vicino a voi di farvi un segnale ogni volta che pronunciate una "non-parola". Che siate consapevoli oppure no di questi "riempitivi", siate sicuri che chi vi ascolta li noterà e che ascoltarli spesso darà fastidio al vostro pubblico.

Quindi, identificate le "non-parole" che utilizzate ed eliminatele.

Infine, vi raccomando di aggiungere un tocco di "umanità" alla vostra presentazione orale: persino se state presentando delle statistiche o dei crudi dati scientifici, non dimenticate che siete una persona che sta parlando ad altre persone. Includere un po' di "humour" (non delle barzellette), una storia breve o un aneddoto, oppure parlare semplicemente in una maniera emozionante, semplice e certa, vi garantirà la possibilità di comunicare con il pubblico a un livello personale.

Pertanto, vi auguriamo buona fortuna nella vostra vita professionale e personale e speriamo che questo libro vi apra una finestra verso l'emozionante mondo dell'Inglese Chirurgico e, cosa più importante, vi aiuti a comunicare in modo efficace.

Printed in the United States
By Bookmasters